SBA MCQs for the MRCS Part A

SBA MCQs for the MRCS Part A

Mr Sri G. Thrumurthy MBChB(Hons), MRCS
Core Trainee in General Surgery
London Deanery, UK

Miss Tania S. de Silva MBChB, MRCS(Ed)
Specialty Registrar in General Surgery
Sheffield Teaching Hospitals NHS Trust
Sheffield, UK

Mr Zia M. Moinuddin MBBS, MRCS
Specialty Registrar in General Surgery
Central Manchester University Hospitals NHS Foundation Trust
Manchester, UK

Professor Stuart Enoch MBBS, MRCS(Ed), PGCert (Med Sci), MRCS(Eng), PhD
Clinical Director, Centre for Study of Wound Care and Burns
Visiting Professor, Department of Biomedical Research, Noorul Islam University, India
Director of Education and Research, Doctors Academy, Cardiff, UK

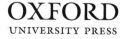

OXFORD
UNIVERSITY PRESS

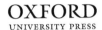

OXFORD

UNIVERSITY PRESS

Great Clarendon Street, Oxford OX2 6DP
United Kingdom

Oxford University Press is a department of the University of Oxford.
It furthers the University's objective of excellence in research, scholarship,
and education by publishing worldwide. Oxford is a registered trade mark of
Oxford University Press in the UK and in certain other countries

British Library Cataloguing in Publication Data
Data available

Library of Congress Cataloging in Publication Data
Library of Control Number: 2012944661

ISBN 978-0-19-964563-3

DEDICATION

To my father and my greatest role model, Thrumurthy; to my loving mother, Sobanah; to my wonderful wife, Ayishwarriyah; and to my baby sister, Sasha, for their unconditional love and endless support. To Mr Muntzer Mughal, for his relentless inspiration.

SGT

To my parents for their love and tireless support.
To Amit, for his endless patience and support over the years.
To Aiya, with love.

TSdS

To my parents, wife, and brothers for their constant encouragement and support.

ZMM

To Sri Thrumurthy, the lead author of this project, whose focus, passion and enthusiasm helped us compile this resource; this endeavour would not have materialized without his great commitment and motivation.

SE

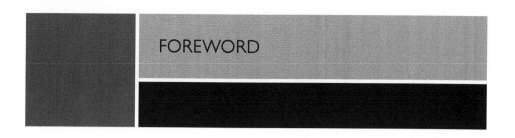

FOREWORD

This book of SBA MCQs will be a valuable resource for trainees preparing for the MRCS examination. The authors have put together 350 questions, which have been carefully crafted to cover the breadth and depth of the MRCS curriculum. The questions cover the different components of the curriculum ranging from basic sciences to the management of common surgical conditions. The authors have been careful about ensuring the right mix of questions in anatomy, physiology, pathology, and surgical conditions. All areas of the curriculum including subjects such as ethics and evidence-based medicine are covered. As each chapter of 50 questions is representative of the MRCS curriculum it can be used as a practice paper. Answers are provided at the end of each chapter with detailed explanations of the salient issues making the book an excellent guide to revision.

Mr Thrumurthy and his colleagues are to be congratulated on producing a book of questions that will enable trainees preparing for the MRCS examination to test their knowledge and identify any gaps. As a result, they will be able to revise more effectively and approach the Part A examination with confidence.

Muntzer Mughal ChM FRCS
Consultant Surgeon and Head of Upper GI Services
University College Hospitals, London

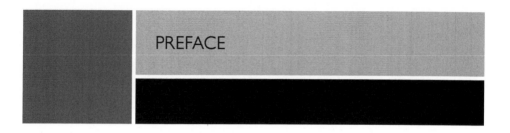

PREFACE

Major reform within the United Kingdom's postgraduate medical education system has necessitated a shift from the traditional true/false multiple questions of the old MRCS Part 1 examination to the 'single best answer' (SBA) and 'extended matching question' (EMQ) format used in the new intercollegiate MRCS Part A examination. Although a thorough understanding of the essential principles of surgery should be obtained from core textbooks and clinical experience, it is vital for candidates to actively recall, apply, and thereby reinforce their knowledge by attempting sample questions in the lead-up to the examination.

SBA MCQs for the MRCS Part A and *EMQs for the MRCS Part A* have been written to provide MRCS candidates with a series of questions preparing them for this new format. As the new format of the Part A paper de-emphasizes the traditional basic science disciplines and accentuates an integrated approach, these books will contain a substantial number of patient-based questions or clinical vignettes that will enable prospective candidates to test their ability to integrate key basic science concepts with relevant clinical problems.

Despite our attempt to comprehensively span the syllabus of the MRCS examination, it needs to be acknowledged that encompassing the full breadth and depth of all curricular topics is beyond the scope of this series. It is hence suggested that these books are used in conjunction with time-honoured surgical textbooks and used as a complementary resource rather than to supplement the reading material recommended by the Royal Colleges of Surgeons.

The detailed approach that these books undertake will not only serve MRCS candidates but will also be an appropriate revision aide for higher surgical trainees preparing for their intercollegiate speciality exit examinations. In addition, although the depth and breadth of this series' content surpasses that of typical undergraduate surgical curricula, these books will nevertheless be an ideal tool for the fervent medical student pursuing an 'honours' or 'distinction' grade in his or her surgical finals.

We sincerely wish all readers the very best of success in their surgical examinations and careers.

SGT
TDS
ZM
SE

HOW TO USE THIS RESOURCE

Paper 1 of the new MRCS Part A examination comprises SBA questions relating to applied basic sciences whilst paper 2 consists of EMQs examining principles of surgery in general.

In keeping with the ethos of the examination, *SBA MCQs for the MRCS Part A* focuses intensively on the application of basic sciences (i.e. applied surgical anatomy, physiology, and pathology) to the management of surgical patients. *EMQs for the MRCS Part A* addresses topics relating to principles of surgery in general (i.e. perioperative care, postoperative management and critical care, surgical technique and technology, management and legal issues in surgery, clinical microbiology, emergency medicine and trauma management, and principles of surgical oncology). Each question has been mapped specifically to the MRCS syllabus as defined by the Intercollegiate Surgical Curriculum Project (ISCP). The explanation following each question aims to span the breadth and depth of the subject matter without overlapping with other explanations of similar themes. The diverse layout and level of detail included within the questions and their explanations will serve to help candidates tackle the MRCS Part A examination by allowing effective self-assessment of knowledge and quick identification of key areas requiring further attention.

We have formatted the questions to encompass various subtypes of questioning modalities to effectively guide candidates through the revision process. These modalities include 'clinical case' questions or 'clinical vignettes' (i.e. basic science applied clinically), positively-worded questions (i.e. requiring selection of the most appropriate of relatively correct answers), 'two-step' or 'double-jump' questions (i.e. requiring several cognitive steps to arrive at the correct answer), as well as factual recall questions (i.e. prompting basic recall of facts). The questions posed within these books will offer more thorough and detailed explanations than the majority of preparatory material currently available on the market. This is imperative because market research demonstrates that the vast majority of MRCS candidates are disappointed with the degree of description offered by most MRCS practice questions currently available (i.e. in books or within online question banks).

We are confident that this series, when used in conjunction with the recommended reading material of the Royal Colleges of Surgeons, will ensure the success of every candidate attempting the MRCS Part A examination.

SGT
TDS
ZM
SE

CONTENTS

Abbreviations   xv

Chapter 1
Questions   1
Answers   17

Chapter 2
Questions   31
Answers   48

Chapter 3
Questions   61
Answers   78

Chapter 4
Questions   93
Answers   110

Chapter 5
Questions   125
Answers   141

Chapter 6
Questions   157
Answers   175

Chapter 7

Questions   191

Answers   210

Index   227

MRI	magnetic resonance
MTC	medullary thyroid carcinoma
Na	sodium
NICE	National Institure for Health and Clinical Excellence
NJT	nasojejunal tube
NO	nitric oxide
NSAID	non-steroidal anti-inflammatory drug
NSGCT	non-seminomatous germ cell tumour
OGD	oesophagogastroduodenscopy
PAS	periodic acid–Schiff
PBC	primary biliary cirrhosis
PCC	prothrombin complex concentrate
PEG	percutaneous endoscopic gastrostomy
PMNL	polymorphonuclear leucocyte
PTH	parathyroid hormone
RAAS	renin–angiotensin–aldosterone system
RLN	recurrent laryngeal nerve
RTA	road traffic accident
RVOTO	right ventricular outflow tract obstruction
SAH	subarachnoid haemorrhage
SAN	sinoatrial node
SIADH	syndrome of inappropriate antidiuretic hormone hypersecretion
SIRS	systemic inflammatory response syndrome
TAPVD	total anomalous pulmonary venous drainage
TB	tuberculosis
TFT	thyroid function test
TGFα	transforming growth factor-alpha
TGFβ	transforming growth factor-beta
TIA	transient ischaemic attack
TIPS	transjugular intrahepatic portosystemic shunting
TOE	transoesophageal echocardiography
TOF	tetralogy of Fallot
TOGA	transposition of great arteries
TPN	total parenteral nutrition
TTE	transthoracic echocardiography
U&E	urea and electrolytes
UV	ultraviolet
VIP	vasoactive intestinal peptide
WCC	white cell count

Basic sciences: Applied anatomy

1. **Which among the following statements regarding the functions of the extraocular muscles is incorrect?**
   A. The inferior oblique muscle abducts the eye and moves it upwards
   B. The superior rectus muscle abducts the eyes and moves it laterally
   C. The superior oblique muscle abducts the eye and moves it downwards
   D. The medial rectus muscle moves the eye medially
   E. The inferior rectus muscle adducts the eye and moves it downwards

Basic sciences: Physiology

2. **From the following statements regarding normal wound healing, choose the one statement which is incorrect.**
   A. Wound healing can proceed in the absence of polymorphonuclear leucocytes
   B. Monocytes are essential for wound healing
   C. Collagen is formed by two polypeptide chains
   D. Type IV collagen is predominantly seen in the basement membrane
   E. The normal ratio of type I to type III collagen in the skin is approximately 4:1

Basic sciences: Pathology

3. **Which among the following statements regarding metaplasia is not true?**
   A. Metaplasia is the transformation of one fully differentiated cell type into another
   B. Metaplasia may be reversible
   C. Barrett's oesophagus is a type of squamous metaplasia
   D. Metaplasia can be a physiological process
   E. Metaplasia characterized by abnormal mitosis, pleomorphism, and a high nuclear/cytoplasmic ratio

Common surgical conditions and the subspecialties: Trauma
and orthopaedics

4. A 54-year-old woman presents with a 1-month history of a painful right
    shoulder. The pain is present on almost all movements and movements
    in the joint are restricted because of the pain. Both active and passive
    movements result in pain. Plain radiographs of the shoulder are
    normal. What is the most likely diagnosis?
    A. Acute calcific tendonitis
    B. Supraspinatus tendonitis
    C. Adhesive capsulitis
    D. Rotator cuff tear
    E. Subacromial bursitis

Common surgical conditions and the subspecialties: General presenting
symptoms or syndromes

5. A 47-year-old alcoholic presents to the Emergency Department with
    central abdominal pain and vomiting. She prefers to sit up as the pain
    aggravates on lying supine and on eating. On examination, her pulse
    rate is 140/min, her temperature is 38.2°C, and there is periumbilical
    discoloration. What is the most likely diagnosis?
    A. Acute pancreatitis
    B. Ruptured ovarian follicle
    C. Crohn's disease
    D. Urinary tract infection
    E. Pyelonephritis

Perioperative care: Intraoperative care

6. When considering the use of anaesthesia for abdominal aortic
    aneurysm (AAA) repair, which of the following statements is incorrect?
    A. Aggressive preoperative fluid resuscitation is contraindicated
    B. Patients should be anaesthetized after their skin is prepared and draped in the
        emergency setting
    C. Vasodilators should be given following infrarenal cross clamping, during elective
        AAA repair
    D. Blood pressure and cardiac output usually increase during aortic cross clamping
    E. Patients with aorto-occlusive disease have an exaggerated hypertension and arterial
        hypertension during cross-clamping

The assessment and management of the surgical patient:
Planning investigations

7. **A 31-year-old woman who is due for an elective cholecystectomy presents to the Emergency Department with sudden-onset right-sided weakness approximately 2 days after returning to the United Kingdom from South East Asia. She has no significant past medical history and physical examination is normal. Chest radiography, electrocardiogram (ECG), and a computed tomography (CT) head scan are entirely normal. Which one of the following investigations is most likely to reveal the cause of her presentation?**
   A. Carotid Doppler ultrasonography
   B. Cerebral angiography
   C. Magnetic resonance imaging (MRI) of the head
   D. Transoesophageal echocardiography (TOE)
   E. Transthoracic echocardiography (TTE)

Basic sciences: Applied anatomy

8. **A 45-year-old jockey falls off his horse and sustains a fracture of his distal tibia involving the ankle joint. After initial resuscitation, a senior orthopaedic review determines that stability will be best achieved by external fixation with a quadrilateral frame. This involves a pin placed in the proximal tibia, linked by rods to another pin which is placed through the calcaneum. The distal pin is inserted from the medial aspect of the calcaneum, about an inch (2.5 cm) superior and towards the toes, away from the heel. Which local nerve is most likely to be damaged by improper pin placement?**
   A. Deep fibular (peroneal) nerve
   B. Lateral plantar nerve
   C. Medial plantar nerve
   D. Saphenous nerve
   E. Superficial fibular (peroneal) nerve

Basic sciences: Physiology

9. **The following are the blood results of a 70-year-old man:**
   Sodium: 128 mmol/L
   Potassium: 4 mmol/L
   Urea: 5 mmol/L
   Creatinine: 89 mmol/L
   Glucose: 13 mmol/L

   What is the serum osmolality (mOsmol/kg)?
   A. 290
   B. 288
   C. 282
   D. 269
   E. 275

Basic sciences: Pathology

10. Which of the following is not true about haemorrhoids?

A. Haemorrhoids are formed by the expansion of the endoanal cushions

B. Portal hypertension may result in haemorrhoids

C. Blood supply is mainly from the superior rectal artery

D. Internal haemorrhoids are lined by columnar and transitional epithelium

E. External haemorrhoids are lined by transitional and squamous epithelium

Common surgical conditions and the subspecialties: Trauma and orthopaedics

11. An 82-year-old woman, who is normally healthy and independently mobile, presents to the Emergency Department complaining of severe hip pain after sustaining a mechanical fall. Plain radiography of her pelvis reveals an undisplaced intracapsular fracture of the femoral neck. No signs of osteoarthritis are visible on the radiograph. What is the best form of treatment for this patient's hip fracture?

A. Cannulated screw fixation

B. Cemented Thompson's hemiarthroplasty

C. Dynamic hip screw

D. Non-surgical management

E. Total hip replacement

Common surgical conditions and the subspecialties: Neurology and neurosurgery

12. A 68-year-old previously healthy woman is brought to the Emergency Department by ambulance in an unconscious state, after having slipped on ice and hitting her head on the pavement. After initial resuscitation, a CT scan of her brain demonstrates a recent right-sided extradural haematoma. However, it also demonstrates the incidental finding of a space-occupying lesion in the left temporal lobe with an enhancing ring around an area of presumed necrosis. The radiologist is concerned that this incidental finding is suggestive of malignancy. What type of malignancy is this lesion most likely to represent?

A. Astrocytoma

B. Ependymoma

C. Glioblastoma multiforme

D. Meningioma

E. Oligodendroglioma

Perioperative care: Coagulation, deep vein thrombosis, and embolism

13. **A 10-year-old boy bleeds excessively after circumcision. Blood tests show a normal platelet count, a normal international normalized ratio (INR) but an elevated activated partial thromboplastin time (APTT). What is the most likely cause of the bleeding?**

    A. Haemophilia A
    B. Protein C deficiency
    C. Factor V deficiency
    D. Von Willebrand's disease
    E. Christmas disease

The assessment and management of the surgical patient: Surgical history and examination (elective and emergency)

14. **A 29-year-old motor cyclist involved in a high-speed road traffic accident (RTA) is brought to the Emergency Department by the paramedics. He is conscious but is complaining of severe discomfort in his lower abdominal region. On examination, he appears to be in hypovolaemic shock with a blood pressure of 100/70 mmHg and a pulse rate of 114/min. Palpation reveals marked tenderness over the suprapubic region and the iliac crests bilaterally. Further examination reveals the pelvis to be unstable, suggesting a fracture. Bruising is noted over the penis, scrotum, and the perineum. A per rectal examination reveals a high riding prostate. What is the most likely diagnosis?**

    A. Injury to the spermatic cord
    B. Injury to the peripheral sacral nerves
    C. Injury to the cauda equina
    D. Injury to the prostate
    E. Injury to the urethra

Basic sciences: Applied anatomy

15. **A vascular surgeon considers the use of cerebrospinal fluid drainage during thoracic endovascular aneurysm repair, to reduce the risk of spinal cord ischaemia. Which of the following statements regarding the blood supply of the spinal cord is true?**

    A. The artery of Adamkiewicz commonly arises from a posterior intercostal artery between T3 and T7
    B. The conus medullaris is the site of anastomosis of the anterior spinal artery with the posterior spinal arteries
    C. The internal carotid arteries give rise to the anterior spinal artery
    D. The paired anterior spinal arteries supply the anterior two-thirds of the spinal cord
    E. The posterior spinal arteries supply the posterior two-thirds of the spinal cord

Basic sciences: Physiology

16. Which of the following is not true about cerebrospinal fluid (CSF)?

A. CSF is produced by the choroid plexus in the lateral and third ventricles

B. CSF passes into the fourth ventricle via the aqueduct of Sylvius

C. CSF enters the subarachnoid space through the two lateral foramina of Magendie and the central foramina of Luschka

D. The total CSF volume is recycled more than once per day

E. CSF is absorbed by the arachnoid villi into the venous blood of the superior sagittal sinus

Common surgical conditions and the subspecialties: Cardiovascular and pulmonary disease

17. Which of the following is governed by the law of Laplace?

A. Blood flow in a vessel

B. Aneurysmal expansion

C. Peripheral arterial occlusive disease

D. All of these

E. None of these

Perioperative care: Preoperative assessment and management

18. Which of the following options is most appropriate for a type II diabetic patient undergoing bilateral hernia repair as a day-case procedure under general anaesthetic?

A. Their usual diabetic medication should be omitted on the night before surgery

B. They should be prescribed an insulin/dextrose sliding scale starting at 6 am on the day of surgery

C. They should be placed first on the operating list whenever possible

D. They should be kept nil by mouth at least 6 hours before the procedure

E. Their usual diabetic medication should be omitted on the evening following surgery

The assessment and management of the surgical patient: Planning investigations

19. A 55-year-old shipyard worker is referred by his general practitioner (GP) to the Ear, Nose, and Throat (ENT) clinic for a lump in the anterior triangle of his neck. The firm 2 cm by 2 cm mass seems to be fixed to the underlying tissue and moves with swallowing but not with tongue protrusion. Which of the following is true of fine-needle aspiration (FNA) of this lesion?

A. A FNA sample containing colloid is suggestive of malignancy

B. A FNA sample containing follicular cells is suggestive of malignancy

C. FNA is useful in the diagnosis of papillary carcinoma

D. FNA is useful in the exclusion of follicular malignancy

E. Reversal of anticoagulation is not usually required before image-guided FNA

Basic sciences: Applied anatomy

20. Which of the following is true about the parotid gland?

A. The parotid gland is a mucus secreting gland contained within the parotid sheath
B. The gland is divided into two lobes in relation to the retromandibular vein
C. Its autonomic nerve supply is via the facial nerve, which passes through the gland
D. The mandibular branch of the facial nerve lies superficial to the parotid gland
E. The parotid duct drains into the buccal mucosa opposite the lower second molar

Basic sciences: Physiology

21. Which among the following statements concerning the mechanics of respiration is incorrect?

A. Lung compliance is greater during the expiration phase compared with the inspiration phase
B. The majority of airway resistance is generated in the trachea and subsequent airway divisions
C. Resistive forces oppose airflow during inspiration
D. The radial traction experienced by the airways is inversely proportional to the lung volume
E. Under conditions of turbulent flow, pressure is proportional to $(flow)^2$

Common surgical conditions and the subspecialties: General presenting symptoms or syndromes

22. Which of the following is not true about a direct inguinal hernia?

A. The sac originates medial to the inferior epigastric vessels
B. The sac passes through the triangle of Hesselbach
C. It occurs due to a defect in the posterior wall transversalis fascia
D. The risk of complications from it is similar to that of indirect inguinal hernias
E. It is not commonly distinguishable from an indirect inguinal hernia in the clinical setting

Perioperative care: Postoperative care

23. A 53-year-old man with a history of Type I diabetes mellitus and hypertension undergoes an uncomplicated anterior resection for rectal malignancy. Three days after his operation, he describes faintness whilst walking to the toilet in the morning. His vital signs include a blood pressure of 78/55 mmHg, heart rate of 130/min and respiratory rate of 27/min. His oxygen saturations are normal. A finger-prick glucose check shows a value of 18 mmol/L. Which of the following is the most appropriate immediate investigation for this patient?

A. Arterial blood gas
B. Chest radiograph
C. ECG
D. Serum lactate
E. Urine ketones

The assessment and management of the surgical patient: Surgical history and examination (elective and emergency)

24. **A 42-year-old woman presents to the Emergency Department with a history of sudden onset severe headache. Examination reveals a temperature of 38.1°C, neck stiffness, and photophobia. Which one of the following would suggest a diagnosis of subarachnoid haemorrhage instead of meningitis?**

    A. Leucocytosis
    B. Fluctuating level of consciousness
    C. History of neurofibromatosis type 1
    D. History of diabetes
    E. History of chronic obstructive pulmonary disease (COPD)

Basic sciences: Applied anatomy

25. **Which one of the following does not form a boundary of Calot's triangle?**

    A. Inferior border of the liver
    B. Common hepatic duct
    C. Cystic artery
    D. Aberrant right hepatic artery
    E. Cystic duct

Basic sciences: Physiology

26. **Which cells are responsible for the remodelling phase of wound healing?**

    A. Platelets
    B. Myofibroblasts
    C. Neutrophils
    D. Monocytes
    E. Fibroblasts

Common surgical conditions and the subspecialties: General presenting symptoms or syndromes

27. **A 44-year-old man who had undergone repair of his perforated duodenal ulcer 3 weeks previously presents to his GP with a 24-hour history of right upper quadrant abdominal pain, fever with chills and rigors, and shortness of breath. He says that the pain is radiating to his right shoulder tip. On examination, his temperature is 39.2° C, pulse rate is 110/min, and blood pressure is 124/78 mmHg. Abdominal examination reveals tenderness over the right hypochondrium. Chest radiography reveals right-sided basal atelectasis and mild pleural effusion. What is the most likely diagnosis?**
   A. Pyonephrosis
   B. Subphrenic abscess
   C. Empyema of right lung
   D. Sclerosing cholangitis
   E. Acute cholecystitis

Perioperative care: Postoperative care

28. **A 60-year-old woman undergoes a right hip hemiarthroplasty for a fracture of the right femoral neck. A few days postoperatively her serum sodium is found to be 124 mmol/L and her urinary sodium is <20 mmol/L. Which of the following is the least likely cause of her hyponatraemia?**
   A. Syndrome of inappropriate antidiuretic hormone hypersecretion (SIADH)
   B. Hypothyroidism
   C. Vomiting
   D. Addison's disease
   E. Diuretic therapy

Basic sciences: Physiology

29. **A 35-year-old female undergoes a laparoscopic cholecystectomy for acute severe cholecystitis. The procedure proves difficult and the surgeon performs a subtotal cholecystectomy without the ligation of the cystic duct and inserts a drain in the gallbladder fossa for expected bile leak. Which of the following statements is incorrect regarding the physiology of bile secretion and the effect of cholecystectomy?**
   A. 5 L of bile is produced by the liver every day
   B. Less than 250 mL of bile can be expected through the drain in 24 hours
   C. 20% of bile is recycled by the terminal ileum
   D. Following cholecystectomy an increased volume of bile released into the duodenum may result in biliary reflux into the stomach with associated biliary gastritis
   E. Fat intolerance and malabsorption of fat may result in colicky abdominal pain and diarrhoea after fatty meals in post-cholecystectomy patients.

Common surgical conditions and the subspecialties: General presenting symptoms or syndromes

30. **A 54-year old man is referred to the general surgical clinic with a 4-week history of epigastric discomfort and fullness. He reports occasional episodes of vomiting and early satiety. He has a previous history of alcohol abuse and was discharged from hospital 2 months previously, following treatment for acute pancreatitis. On examination he appears clinically well, with a soft abdomen and mild epigastric tenderness and fullness. Preliminary investigations reveal a normal full blood count and biochemistry, with a serum amylase of 100 IU. What is the most likely diagnosis in this patient?**

    A. Acute pancreatitis
    B. Pancreatic pseudocyst
    C. Pancreatic cancer
    D. Chronic pancreatitis
    E. Gastric cancer

Basic sciences: Applied anatomy

31. **Which of the following tendons are contained in the second compartment of the extensor retinaculum?**

    A. Extensor digitorum communis and extensor indicis proprius
    B. Abductor pollicis longus and extensor pollicis brevis
    C. Extensor carpi radialis longus and brevis
    D. Extensor carpi ulnaris
    E. Extensor digiti minimi

Basic sciences: Physiology

32. **Which one of the following is not true about the cell cycle?**

    A. Neurons remain in G1 phase of the cell cycle
    B. S phase is where DNA synthesis occurs
    C. G1 is a gap phase under the influence of p53
    D. The restriction point (R) is where the cell decides whether to complete the cycle
    E. G2 phase is where cell growth and differentiation occur before division

Basic sciences: Applied anatomy

33. **An orthopaedic specialist registrar decides to revise the posterolateral approach to the hip for her next total hip replacement. Which of the following muscles is not normally divided to expose the joint capsule in this approach?**

    A. Inferior gemellus
    B. Obturator externus
    C. Obturator internus
    D. Piriformis
    E. Superior gemellus

Common surgical conditions and the subspecialties:
Gastrointestinal disease

34. **A 65-year-old male presents to hospital with obstructive jaundice, vomiting, and vague epigastric tenderness and fullness. He undergoes an ultrasound scan which excludes the presence of gallstones or duct dilatation. This is followed by a CT scan which confirms the presence of an irregular circumferential mass extending from the second to the fourth part of the duodenum. Tissue biopsies taken from the mass reveals dense infiltration of the epithelium by lymphocytes and atypical binucleate and trinucleate lymphoid cells. Which of the following disease processes would have predisposed to the development of this type of tumour?**

   A. Coeliac disease
   B. Crohn's disease
   C. Duodenal adenomatous polyps
   D. Small bowel tuberculosis
   E. Ulcerative colitis

Basic sciences: Applied anatomy

35. **Which one of the following structures lies parallel and immediately deep to the carotid sheath in the neck?**

   A. Vagus nerve
   B. Recurrent laryngeal nerve
   C. Scalenus anterior
   D. Trachea
   E. Sympathetic trunk

Common surgical conditions and the subspecialties: General presenting symptoms or syndromes

36. **A 91-year-old man living in residential care is brought to the Emergency Department with a 24-hour history of sudden-onset abdominal pain. On examination, he appears pale, cold, and clammy. His blood pressure is 98/68 mmHg and his pulse is 94/min and irregular. Examination reveals a soft abdomen with mild central tenderness and absent bowel sounds. Digital rectal examination reveals soft stool mixed with dark red blood. Arterial blood gas analysis reveals a pH of 7.22, bicarbonate of 18 mmol/l, and base excess of -10 mEq/L. Which of the following options best reflects this clinical picture?**

   A. Mesenteric infarction
   B. Sigmoid volvulus
   C. Acute small bowel obstruction
   D. Toxic megacolon
   E. Leaking abdominal aortic aneurysm

Basic sciences: Applied anatomy

37. A 23-year-old man is brought to the Emergency Department with a gunshot injury to his right upper thigh. On examination, the wound lies about 4 cm below the inguinal ligament. The vascular status of the limb is normal. Local neurological examination reveals numbness over the anterior thigh and medial aspect of his leg. Although he is able to flex the hip, he is unable to extend the knee on the affected side. The knee jerk is diminished but the ankle jerk is preserved. Which nerve is most likely to be affected in this patient?

   A. Sciatic nerve
   B. Tibial nerve
   C. Saphenous nerve
   D. Common peroneal nerve
   E. Femoral nerve

Common surgical conditions and the subspecialties:
Gastrointestinal disease

38. A 24-year-old male presents to the surgical assessment unit with a 48-hour history of constant right iliac fossa pain associated with loose stools and vomiting. He has had similar episodes before, having been admitted twice recently for conservative management. He also describes malaise and weight loss which he attributed to his recent mouth ulcers. On examination he is apyrexial, with a pulse rate of 90/min and blood pressure of 110/80 mmHg. His abdomen is soft but tender over McBurney's point with no signs of peritonism. Blood tests reveal a white cell count (WCC) of 13×10^9/L and C-reactive protein (CRP) of 15 mg/L. Which of the following is the most likely diagnosis?

   A. Acute appendicitis
   B. Crohn's disease
   C. Gastroenteritis
   D. Mesenteric adenitis
   E. Tuberculosis (TB) ileitis

Basic sciences: Applied anatomy

39. A 23-year-old student is referred to the urology clinic with unilateral testicular enlargement and a dragging sensation in his left testis. Examination reveals a firm mass in the body of the left testes. Together with preliminary blood results including an elevated alpha fetoprotein level, a clinical diagnosis of testicular cancer is made. Staging CT scans were performed of his chest, abdomen, and pelvis, indicating Royal Marsden classification stage 2 disease. Which of the following is the primary site of lymphatic spread?
    A. Axillary lymph nodes
    B. Cervical lymph nodes
    C. Pulmonary hilar lymph nodes
    D. Inguinal lymph nodes
    E. Para aortic lymph nodes

Common surgical conditions and the subspecialties: Genitourinary disease

40. A 67-year-old man is referred to the urology clinic with painless haematuria. There are no other significant findings in his history and examination. He undergoes a cystoscopy which reveals a transitional cell carcinoma. Which of the following is not a risk factor for bladder cancer?
    A. Smoking
    B. Schistosomiasis
    C. Cyclophosphamide
    D. Renal stones
    E. Aniline dye

Basic surgical skills: Wounds, scars, and contractures

41. Which among the following treatment options is not used in the management of Keloid scars?
    A. Topical silicone gel
    B. Steroid injections
    C. Radiotherapy
    D. Intralesional surgical excision
    E. Systemic steroids

Common surgical conditions and the subspecialties: General presenting symptoms or syndromes

42. From the following statements regarding abdominal compartment syndrome, choose the one statement which is incorrect:

A. The incidence of intra-abdominal compartment syndrome is grossly overestimated in the critically ill population

B. An intra-abdominal pressure between 15–25 mmHg is thought to normal

C. Intra-abdominal pressure can be measured by placing a pressure transducer in the femoral vein or within the stomach

D. The incidence of abdominal compartment pressure is increased after emergency aortic aneurysm repairs

E. Abdominal compartment syndrome maybe complicated by disseminated intravascular coagulation

Basic sciences: Applied anatomy

43. A 24-year-old construction worker was brought into the Emergency Department having suffered a crush injury to his left lower leg. Plain radiography performed on admission excluded a fracture. However, his pain increased overnight, requiring a large quantity of opioid analgesia. Examination revealed an erythematous, swollen, and shiny leg that was tender to palpation. Increased pain was elicited upon passive extension of the foot and great toe. In which of the following compartments of the leg was raised pressure most likely to have developed?

A. Anterior

B. Lateral

C. Deep posterior

D. Superficial posterior

E. Popliteal fossa

Common surgical conditions and the subspecialties: Neurology and neurosurgery

44. A 29-year-old mechanic presents to his GP with an acute-onset of back pain whilst lifting a 35-kg load in his garage. Which of the following options would support a diagnosis of prolapsed intervertebral disc?

A. Bilateral symmetrical nerve involvement

B. Loss of sensation over the left outer upper thigh

C. No evidence of nerve compression

D. Pain which is unremitting in character

E. Pain which is worse on resting

Basic sciences: Applied anatomy

45. A 29-year-old male was accidentally struck on the side of his head by a cricket bat. On arrival at the Emergency Department he was unconscious, with bruising over the region of his right pterion and an ipsilateral dilated pupil. Which of the following arteries is most likely to have been damaged?

A. Anterior cerebral artery

B. Posterior cerebral artery

C. Middle cerebral artery

D. Middle meningeal artery

E. Internal carotid artery

Common surgical conditions and the subspecialties: General presenting symptoms or syndromes

46. A 26-year-old female in her third trimester of her pregnancy has presented to the obstetric ward with a 24-hour history of worsening abdominal pain and vomiting. The obstetric team has requested for a surgical review as they suspect she might have appendicitis. Which of the following statements is incorrect regarding appendicitis in pregnancy?

A. Mortality risk for the fetus from appendicitis may rise to high as 20% in the third trimester

B. Perforation and abscess formation is more likely to occur in pregnant patients with appendicitis than in non-pregnant patients with appendicitis

C. Diagnostic laparoscopy may be performed safely before 26 weeks of pregnancy

D. A high WCC of 15,000/mm³ is indicative of appendicitis

E. Pain due to appendicitis in the third trimester is usually felt in the right upper quadrant or more diffusely

Common surgical conditions and the subspecialties: Gastrointestinal disease

47. A 4-year-old boy is brought to the Emergency Department with vomiting and abdominal pain. His parents say that he has been unwell for the past 3 days with intermittent abdominal pain, vomiting, and diarrhoea. He has not passed urine for more than 8 hours. On questioning, he points to pain in the region of the right iliac fossa. On examination, his abdomen is rigid and tender. Bowel sounds are absent. His temperature is 38.3°C, blood pressure 80/60 mmHg, and pulse rate 190/min. What is the most likely diagnosis in this patient?

A. Acute gastroenteritis

B. Bacterial peritonitis

C. Caecal volvulus

D. Meconium peritonitis

E. Necrotizing enterocolitis

Common surgical conditions and the subspecialties:
Gastrointestinal disease

48. Which among the following statements concerning pyloric stenosis is correct?

A. Its incidence is around 1 in 80,000 live births

B. It usually presents at about 3–5 weeks after birth

C. It results from a constricting band around the gastric antrum

D. It may be clinically suggested by projectile bilious vomiting

E. It leads to hyperkalaemic metabolic acidosis

Basic sciences: Microbiology

49. A 60-year-old male is admitted under the care of the physicians with a 4-week history of fever, joint pains, and night sweats. He had taken a 2-week course of co-amoxiclav prescribed by his GP but with little effect. On examination, his temperature is 39.2°C and his heart rate is 104/min. He is noted to have tender nodules on his hands and a bluish discoloration of his left second toe. On auscultation, a loud pan-systolic murmur is heard in the mitral area. Urinalysis is positive for leucocytes and red cell casts. He does not have any significant past medical history but he states that he had a root canal treatment from his dentist about 6 weeks ago. Which is the most likely organism causing his condition?

A. *Staphylococcus aureus*

B. *Streptococcus viridans*

C. *Enterococci*

D. *Staphylococcus epidermidis*

E. *Pseudomonas aeruginosa*

Professional behaviour and leadership: Medical consent

50. A 45-year-old bus driver is disorientated and confused on arrival to the Emergency Department after a RTA. It is believed that the bus that he was driving collided into a building, seriously injuring two passers-by. Although the police are keen to obtain a blood sample for alcohol measurement, the patient is neither keen nor competent enough to provide consent to have this procedure. What is the most appropriate action in these circumstances?

A. Obtain a blood sample now but analyse it only when the patient is competent and willing to consent

B. Obtain a blood sample now but analyse it after informing the patient once he is competent, regardless of his willingness to consent

C. Obtain a blood sample for immediate analysis

D. Inform the police that you may only take blood samples on medical grounds, and in your patient's best interests

E. Obtain consent from the patient's next of kin to draw the blood sample

1. Answer: B

There are six extraocular muscles which act to rotate an eye about its vertical, horizontal, and anteroposterior axes. They are the inferior oblique, and the superior oblique, the medial rectus, the lateral rectus, the superior rectus, the inferior rectus. The inferior oblique abducts the eye and moves it upwards; the superior oblique abducts the eye and moves the eye downwards; the medial rectus moves the eye medially; the lateral rectus moves the eye laterally; the superior rectus primarily adducts the eyes and moves it upwards (not abduct the eye and move it laterally); and the inferior rectus adducts the eye and moves it downwards.

2. Answer: C

Acute wound healing occurs as a sequential cascade of overlapping processes that requires the coordinated completion of a variety of cellular activities including phagocytosis, chemotaxis, mitogenesis, and the synthesis of extracellular matrix (ECM) components. These activities do not occur in a haphazard manner but in a carefully regulated and systematic cascade that correlates with the appearance of different cell types in the wound during various stages of the healing process. Although polymorphonuclear leucocytes (PMNLs) are important in the early stages of the wound healing process, healing can nevertheless proceed in the absence of PMNLs (and also lymphocytes), but monocytes are essential for wound healing. Blood monocytes on arriving to the wound site undergo a phenotypic change to become tissue macrophages. Collagen is a rod-shaped molecule composed of three polypeptide chains that form a rigid triple helical structure (that is 15 Å in diameter and 3000 Å in length). Collagen is also peculiar in that it is almost devoid of sulphur-containing amino acids, such as tryptophan and cysteine, but is rich in hydroxylysine and hydroxyproline. There are five main types of collagen in the human body. Their common distribution is as follows:

Type I: bone, skin, tendon, uterus, arteries
Type II: hyaline cartilage, eye tissues
Type III: skin, arteries, uterus, and bowel wall
Type IV: basement membrane
Type V: basement membrane and other tissues

The normal ratio of type I to type III collagen in the skin is approximately 4:1.

3. Answer: E

Metaplasia is defined as the transformation of one fully differentiated cell type into another. Metaplasia usually occurs in response to an environmental stimulus; it is an adaptive process and is usually reversible. However, metaplasia can progress to dysplasia (e.g. of bronchial epithelium in smokers) and eventually malignancy if the agent that caused the metaplastic transformation persists. Barrett's oesophagus—replacement of squamous epithelium by gastric epithelium in patients with reflux oesophagitis—is a type of epithelial metaplasia. Metaplasia can also be a physiological process as seen in squamous metaplasia occurring in the endocervix in response to hormonal surges during puberty. Abnormal mitosis and cellular atypia including pleomorphism, hyperchromatism, and a high nuclear/cytoplasmic ratio are features of dysplasia or malignancy, and are not seen in metaplasia.

4. Answer: C

Adhesive capsulitis (frozen shoulder) is characterized by a progression through pain, stiffness, and resolution over a period of 12–18 months. The cause is unknown but is thought to be autoimmune and is particularly prevalent in diabetics. The patient is usually 40–60 years old. The pain in the shoulder gradually increases over several months and is worse on all movements (distinguishing it from supraspinatus tendinitis where pain occurs in a small arc between 60–120° degrees of abduction). Plain radiographs are normal as opposed to calcific tendinitis, which shows a calcification in the area of the supraspinatus tendon. Treatment is usually by physiotherapy.

5. Answer: A

Recognized causes of acute pancreatitis include gallstones (50%), alcohol (25%), trauma, certain drugs (e.g. steroids, azathioprine, and thiazide diuretics), mumps, autoimmune pancreatitis, scorpion venom (rare), hyperlipidaemia, hypercalcaemia, and endoscopic retrograde cholangiopancreatography (ERCP). Pancreatitis results from the early activation of pancreatic enzymes, producing autodigestion of the pancreas and surrounding tissues. Exposure of trypsinogen to lysosomal enzymes such as cathepsin B has been elucidated as a mechanism for early trypsin activation. Digestive enzyme release is amplified as acinar cells lyse, leading to a vicious cycle of inflammation and necrosis. The common presentations include central abdominal pain that starts at a low intensity and gradually increases in severity. The pain may radiate to the back, may be associated with nausea and vomiting, and may be improved by sitting forward. On examination, the patient may be tachycardic with fever and jaundice; in acute haemorrhagic pancreatitis, there may be periumbilical discoloration (Cullen's sign) or bruising of the flanks (Grey–Turner's sign). Blood tests will usually show significantly raised serum amylase levels. Management includes keeping the patient nil by mouth. Consider administering intravenous (IV) fluids and plasma expanders if the urine output falls to less than 30 mL/hour. For analgesia, give morphine and ensure that the vital signs are recorded regularly. Complications include intra-abdominal sepsis, pseudocyst, shock, renal failure, and pancreatic necrosis.

6. Answer: E

When considering anaesthesia for elective AAA repair, epidural anaesthesia have not been shown to decrease mortality when compared to general anaesthesia. However, it provides a better form of postoperative analgesia leading to early extubation and fewer pulmonary complications. Patients will usually have arterial and central venous pressure monitoring as well as temperature, urine output and five-lead ECG measurements. Cardiac output monitoring is not performed routinely. A prophylactic dose of heparin is given prior to cross clamping as this has been shown to reduce thrombotic and embolic complications. Infra-renal aortic cross clamping performed during open AAA repair results in increased vascular resistance and hypertension as BP = CO × SVR. Patients with coronary artery disease may struggle with this increased cardiac workload and develop cardiac failure, which may be amenable to vasodilator therapy at this stage. Patients with severe aorto-iliac disease would have a developed collateral circulation and show minimal response to cross clamping. Unclamping results in dramatic falls in systemic vascular resistance and BP due to the release of vasoactive cytokines and toxic metabolites from ischaemic tissue. In the emergency setting, the patient's skin should be prepared and draped prior to rapid sequence induction. This is because the loss of abdominal tone and the negatively inotropic and vasodilatory effects of anaesthetic agents may result in severe hypotension upon induction.

7. Answer: D

This patient's history (i.e. acute onset cerebrovascular symptoms on a background of recent travel) suggests a lower limb deep vein thrombosis with peripheral embolus through a patent foramen ovale, leading to a left-sided cerebrovascular event (i.e. a 'paradoxical embolus'). TOE is the imaging of choice for investigation of a patent foramen ovale, although TTE with contrast may be a more practical alternative (due to the better availability and non-invasive nature of TTE). Upon confirmation of the diagnosis, patients with a patent foramen ovale do not require treatment if asymptomatic. Anticoagulation may be considered after the first presentation of stroke or transient ischaemic attack (TIA) to prevent recurrent episodes. Closure of the defect (i.e. if recommended by a cardiologist) is most frequently performed percutaneously, rather than via an open approach. Cardiac catheterization is first performed to assess suitability for this.

8. Answer: C

This patient has sustained a tibial plafond fracture (also known as a tibial pilon fracture) at the distal tibia and involving the ankle joint. As is the case with tibial plateau fractures, these injuries occur close to the joint surface and must be treated with the joint cartilage surface in mind. The various management options for tibial plafond fractures include casting, external fixation, limited internal fixation, internal fixation, and ankle fusion. In this case, external fixation is the treatment of choice and this involves insertion of a distal pin in the region of the medial calcaneum, where the medial plantar nerve runs and this may potentially be damaged. The medial plantar nerve is the larger of the two terminal divisions of the tibial nerve and accompanies the medial plantar artery along its course.

9. Answer: C

The intracellular and extracellular compartments are separated by cell membranes which are extremely permeable to water but less so to electrolytes. Sodium pumps in the cell membrane pump sodium out of the cell. This means that the distribution of water between the two compartments is largely determined by the osmotic effect of electrolytes in the extracellular fluid and the proteins within the cell.

Osmotic pressure is the pressure required to prevent osmosis and is directly proportional to the concentration of osmotically active particles in the solution. 'Osmoles' refers to the number of osmotically active particles in a solution; it is the standard unit of osmotic pressure.

Osmolality is the number of osmoles of solute per kilogram solvent (mOsmol/kg). Osmolarity is the number of osmoles of solute per litre solution (mOsmol/L).

Plasma osmolality (mOsmol/kg) is estimated by: 2(Na + K) + urea + glucose, which in this case, is approximately equal to 282 mOsmol/kg.

10. Answer: B

Anorectal vascular cushions are normally present in the anal canal. They commonly form three prominent cushions and help maintain continence for liquid and gas. They are formed from mucosa, submucosal connective tissue, and associated blood vessels. Expansion of the endoanal cushions (vascular and associated connective tissue) results in haemorrhoids. Arterial supply to the endoanal cushions mainly comes from the lower rectal submucosal vascular network (from the superior rectal artery) reinforced by perforating branches from the inferior rectal artery (from the pudendal artery). Precipitating factors include: constipation, prolonged straining at stool, obesity, family history, and previous rectal surgery. Portal hypertension may result in rectal varices but not haemorrhoids.

11. Answer: A

It is common that patients with fractured femoral necks, who are also eligible for surgery, would proceed to have surgical fixation of their injuries. This relatively fit patient (i.e. advanced age alone should not preclude surgical intervention in any patient) has an undisplaced intracapsular fracture of her femoral neck and so fixation with cannulated screws would be the most appropriate therapeutic option for her. If the patient had an osteoarthritic hip and was independently mobile, a total hip replacement would be more appropriate. Dynamic hip screws are employed for extracapsular fracture fixation.

12. Answer: C

Glioblastoma multiforme is the most common and most aggressive type of primary brain tumour in humans, involving glial cells and accounting for over 50% of all parenchymal brain tumours and about 20% of all intracranial tumours. They have a peak incidence between 55–65 years of age. The CT findings described in this scenario are also typical of glioblastoma (i.e. a 'ring-enhancing' lesion, although this is not specific; other pathologies such as abscesses, metastases, tumefactive multiple sclerosis, etc. may demonstrate similar appearances). The site of this patient's tumour excludes a meningioma, as it is reported to be in the temporal lobe and is therefore intrinsic. Ependymomas are tumours arising from the ependyma, a tissue of the central nervous system; they usually arise in the fourth ventricle. Astrocytomas account for about 10% of primary brain tumours in adults but are more common in children. Oligodendrogliomas occur primarily in adults (9%) of all primary brain and central nervous system tumours) but are also found in children (4%).

13. Answer: D

Von Willebrand's disease is an autosomal dominant disorder that causes a deficiency of von Willebrand factor, resulting in reduced platelet adherence to exposed vascular endothelium and instability of factor VIII:C. It is the most common inherited disorder, with some degree of deficiency detectable in 1% of the population. Clinical features are usually mild, and include bleeding that follows minor trauma or surgery. Platelet count, INR, fibrinogen levels are normal, while APTT and bleeding time are prolonged. Factor VII levels and von Willebrand factor are found to be low. Perioperative management of this condition includes desmopressin being given preoperatively and a short course of anti-fibrinolytic therapy given postoperatively.

14. Answer: E

The signs and symptoms in this patient are highly suggestive of a urethral injury. Hypovolaemia is due to the loss of blood from the associated pelvic fracture. Urethral injury should be suspected in the setting of pelvic fractures, straddle-type injuries, traumatic catheterization, or any penetrating injury to the perineal region. Amongst others, the important symptoms of urethral injury include pain, inability to pass urine, and haematuria (macroscopic or microscopic). Physical examination may reveal blood at the urethral meatus and a high-riding prostate may be identified upon rectal examination. Extravasation of blood may occur along the fascial planes leading to bruising in the perineum, scrotum, and penis. The urethra may be injured anywhere along its course. The membranous urethra is more prone to injury from pelvic fractures because the puboprostatic ligaments fix the apex of the prostate gland to the bony pelvis and thus cause shearing of the urethra when the pelvis is displaced. The bulbar urethra is susceptible to blunt force injuries because of its path along the perineum. Straddle-type injuries from falls or kicks to the perineal area can result in injury to the bulbar urethra. The penile urethra is less likely to be injured from external trauma because of its mobility, but iatrogenic injury may occur during catheterization or cystoscopy. If urethral injury is suspected, the patient should be discouraged from passing urine. Urethral catheterization should be avoided. Retrograde urography is the investigation of choice in suspected urethral injuries. If surgical intervention is required, then suprapubic catheterization may be required. Complications of urethral injuries include infection, bleeding, stricture, erectile dysfunction, and urinary incontinence.

15. Answer: B

The artery of Adamkiewicz (i.e. the 'greater radicular artery') usually arises from a left intercostal branch of the aorta between T8 and T12, and supplies the anterior spinal artery and distal spinal cord.

The anterior spinal artery is an unpaired vessel that arises from the vertebral arteries (i.e. not the carotids), which unite below the foramen magnum to form a single anterior spinal artery. This artery then supplies the pia mater and anterior two-thirds of the spinal cord, including the anterior and lateral columns (i.e. the major motor tracts). It anastomoses with the posterior spinal arteries over the conus medullaris.

The posterior spinal arteries arise from the vertebral arteries. They pass down the spinal cord individually and supply the posterior one-third of the spinal cord (i.e. including the major sensory tracts).

The blood supply of the anterior and posterior spinal arteries is augmented by collateral radicular arteries—the most important of these are the branches of the posterior intercostal arteries at the sites of the cervical and lumbar cord enlargements.

16. Answer: C

CSF is produced by a combination of ultrafiltration and active ion transport. Eighty per cent of the CSF is secreted by the choroid plexus of the lateral ventricles. It is produced at the rate of 20 mL/hour. The total volume of CSF in an adult is approximately 150 mL. This means that the total CSF volume is recycled over three times a day. CSF passes from the third ventricle via the aqueduct of Sylvius into the fourth ventricle. From the fourth ventricle CSF enters the subarachnoid space through the two lateral foramina of Luschka and the central foramen of Magendie. The fluid circulates throughout the ventricles and the subarachnoid space of the brain and spine before the majority is absorbed into the superior sagittal venous sinus via the arachnoid villi.

17. Answer: B

Aneurysmal expansion is governed by the law of Laplace. This states that the wall tension is proportional to the pressure multiplied by the radius. With increasing diameter, there is further increase in wall tension and diameter, leading to an increased risk of rupture.

$$T = PR$$

T = wall tension, P = pressure, R = radius.

Poiseuille's law describes the relationship of flow to pressure, viscosity, vessel radius, and vessel length.

18. Answer: C

Diabetic patients are suitable for most procedures performed in the day-case (day-surgery) unit although it is important for them to have good glycaemic control in the days and weeks before surgery. Type II diabetic patients can take their usual diabetic medications on the night before surgery. If the surgery is in the morning, then it is preferable to keep them nil by mouth for at least 6 hours preoperatively (with clear fluids allowed until 2 hours before surgery). In the morning, their blood glucose level has to be checked by finger prick and if it is high then they can be given small doses of soluble insulin (note that for major surgery or where there is prolonged postoperative starvation, insulin sliding scales should be considered). If they are known to have poor glycaemic control, then it may be advisable to monitor their blood glucose hourly (by finger prick) until the time of surgery. However, patients with type I diabetes should ideally be prescribed an insulin/dextrose sliding scale starting at 6 am on the day of surgery and have their blood glucose monitored closely. It is not essential that patients with type II diabetes are placed first on the list but this is nonetheless recommended whenever possible. Following day-case surgery, patients should be encouraged to eat as soon as they can tolerate it; and they can be recommenced on their diabetic medication as usual.

19. Answer: C

FNA biopsy has become a useful tool in the investigation of patients with a solitary thyroid nodule. Despite a false negative rate of between 1–6%, FNA is extremely accurate at diagnosing papillary carcinoma. Follicular cells, however, can be found with both follicular adenoma and carcinoma, and so the diagnosis of follicular carcinoma cannot be made solely with FNA; such patients are normally referred for surgery. Colloid and macrophages in the aspirate are highly suggestive of benign disease. During the procedure, any inherent coagulopathy is of concern because an uncontrolled haematoma is likely to compress local structures and may compromise the airway. As most FNA procedures are elective, efforts should be directed at reversing the coagulation defect. In patients who are anticoagulated, some reversal of the drug is usually done before the procedure.

20. Answer: B

The parotid gland is a serous gland contained in the parotid sheath. It has two lobes, superficial and deep in relation to the facial nerve and retromandibular vein. The facial nerve divides into its terminal motor branches within the substance of the parotid gland. The salivary flow is regulated by the parasympathetic nervous system. The parotid gland receives autonomic supply via the auriculotemporal nerve. Misdirected re-innervation of these autonomic nerve fibres after superficial parotidectomy leads to Frey's syndrome. This typically develops about 6 months after surgery and mainly features sweating and vasodilatation of the skin supplied by the auriculotemporal nerve. The parotid duct drains in the buccal mucosa opposite the upper second molar tooth.

21. Answer: D

During inspiration, a greater pressure is required to inflate the lungs to a given volume than that is required to achieve the same volume during the expiratory phase. This is the phenomenon of hysteresis and reflects the fact that work must be done during inspiration to overcome resistive forces such as the resistance of the airways and pulmonary tissue. Approximately 30% of airway resistance is located in the nose, pharynx, and larynx, and the remaining 70% of airway resistance is generated by the trachea and subsequent airway divisions. As the lungs inflate, increased radial traction is exerted on the airways, allowing them to expand such that radial traction is directly proportional to lung volume. The relationship between laminar flow and pressure is one of direct proportionality. However, during conditions of turbulent flow, pressure is indeed proportional to the square of the flow rate. Note: a full understanding of airway resistance and air flow involves consideration of several key principles of physics including Poiseuille's and Bernoulli's laws, and is a complex issue. The interested reader may wish to start with chapter 4 of Schwartzstein and Parker's Respiratory Physiology: A Clinical Approach (Baltimore: Lippincott Williams & Wilkins, 2006).

22. Answer: D

A direct inguinal hernia passes through the triangle of Hesselbach, the boundaries of which are as follows: laterally the inferior epigastric vessels; medially the lateral edge of the rectus; and inferiorly the inguinal ligament. Direct inguinal hernias therefore originate medial to the deep ring and inferior epigastric vessels. They usually occur due to a defect in the posterior wall of the transversalis fascia. They are wide necked, increase in size over time, and are at low risk (0.5% per annum) of acute complications (obstruction and strangulation) when compared to indirect hernias, which are at a medium to high risk of complications (2–5% per annum).

23. Answer: C

Patients presenting with cardiorespiratory dysfunction in the early postoperative period must urgently be assessed for cardiac complications of surgery. It has been demonstrated that the highest incidence of myocardial infarction is at 72 hours post-surgery. It must also be remembered that patients with diabetes mellitus and elderly patients may present with 'silent myocardial infarction' due to autonomic dysfunction—this is why careful monitoring of vital signs is crucial in such individuals. The patient in this case has two major cardiovascular risk factors and so a cardiac cause of his symptoms must be excluded. Although there may be many differential diagnoses (e.g. pulmonary embolus), the most appropriate immediate investigation in this scenario would be an ECG (and serum markers of cardiac ischaemia, e.g. troponin T).

24. Answer: C

Genetic and environmental factors have a role in the development of cerebral aneurysms and their risk of rupture:

- Family history of intracranial aneurysms.
- Smoking and hypertension both independently increase the risk of developing cerebral aneurysms.
- Several rare connective tissue disorders are associated with cerebral aneurysms, including autosomal dominant adult polycystic kidney disease, Ehlers–Danlos type IV, neurofibromatosis type 1 and Marfan's syndrome.

Sudden onset of severe headache without warning ('thunderclap headache') warrants urgent exclusion of a subarachnoid haemorrhage. Subarachnoid haemorrhage may occasionally present less overtly as a seizure or as a loss of consciousness. Delayed presentation may be with symptoms of meningeal irritation.

Fluctuating consciousness is also seen with bacterial meningitis and is not immediately suggestive of subarachnoid haemorrhage.

25. Answer: C

Calot's triangle is formed by the cystic duct inferiorly, the common hepatic duct medially, and the inferior edge of the liver superiorly. The triangle contains the cystic artery and a lymph node (Lund's node or Mascagni's lymph node). An aberrant right hepatic artery running medial to the common hepatic duct and arising from the superior mesenteric artery is seen in approximately 15% of patients. Numerous anatomical variations and anomalies can occur in this region. Surgeons should therefore appreciate that meticulous dissection of Calot's triangle and recognition of anatomy is vital during cholecystectomy.

26. Answer: B

Wound healing by primary intention can be divided in to four phases:

- Coagulation (fibrin–fibronectin clot formation): a wound invariably causes blood vessel injury and bleeding. This stimulates vasoconstriction and haemostasis. Platelets release cytokines, which stimulate inflammation. The resulting clot protects the wound as well as providing a matrix through which the inflammatory cells can migrate.

- Inflammatory cell recruitment: neutrophils and monocytes are rapidly recruited to the wound by chemotactic signals.
- Proliferation: this phase can be summarized by fibroplasia, matrix deposition, angiogenesis, and re-epithelialization. It begins within hours of the injury and continues until the wound is fully covered.
- Remodelling: remodelling results in wound contracture and gradual increase in tensile strength. Some fibroblasts become myofibroblasts which pull the opposing dermis and adipose tissue together.

27. Answer: B

Subphrenic abscess usually arises 3–6 weeks following abdominal surgery, mainly to the biliary tract, duodenum, or stomach, or following a perforated viscus or anastomotic leakage. The subphrenic space is in direct contact with the paracolic gutter, thereby facilitating the spread of peritoneal contaminants such as bile, blood or bowel contents in the paracolic gutter spread to this space. Subphrenic abscesses are right-sided in about 50%, left-sided in 25%, and bilateral in 25% of patients. Some clinical features of subphrenic abscess include pyrexia with chills and rigors, tachycardia, anorexia, loss of appetite, and loss of weight. Diaphragmatic irritation may affect the lung, resulting in chest pain, dyspnoea, and non-productive cough. Basal atelectasis, pneumonia, and pleural effusion are recognized complications of this condition. Abdominal CT imaging (or ultrasound scanning if CT is not readily available) is the investigation of choice to diagnose subphrenic abscess, and, if an abscess is identified, a CT-guided (or ultrasound-guided) percutaneous drainage catheter may be placed at the same time.

28. Answer: C

Hyponatraemia is a common finding in postoperative patients; any abnormal trends in serum sodium levels must therefore be monitored carefully. An assessment of the extracellular fluid (ECF) volume (i.e. reflected by the patient's hydration status) and plasma osmolality is crucial for diagnosis.

- Reduced ECF: dehydrated patients with urinary sodium >20 mmol/L suggests renal loss of sodium (e.g. Addison's, renal failure, diuretics). Sodium <20 mmol/L suggests losses elsewhere (sweating, gastrointestinal (GI) tract).
- Normal ECF: syndrome of inappropriate antidiuretic hormone (ADH) secretion or hypothyroidism.
- Increased ECF: excessive water administration, heart failure, renal failure.

29. Answer: B

Approximately 5 L of bile is produced by the liver every day. It consists of 97% water, 1.8% bicarbonate, 0.7% bile salts, 0.2% glucuronidated bilirubin, 0.3% cholesterol, fatty acids, and lecithin. The gallbladder concentrates this 5 L into 500 mL per day by gradually extracting the water into its mucosal lining. In the absence of a gallbladder to concentrate bile, large volumes of it will flow into the duodenum and may cause biliary reflux. Similarly, a bile leak as previously described may result in litres of bile being leaked daily. Production of bile salts is stimulated by secretin, cholecystokinin, and vagal innervation. It is suppressed by fasting and sympathetic alpha agonists. Ninety per cent of the bile is recycled in the terminal ileum.

30. Answer: B

The presentation of this patient is most consistent with a diagnosis of pseudocyst of the pancreas. Pancreatic pseudocyst is defined as a localized collection of pancreatic secretions, usually rich in digestive enzymes, that is enclosed by a non-epithelialized wall and persists for more than 4 weeks. Treatment is either conservative or drainage of the pseudocyst. Small pseudocysts (<5 cm) usually resolve spontaneously. Larger pseudocysts (5–6 cm or more) and those causing symptoms, i.e. gastric outlet obstruction, pain, bleeding, or infection, should be considered for drainage. Drainage can either be surgical, percutaneous, or endoscopic (cystogastrostomy or the commoner cystoenterostomy).

31. Answer: C

The fascia surrounding the extensors condenses at the wrist to form the extensor retinaculum. The space below is divided into six compartments, as follows (radial to ulnar):

1. Abductor pollicis longus and extensor pollicis brevis (forming the radial border of the ana-tomical snuff box)
2. Extensor carpi radialis longus and brevis through the floor of the anatomical snuff box
3. Extensor pollicis longus bends around the Lister's tubercle, which separates it from the second compartment
4. Extensor digitorum communis and extensor indicis proprius.
5. Extensor digiti minimi
6. Extensor carpi ulnaris.

32. Answer: A

The cell cycle is divided into the M (mitosis) phase and interphases G1 (gap 1), S (synthesis) and G2 (gap 2) phases. G0 is a resting phase of variable duration and is permanent for terminally dif-ferentiated cells like neurons. G1 has a high rate of biosynthetic activity. At the restriction point (R) the cell decides whether to complete the cycle. DNA synthesis occurs in the S phase. Further cell growth and differentiation occurs in G2 followed by cell division (both nuclear and cytoplas-mic) in the M (Mitosis) phase. G1 phase is under the influence of p53. Cyclins and cyclin-depend-ent kinases are the two main classes of molecules involved in regulating the cell cycle.

33. Answer: B

The posterolateral approach to the hip involves dividing the short external rotators of the hip (i.e. from superior to inferior: piriformis, gemellus superior, obturator internus, gemellus inferior and quadratus femoris) to expose the joint capsule. In contrast to these muscles, the obturator externus covers the outer surface of the anterior wall of the pelvis and is part of the medial compartment of the thigh. The anterior approach (Smith–Petersen) and anterolateral approach (Watson–Jones) are other methods of accessing the joint for procedures like the total hip replacement.

34. Answer: A

In the presence of obstructive jaundice and the absence right upper quadrant pain, gallstones remain an unlikely diagnosis. Other causes of biliary obstruction such as carcinoma of the head of the pancreas, lymphoma, cholangiocarcinoma, and malignancy of the duodenum should be consid-ered particularly in the elderly. Patients with coeliac disease are at five times the risk of the general population in developing enteropathy-associated T-cell lymphoma (EATL) which is a rare form of T-cell non-Hodgkin's lymphoma. These patients usually have a poor prognosis. Diagnosis involves investigations such as barium studies, CT scans, and endoscopic biopsy. Discrete bulky tumours may be amenable to surgery with subsequent radiotherapy, chemotherapy or both. Steroids are often used to shrink these tumours to assist with symptom control and further intervention.

35. Answer: E

Within the neck, the sympathetic trunk lies parallel and immediately deep to the carotid sheath, which itself contains the common carotid (and cranially, the internal carotid) artery, internal jugular vein, vagus nerve, and deep cervical lymph nodes. The sympathetic trunk lies ventral to the cervical muscles and transverse processes of the cervical vertebrae. It travels downward from the skull, just lateral to the vertebral bodies, and communicates with the spinal nerves (or their ventral roots) by means of rami communicantes. The superior end of the trunk enters the skull via the carotid canal and forms a plexus on the internal carotid artery. The inferior end descends in front of the coccyx, converging with the contralateral sympathetic trunk at the ganglion impar. Paravertebral ganglia are present along the length of the sympathetic trunk.

36. Answer: A

The history, signs, and symptoms in this scenario are typical of mesenteric infarction—a complication of ischaemic bowel disease. The majority of the patients who develop ischaemic bowel disease are elderly and a significant number of them will be in atrial fibrillation (i.e. increasing the risk of emboli entering the systemic circulation). Clinical features of this condition vary with some patients being asymptomatic or manifesting minimal symptoms during the initial period of bowel ischaemia; other patients may present with persistent, generalized abdominal pain. Vomiting may occasionally be present. Some patients may present with shock that is out of proportion to the clinical picture. The ischaemic bowel may shed the non-viable mucosa, which when mixed with mucus, results in dark-coloured (also known as 'plum-coloured) stools. Inflammatory markers such as the WCC and CRP may be elevated. Arterial blood gas analysis is a very useful investigation, potentially revealing a metabolic acidosis and raised serum lactate. This condition is a surgical emergency as the patient rapidly becomes toxic and may die from septic shock unless the infarcted bowel ('dead gut') is removed.

37. Answer: E

The femoral nerve arises from the lumbar plexus (L2–L4). It exits the pelvis by passing beneath the medial inguinal ligament to enter the femoral triangle after penetrating the psoas muscle. Within the femoral triangle, it lies lateral to the femoral artery and vein. It may be injured by gunshot wounds, direct penetrating wounds, traction during surgery, catheterization of the femoral artery, haematoma within the thigh, nerve injury secondary to femoral nerve block, psoas abscess, fractured pelvis, or by dislocation of the hip. Apart from trauma, it may be affected in patients with diabetes mellitus (diabetic neuropathy) and lumbar spondylosis. The femoral nerve innervates the iliopsoas, which helps in flexion of the hip, and the quadriceps, which act to extend the knee. The motor branch to the iliopsoas originates in the pelvis proximal to the inguinal ligament and injury at or above this level leads to loss of hip flexion. The sensory branch of the femoral nerve, the saphenous nerve, innervates the skin over the medial aspect of the thigh and the anteromedial aspect of the calf. Hence, femoral nerve injury results in numbness over the medial aspect of the thigh and the anteromedial aspect of the leg. Motor loss includes weakness of the quadriceps and decreased patellar reflex (knee jerk) (the ankle jerk is preserved since it is innervated by the tibial nerve (S1–S2)). In long-standing, subacute injuries, the patient finds that the knee gives way on walking and has difficulty climbing stairs.

38. Answer: B

Right iliac fossa pain has been the hallmark for acute appendicitis but making this diagnosis can sometimes be tricky. The Alvarado score (remembered by the acronym MANTRELS in Table 1.1) was developed to help with this process.

Table 1.1 The Avarado Score

	Score
M = migration of the pain from central to right iliac fossa	1
A = anorexia	1
N = nausea and vomiting	1
T = tenderness in the RLQ	2
R = rebound tenderness	1
E = elevated temperature	1
L = leucocytosis	2
S = shift of WCC to the left	1
Total	10

Reprinted from *Annals of Emergency Medicine*, 15, 5, Alfredo Alvardo. 'A practical score for the early diagnosis of acute appendicitis', pp. 557–64. Copyright 1986, with permission from Elsevier.

Score 1–4: acute appendicitis is very unlikely; keep under observation. Score 5–6: may be appendicitis; keep under regular observation. Score 7–8: probable acute appendicitis; operate. Score 9–10: definite acute appendicitis; operate.

The patient described in the question scores 3–4 so acute appendicitis becomes an unlikely diagnosis. Considering the recurrent nature of the pain, weight loss and mouth ulcers, Crohn's disease is a more likely possibility. The patient should undergo colonoscopy and biopsy of the terminal ileum to confirm the diagnosis.

39. Answer: E

About 1 in 500 men develop testicular cancer in the UK. They usually present between 20–45 years of age. These tumours can be classified into seminomas or non-seminomatous germ cell tumours (NSGCTs). NSGCTs include teratomas, yolk sac tumours, and choriocarcinomas. Occasionally Leydig cell or Sertoli cell tumours can arise from sex cord stroma.

Upon diagnosis, patients will have a staging CT of the chest, abdomen, and pelvis. The primary site of lymphatic metastasis is the para-aortic lymph nodes. The extent of spread is classified using the Royal Marsden staging system as follows:

Stage 1: tumour confined to testis
Stage 2: abdominal lymphadenopathy
Stage 3: supra-diaphragmatic disease
Stage 4: extralymphatic spread (e.g. lungs, liver)

40. Answer: D

The most common type of bladder cancer is transitional cell carcinoma. About 10% are squamous cell carcinoma which is associated with chronic irritation with long-term catheterization and schistosomiasis. Risk factors for developing bladder cancer include smoking, cyclophosphamide, radiation, and industrial exposure to aniline dye and rubber industry chemicals.

Genetic factors which predispose one to bladder cancer include abnormalities in chromosomes 9 or 17 and tumour suppression gene *p53*.

41. Answer: E

Keloid scars are benign dermal proliferative tumours unique to humans. They represent a dysregulated response to cutaneous wounding in genetically susceptible individuals, resulting in the excessive deposition of extracellular matrix, especially collagen. Although the exact mechanism remains unclear, various theories have been purported regarding its aetiology including: familial tendency, such as an autosomal dominant or recessive inheritance; abnormality of keratinocyte control over fibroblasts (epithelial–mesenchymal interactions); hormonal influence; altered immunological response; enhanced role of transforming growth factor β (TGFβ); and downregulation of apoptosis-related genes. In addition, keloids are also associated with various connective tissue diseases and some research has found a relationship with cell membrane proteins such as human leucocyte antigens. The management of keloid scars remains challenging. Various treatment options such as topical silicone gel application, intralesional excision (excision through the substance of the keloid), steroid injections, and radiotherapy have been attempted and widely used but none has gained lasting or universal acceptance. However, a combination of these treatment options is generally considered to produce the most promising results. Systemic steroids do not have any role in the treatment of keloid scars.

42. Answer: B

Normal intra-abdominal pressure (IAP) relates to intrathoracic pressure and is either 0 or subatmospheric. Following abdominal surgery or during mechanical ventilation IAP will be between 3–15 mmHg. Abdominal compartment syndrome occurs when the IAP rises to a level where the blood flow to the intra-abdominal viscera is compromised. However, this may vary widely with the intravascular pressure and the abdominal wall compliance. At pressures above 25 mmHg cardiovascular, pulmonary, and renal dysfunction develops. IAP can be measured either laparoscopically or via pressure transducers placed in the femoral vein, stomach, rectum, or bladder, the last being the most popular method. Some causes of abdominal compartment syndrome are blunt trauma, traumatic haemorrhage, pancreatitis, and, commonly, ruptured aortic aneurysm.

43. Answer: A

The bones, interosseous membranes, and fascia divide the lower leg into distinct compartments.

Anterior compartment: lies between the deep fascia and the interosseous membrane, with the tibia medially and the fibula laterally. It is also known as the extensor compartment as it contains tibialis anterior, extensor hallucis longus, extensor digitorum longus, peroneus tertius, the deep peroneal nerve and the anterior tibial vessels.

Lateral compartment: lies between the deep fascia, peroneal surface of the fibula and the anterior and posterior intermuscular septa. Within it lies peroneus longus, peroneus brevis and the superficial peroneal nerve.

The posterior compartment is divided into deep and superficial compartments. The deep posterior compartment contains the tibialis posterior, flexor hallucis longus, flexor digitorum longus, popliteus, posterior tibial vessels and the tibial nerve.

The superficial posterior compartment contains the gastrocnemius, soleus and plantaris muscles; and the medial sural cutaneous nerve.

44. Answer: B

The commonest presentation of prolapsed intervertebral disc is with pain and neurological deficit in a single nerve root. Roots of the sciatic nerve are more frequently affected as it is the lumbosacral region of the spine that is most likely to sustain disc prolapse. Clinical signs of multiple nerve root compression would allude to an alternative diagnosis. Similarly, pain at rest would suggest an alternative diagnosis such as infection, tumour, or metabolic disease, as would unremitting pain. Bilateral symmetrical nerve root involvement in the legs can be a feature of cauda equina syndrome, especially if other characteristic features (e.g. loss of perianal sensation and anal tone) are present.

45. Answer: D

The middle meningeal artery is a branch of the maxillary artery, which in itself is a terminal branch of the external carotid artery. It supplies only the bones of the skull and not any intracranial structures. The anterior branch of the middle meningeal artery lies beneath the pterion, which is formed at the site of fusion of the frontal, parietal, temporal, and sphenoidal bones. The surface marking for this is two finger breadths behind the zygomatic arch and a thumb's breadth behind the frontal process of the zygomatic bone. It is important to know this landmark as it is the site where an emergency burr hole may be created to drain an extradural haematoma.

46. Answer: D

The incidence of appendicitis is not increased with pregnancy, but the severity of appendicitis is certainly greater. The incidence of perforation of the appendix during pregnancy is as high as 25%; if the diagnosis is delayed this may rise to 66%. As the uterus enlarges, it displaces the appendix upwards and therefore although pain from appendicitis in the first trimester is felt in the right iliac fossa, it is felt more centrally in the second trimester and in the right upper quadrant or more generally in the third trimester. The normal WCC in pregnancy can be as high as 15,000/mm^3; this increased reference range limits the usefulness of an elevated WCC in pregnancy. Diagnostic laparoscopy may be indicated in some cases but may be technically difficult beyond 26 weeks of pregnancy.

47. Answer: B

Bacterial peritonitis in children and neonates may occur as a result of ruptured appendicitis, ruptured viscus, or as a complication of any abdominal surgery. The child or baby may have classical signs of peritonitis such as abdominal pain, pyrexia, nausea, vomiting, tachycardia, hypotension, and decreased urine output. Abdominal examination may reveal board-like rigidity, rebound tenderness, and absent bowel sounds. An erect chest radiograph may reveal free gas under the diaphragm, alluding to perforation of the GI tract. Blood cultures and diagnostic paracentesis with culture of the peritoneal fluid may help with the diagnosis. Plain abdominal radiography should be undertaken and may demonstrate the affected (e.g. dilated) bowel segments, possibly excluding conditions such as caecal or sigmoid volvulus. Occasionally, the possibility of primary peritonitis may seem high enough to warrant aspiration and Gram stain of the peritoneal fluid. Laparotomy is the most important means of diagnosis. The common organisms responsible for bacterial peritonitis include *Escherichia coli*, *Klebsiella pneumoniae*, and *Pseudomonas* species. Although local policies may vary, the antibiotics commonly used to treat this condition include IV cefotaxime and oral ofloxacin.

48. Answer: B

Pyloric stenosis, also known as infantile hypertrophic pyloric stenosis, is the most common cause of intestinal obstruction in infancy. The incidence is estimated to be about 2–4 per 1000 live births. Pyloric stenosis has a male-to-female predominance of 4:1, with 30% of babies being first-born males. The condition is not present at birth but develops over a number of weeks after birth (and is therefore 'acquired' and not a congenital condition, as once believed). The pathophysiology of the condition represents a marked hypertrophy and hyperplasia of the circular and longitudinal muscular layers of the pylorus, leading to a narrowing of the gastric antrum. Palpation of the abdomen on 'test feeding' may reveal an olive-shaped mass just below the right costal margin (i.e. the hypertrophied pylorus), and a distended stomach. Visible peristalsis may be seen on inspection of the abdomen. The vomit is not bilious in nature since the stenosis occurs proximal to the ampulla of Vater (i.e. where the pancreatic duct opens into the duodenum). This condition leads to hypokalaemia, hypochloraemia, and metabolic alkalosis due to the loss of hydrogen, potassium, and chloride ions in the vomit, but more importantly, because the kidneys continue to exchange hydrogen and potassium for sodium in an effort to conserve sodium and water in the presence of dehydration.

49. Answer: B

This patient is most likely to have infective endocarditis. He has at least three Duke minor criteria: Osler's nodes, embolic episode in the extremities, temperature >39°C, evidence of glomerulonephritis, and a (new) cardiac murmur. *Streptococcus viridans* is the most likely organism to cause native valve endocarditis. *Staphylococcus aureus* and *Staphylococcus epidermidis* are the commonest organisms causing endocarditis following early prosthetic valve replacement. Endocarditis due to enterococci is associated with genitourinary and GI procedures.

50. Answer: A

The British Medical Association has provided clear guidance on consent for investigation under such challenging circumstances. Following the Police Reform Act, it is no longer necessary to obtain consent from unconscious or incapacitated drivers. However, the sample cannot be tested until the patient regains competence and provides valid consent to it being tested. A competent patient who refuses to allow his or her sample to be tested in accordance with these legal obligations might be liable to prosecution. In this way, the new law recognizes the clinician's duty to justice.

Basic sciences: Applied anatomy

1. **Which among the following statements concerning the lymphatic drainage of the colon is incorrect?**
   A. Lymph from the intermediate mesocolic lymph nodes drain to the principal nodes
   B. Lymph from the caecum drains into the principal nodes at the origin of the inferior mesenteric artery
   C. Lymph from the ascending colon passes to the superior mesenteric lymph nodes
   D. Lymph from the descending colon passes to the intermediate colic lymph nodes along the left colic artery
   E. Lymph from the transverse colon passes to the lymph nodes that lie along the middle colic artery

Basic sciences: Physiology

2. **Which of the following statements regarding renal function is correct?**
   A. The optimum urine output in an adult in the postoperative period should be 0.1 mL/kg/hour
   B. Oliguria in the postoperative period is defined as a urine output of less than 25 mL/hour for 2 consecutive hours
   C. Intravenous furosemide should be promptly instituted in a postoperative surgical patient with low urine output for more than 3 hours
   D. A rise in serum creatinine is one of the earliest signs of impending renal failure
   E. Pre-existing renal disease is an important cause for postoperative renal dysfunction

Basic sciences: Pathology

3. **Which of the following is not a histological feature of malignant tumours?**
   A. Increased mitosis
   B. Pleomorphism
   C. Hyperchromatism
   D. A decrease in the nuclear:cytoplasmic ratio
   E. Focal areas of haemorrhage and necrosis

Common surgical conditions and the subspecialties:
Trauma and orthopaedics

4. A 5-year-old girl is thrown off a swing and lands on her right leg,
    which becomes tender and swollen. She is brought to the Emergency
    Department where radiography demonstrates a fracture of the distal
    tibia, which seems to be through a well-defined radiolucent area with
    sclerotic edges. What is the most likely diagnosis?

    A. Bone cysts
    B. Bone metastasis
    C. Chondrosarcoma
    D. Ewing's tumour
    E. Osteosarcoma

Common surgical conditions and the subspecialties: General presenting
symptoms or syndromes

5. A 70-year-old lady presents to the Emergency Department with
    sudden-onset epigastric pain. Her blood pressure is 110/80 mmHg and
    her pulse rate is 110/min (regular). The only ailment in her medical
    history is osteoarthritis. Plain abdominal radiography is normal. An
    erect chest radiograph shows gas under the diaphragm. A rectal
    examination reveals melaena. What is the most likely diagnosis?

    A. Ureteric colic
    B. Crohn's disease
    C. Adhesive small bowel obstruction
    D. Perforated peptic ulcer
    E. Acute pancreatitis

Perioperative care: Postoperative care

6. Which of the following statements is incorrect regarding the
    physiological effects following trauma/surgery?

    A. A raised basal metabolic rate results in proteolysis in the absence of calorific intake
    B. In sepsis or shock, hypoglycaemia may ensue in the diabetogenic state
    C. Serum ketone levels are usually high
    D. Proteolytic states result in a negative nitrogen balance
    E. There is a tendency towards sodium retention

The assessment and management of the surgical patient:
Clinical decision-making

7. A 38-year-old man sustains major trauma to multiple organs in a
    road traffic accident. He is admitted to intensive care, where he
    is fully ventilated. His presentation is soon complicated by septic
    shock, for which he is commenced on noradrenaline, continuous
    veno-venous haemofiltration and intravenous antibiotics. His mean
    arterial pressure remains at 60 mmHg and does not improve after
    his noradrenaline is changed to adrenaline. There is no evidence of
    myocardial dysfunction. What would be the most appropriate next
    step in managing this patient?
    A. Activated protein C
    B. Change of inotropes
    C. Dexamethasone
    D. Hydrocortisone
    E. Nitric oxide

Basic sciences: Applied anatomy

8. A 34-year-old secretary presents to the Emergency Department
    after sustaining multiple penetrating injuries to her right upper limb.
    Careful examination reveals no vascular injury to the limb, and sensory
    function remains intact. On examination of motor function, however,
    finger extension is severely limited. Which nerve is most likely to have
    been damaged?
    A. Anterior interosseous nerve
    B. Medial antebrachial cutaneous nerve
    C. Musculocutaneous nerve
    D. Posterior interosseous nerve
    E. Radial nerve

Basic sciences: Physiology

9. Which of the following is not true about insulin?
    A. It increases glucose uptake in tissues
    B. It increases the uptake of amino acids and lipids in tissues
    C. It stimulates glycogenesis
    D. It increases protein catabolism
    E. It stimulates lipid oxidation

Basic sciences: Pathology

10. **A 60-year-old smoker with apical lung cancer has signs and symptoms of Horner's syndrome. Which of the following is not a feature of Horner's syndrome?**
    A. Ptosis
    B. Miosis
    C. Enophthalmos
    D. Loss of ciliospinal reflex
    E. Loss of lacrimation

Common surgical conditions and the subspecialties: Trauma and orthopaedics

11. **A 5-year-old boy presents to his GP with a 1-week history of progressively worsening left hip pain and limping. The GP suspects Perthes' disease and reassures the boy and his parents. Which imaging modality is most likely to detect the earliest changes of Perthes' disease?**
    A. Plain radiography
    B. Computed tomography
    C. Magnetic resonance imaging
    D. Ultrasonography
    E. Radioisotope bone scanning

Common surgical conditions and the subspecialties: Gastrointestinal disease

12. **A 45-year-old diabetic man is referred to the Emergency Department by his GP for recurrence of a previously drained perianal abscess. He is admitted for examination under anaesthesia, which reveals the presence of a fistula draining the abscess cavity. The abscess is clearly visible at 7 o'clock in the lithotomy position. What is the most likely location of the internal opening of the fistula tract?**
    A. At 12 o'clock (i.e. anterior to the anus)
    B. At 3 o'clock (i.e. left of the anus)
    C. At 6 o'clock (i.e. posterior to the anus)
    D. At 7 o'clock (i.e. the fistula tract is in a straight line from the abscess cavity)
    E. At 9 o'clock (i.e. right of the anus)

Perioperative care: Postoperative care

13. **A 30-year-old female undergoes a total pancreatectomy for severe necrotizing pancreatitis that does not respond to conservative therapy. Which of the following statements is incorrect regarding the physiological effects of total pancreatectomy on this patient?**

A. Protein malnutrition and negative nitrogen balance ensues from a loss of proteolytic proenzymes

B. The patient is likely to develop diabetes mellitus

C. Loss of fat emulsification will result in the malabsorption of vitamins A, C, D, and K

D. The patient is at a higher risk of developing iron deficient anaemia

E. The patient has a higher risk of developing osteoporosis

The assessment and management of the surgical patient: Consent

14. **Which of the following is not a necessary topic when obtaining informed consent from a patient before an invasive investigation or intervention?**

A. Explanation of the likely benefits and the probabilities of success

B. The purpose of a proposed investigation or treatment

C. Advice about whether the proposed treatment is experimental

D. Comparative figures of the surgeon's rate of complications against the national rate of complications

E. Other options for investigation or management of the condition

Basic sciences: Applied anatomy

15. **A urologist performs a radical cystectomy for locally advanced bladder malignancy in an elderly gentleman. Which of the following statements about the anatomy of the urinary bladder is correct?**

A. A peritoneal fold separates the bladder from the pubic symphysis

B. The bladder is related superomedially to the levator ani muscle

C. The external iliac veins drain the venous plexus of the bladder

D. The transitional cell epithelium of the bladder is derived from ectoderm

E. The bladder is located in the abdomen in young children

Basic sciences: Physiology

16. **Which of the following statements is not true regarding the secretion of antidiuretic hormone (ADH)?**
    A. Osmoreceptors situated in the hypothalamus are sensitive to increasing plasma osmolarity
    B. Baroreceptors situated in the atria of the heart are sensitive to circulating blood volume
    C. Stretch receptors situated in the carotid arteries are stimulated when the blood pressure rises
    D. Head injury stimulates ADH secretion
    E. Prolonged hypoxia can lead to oliguria and hyponatraemia

Common surgical conditions and the subspecialties: Genitourinary disease

17. **A 70-year-old male presents with lower urinary tract symptoms. A diagnosis of benign prostatic hyperplasia is made. Which of the following could be a likely presenting feature in the patient?**
    A. Phimosis
    B. Enlarged posterior lobes of prostate
    C. Retrograde ejaculation
    D. Vaginal hydrocoele
    E. Detrusor atony

Perioperative care: Preoperative assessment and management

18. **A 79-year-old gentleman with multiple medical comorbidities is undergoing excision of a basal cell carcinoma from his periorbital region under local anaesthesia. Which of the following medications should preferably be stopped prior to surgery?**
    A. Prednisolone
    B. Aspirin
    C. Propranolol
    D. Gliclazide
    E. Bendrofluazide

The assessment and management of the surgical patient:
Clinical decision-making

19. **An 83-year-old gentleman with a history of hypertension, hypercholesterolaemia, insulin-dependent diabetes mellitus and peripheral vascular disease, suffers a transient ischaemic attack involving temporary weakness of his left arm and left leg. Initial investigations including ECG and transthoracic echocardiography are normal. After complete recovery of his motor function, a carotid duplex ultrasound scan reveals complete stenosis of his left internal carotid artery and a 71% stenosis of his right internal carotid artery. Which of the following treatment options would be most appropriate for this patient?**
    A. Right carotid bypass
    B. Right carotid endarterectomy
    C. Bilateral carotid endarterectomy
    D. Left carotid angioplasty
    E. Left carotid endarterectomy

Basic sciences: Applied anatomy

20. **A 30-year-old male undergoes a right superficial parotidectomy. Eight months later he presents to the outpatient department complaining of flushing and sweating of the right side of his face on eating. He is diagnosed as having Frey's syndrome and is listed for botulinum toxin injections. Misdirected re-innervation of which nerve is responsible for this syndrome?**
    A. Greater auricular nerve
    B. Facial nerve
    C. Trigeminal nerve
    D. Auriculotemporal nerve
    E. Greater petrosal nerve

Basic sciences: Physiology

21. **Which of the following statements is incorrect regarding the action of nitric oxide (NO)?**
    A. NO causes vasoconstriction by causing contraction of smooth muscle cells
    B. NO regulates vascular remodelling
    C. NO is responsible for penile erection by causing relaxation of the corpus cavernosum
    D. NO prevents platelet aggregation and adhesion
    E. NO plays an important function in the relaxation of the anal sphincter

Common surgical conditions and the subspecialties: Genitourinary disease

22. **A 30-year-old man presents with severe right loin pain radiating to his groin. He undergoes a CT scan of his kidneys, ureters and bladder, and is diagnosed with a ureteric stone. At which anatomical site may the stone have been impacted?**
    A. Pelviureteric junction
    B. Point at which the iliac vessels cross the ureter
    C. Vesicoureteric junction
    D. All of the above
    E. None of the above

Perioperative care: Haemostasis and blood products

23. **An 85-year-old retired gentleman is referred to the Emergency Department by his GP for a 24-hour history of melaena. The patient was commenced on warfarin 4 weeks previously, after a new diagnosis of atrial fibrillation. The gentleman's blood pressure is 84/59 mmHg, his heart rate is 110/min, and his respiratory rate is 20/min. Cardiorespiratory and abdominal examinations are otherwise normal; a rectal examination confirms melaena. Initial blood tests reveal a Hb of 8.5 g/L, MCV of 80 fL, and INR of 6.3. Which of the following options is most appropriate for managing this patient's coagulopathy?**
    A. Fresh frozen plasma only
    B. Intravenous vitamin K only
    C. Stop warfarin
    D. Stop warfarin and administer intravenous vitamin K
    E. Stop warfarin and administer intravenous vitamin K with prothrombin complex concentrate

The assessment and management of the surgical patient:
Clinical decision-making

24. **A 42-year-old asymptomatic woman undergoes an ultrasound scan of her abdomen as part of a routine private health check-up. The ultrasound scan shows gallstones, and she is subsequently referred to the surgical outpatient clinic. What is the treatment of choice?**
    A. Laparoscopic cholecystectomy
    B. Repeat ultrasound
    C. No treatment—reassurance and discharge
    D. Magnetic resonance cholangiopancreatography (MRCP)
    E. Endoscopic retrograde cholangiopancreatography (ERCP)

Basic sciences: Applied anatomy

25. **A 30-year-old man with a history of alcoholic liver cirrhosis and portal hypertension presents with sudden-onset massive haematemesis. Gastroscopy reveals bleeding oesophageal varices, which are then banded. Which one of the following is true about the anatomy of the portal venous system?**

    A. The portal vein arises from the confluence of the splenic and the inferior mesenteric veins

    B. The portal vein arises behind the neck of the pancreas.

    C. Porto-systemic anastomoses are found only in the lower oesophagus and around the umbilicus.

    D. The portal vein drains the GI tract from the upper oesophagus to the anorectal junction

    E. The portal vein lies anterior to the common bile duct and hepatic artery in the lesser omentum

Basic sciences: Physiology

26. **Which of the following is not true about the cardiac cycle?**

    A. The cardiac cycle lasts about 0.8 seconds

    B. Atrial contraction contributes to about 30% of atrial filling

    C. During exercise there is disproportionate shortening of ventricular relaxation

    D. Isovolumetric contraction is initiated by the QRS complex

    E. The T wave corresponds to reduced ventricular ejection

Common surgical conditions and the subspecialties: Skin, Head, and Neck

27. **A 19-year-old man is brought to the Emergency Department after being found unconscious outside a pub. On examination he has a GCS of 3 with a blood pressure of 116/84 mmHg and pulse rate of 94/min. He smells heavily of alcohol. He is noted to have bilateral periorbital haematomas and bruising over the right mastoid process. There appears to be serosanguinous discharge from his right nostril and right ear. Otoscopic examination of the right ear reveals blood behind the tympanic membrane. What is the most likely diagnosis in this patient?**

    A. Le Fort I fracture

    B. Le Fort II fracture

    C. Le Fort III fracture

    D. Basal skull fracture

    E. Extradural haemorrhage

Basic sciences: Applied anatomy

28. **A 45-year-old male presents to his GP with groin lumps on both sides. Examination reveals firm bilateral inguinal lymphadenopathy. The GP attempts to recall the lymphatic drainage of the region in order to suggest potential causes for this. Which one of the following anatomical structures does not drain to the superficial inguinal lymph nodes?**

    A. Perineum
    B. Feet
    C. Scrotum
    D. Testicle
    E. Lower anal canal

Basic sciences: Physiology

29. **A 55-year-old patient presents to her GP with a longstanding history of nausea. Which of the following statements is incorrect regarding the mechanisms associated with mediating nausea?**

    A. Stimulation of chemoreceptors and stretch receptors of the gut are transmitted by the afferent vagal nerves to produce nausea
    B. The chemoreceptor trigger zone senses potentially toxic chemicals in the gut
    C. Motion sickness is mediated through vestibular apparatus
    D. Disequilibrium caused by alcohol is mediated via the vestibular apparatus
    E. Chemoreceptor trigger zone modulates complex experiences such as taste, sight, smell, memory, and emotion involved in anticipatory nausea

Common surgical conditions and the subspecialties: Genitourinary disease

30. **A 10-year-old boy presents to the Emergency Department with a 24-hour history of progressive right testicular pain. Examination reveals normal lying testes and some scrotal erythema and swelling. The right testes, epididymis, and spermatic cord are tender, and Prehn's manoeuvre leads to some relief of the pain. What is the most likely diagnosis in this patient?**

    A. Testicular torsion
    B. Epididymitis
    C. Epididymo-orchitis
    D. Orchitis
    E. Idiopathic scrotal oedema

Basic sciences: Applied anatomy

31. **A 35-year-old-man is brought to the Emergency Department following a road traffic accident. He demonstrates signs and symptoms of a simple pneumothorax, which is confirmed on chest radiography. Which of the following anatomical landmarks is not useful for delineating the 'safe triangle' for chest drain insertion in this patient?**
    A. Apex of axilla
    B. Inferolateral border of pectoralis major
    C. Anterior border of the latissimus dorsi
    D. Nipple
    E. Mid-clavicular line

Basic sciences: Pharmacology

32. **Which among the following statements concerning atropine is incorrect?**
    A. It is a muscarinic receptor agonist
    B. it leads to an increased heart rate
    C. It is mostly excreted in the urine
    D. It has a half-life of about 2–3 hours
    E. It decreases bronchial and salivary secretions

Basic sciences: Applied anatomy

33. **Before dissection of a gastric tumour, a surgeon identifies the communicating cavity between the greater and lesser sacs in the abdomen. Which of the following forms the inferior boundary of this area?**
    A. Caudate lobe of the liver
    B. First part of duodenum
    C. Gastroduodenal artery
    D. Hepatic portal vein
    E. Third part of the duodenum

Common surgical conditions and the subspecialties:
Gastrointestinal disease

34. **A 47-year-old male presents with pruritis and lethargy over the past 6 months. On examination he is mildly jaundiced and has scratch marks over his lower limbs. Examination reveals a palpable liver edge 2 cm below the costal margin and mild tenderness in the right upper quadrant. Blood tests reveal a normal FBC, bilirubin 30µmol/L, ALT 115 U/L, AST 150 U/L, GGT 110 U/L, cholesterol 7.2 mmol/L, negative hepatitis serology, a negative antinuclear antibody level, and a positive antimitochondrial antibody level. He undergoes an ultrasound scan which shows diffuse parenchymal changes with no duct dilatation or gallstones. What is the most likely diagnosis?**

    A. Cholangiocarcinoma
    B. Haemochromatosis
    C. Primary biliary cirrhosis
    D. Primary sclerosing cholangitis
    E. Wilson's disease

Basic sciences: Applied anatomy

35. **During open hepatobiliary surgery, the surgeon accidentally injures the structure directly posterior to the second part of the duodenum whilst attempting to mobilize this segment of bowel. Which one of the following structures is most likely to have been injured?**

    A. Fundus of the gallbladder
    B. Hepatic portal vein
    C. Hilum of the right kidney
    D. Superior mesenteric artery
    E. Gastric pylorus

Common surgical conditions and the subspecialties:
Gastrointestinal disease

36. **A 10-month-old baby boy is brought to the Paediatric Surgical Emergency unit by his parents with a 24-hour history of intermittent episodes of crying, vomiting, and refusal to feed. The parents say that they have noticed the baby's stools to be mixed with blood. On examination, a 'sausage-shaped' mass is palpable over the right side of abdomen. Per rectal examination reveals an empty rectum but blood is noticed in the glove of the examining finger. What is the most likely diagnosis in this patient?**

    A. Hirschsprung's disease
    B. Intussusception
    C. Duodenal atresia
    D. Meconium ileus
    E. Infantile hypertrophic pyloric stenosis

Basic sciences: Applied anatomy

37. Which of the following nerves does not arise from the posterior cord of brachial plexus?

A. Upper subscapular nerve

B. Long thoracic nerve

C. Thoracodorsal nerve

D. Axillary nerve

E. Radial nerve

Common surgical conditions and the subspecialties:
Gastrointestinal disease

38. A 65-year-old man is referred to the colorectal clinic with a 2-month history of faecal urgency, tenesmus, and diarrhoea with occasionally fresh rectal bleeding. A screening colonoscopy performed 6 months previously was reported as normal. He has had no recent weight loss or loss of appetite. His past medical history includes hypertension and prostate cancer, for which he received external beam radiotherapy one year previously. Abdominal examination is unremarkable and rectal examination does not reveal fissures, haemorrhoids, or rectal polyps. What is the most likely diagnosis in this patient?

A. Anal fistula

B. *Clostridium difficile* proctitis

C. Diverticular disease

D. Radiation proctitis

E. Ulcerative colitis

Basic sciences: Applied anatomy

39. A 45-year-old male presented to the Emergency Department complaining of a fish bone stuck in his throat. Despite soft tissue radiographs of the neck confirming the presence of the bone, it could not be detected during examination of the larynx with a laryngeal mirror. Eventually, endoscopic examination of the laryngopharynx allowed for the bone to be visualized and retrieved. Which structure may have been injured if the fish bone had pierced the mucous membrane?

A. Aryepiglottic fold

B. Internal laryngeal nerve

C. Larynx

D. Recurrent laryngeal nerve

E. Vocal cords

Common surgical conditions and the subspecialties: General presenting symptoms or syndromes

40. **A 55-year-old lady with polymyalgia rheumatica is brought to the Emergency Department by ambulance for sudden onset chest pain, which started while she was driving. The pain was described as being 'ripping' in nature and radiated to her back and jaw. Her pulse rate is 110/min, and blood pressure from her right and left arms are 142/70 mmHg and 167/82 mmHg respectively. A portable CXR reveals a widened mediastinum and a small pleural effusion. What is the most likely diagnosis?**
    A. Aortic dissection
    B. Acute myocardial infarction
    C. Boerhaave's syndrome
    D. Cardiac tamponade
    E. Leaking abdominal aortic aneurysm

Basic surgical skills: Principles of safe surgery

41. **Which of the following statements concerning universal precautions in surgical practice is not true?**
    A. Water-repellent gowns reduce the risk of transmission of blood-borne diseases
    B. Wearing rubber gloves does not protect against sharps injury
    C. Needles should be re-sheathed before handing back to the scrub nurse
    D. Scalpels should be passed in a kidney bowl
    E. Fixed retraction devices reduce the risk of injury due to sharp objects

Common surgical conditions and the subspecialties: Gastrointestinal disease

42. **A 35-year-old male undergoes a terminal ileal resection for Crohn's fistulation. Which of the following conditions is least likely to occur as a result of his operation?**
    A. Vitamin C deficiency
    B. Gallstones
    C. Subacute combined degeneration of the spinal cord.
    D. Macrocytic anaemia
    E. Diarrhoea

Basic sciences: Applied anatomy

43. An 80-year-old osteoporotic female presents to the Emergency Department after having slipped and fallen on her outstretched right arm. After she is diagnosed with a Colles' fracture, she undergoes manipulation under anaesthesia and is eventually discharged home in a cast. At her two-week follow-up in the fracture clinic, she is found to be unable to move her thumb away from the rest of her hand (i.e. in the same plane as her hand), whilst her palm is resting flat on the table. Which of the following structures is she most likely to have damaged?

    A. Abductor pollicis longus
    B. Extensor pollicis longus
    C. Abductor pollicis brevis
    D. Radial nerve
    E. Median nerve

Common surgical conditions and the subspecialties: Endocrine disease

44. Which of the following options represents the commonest clinical manifestation of primary hyperparathyroidism?

    A. Bone disease
    B. Constipation
    C. Pancreatitis
    D. Polyuria
    E. Renal stone disease

Assessment and management of patients with trauma (including the multiply injured patient): Fractures

45. A 3-year-old boy is brought to the Emergency Department after a television fell onto his right knee. The child is in a lot of pain and the right knee appears swollen. Radiography of the right knee reveals a fracture of the distal femur extending through the epiphysis, physis, and metaphysis. Which type of epiphyseal injury has the child sustained, according to the Salter–Harris classification?

    A. Type I
    B. Type II
    C. Type III
    D. Type IV
    E. Type V

Common surgical conditions and the subspecialties:
Gastrointestinal disease

46. **A 35-week-old premature infant is brought to the Emergency
   Department, having had coffee ground vomiting and abdominal
   distension. Examination reveals a peritonitic abdomen and necrotizing
   enterocolitis is suspected. Which of the following is not a feature of
   necrotizing enterocolitis?**

   A. Feeding intolerance
   B. Rectal bleeding
   C. Haematemesis
   D. Metabolic acidosis
   E. Disseminated intravascular coagulopathy

Common surgical conditions and the subspecialties:
Gastrointestinal disease

47. **A newborn baby boy is brought to the neonatal clinic with gross
   abdominal distension and vomiting. His parents describe the vomitus
   as being green in colour, and are concerned that the child has not
   opened his bowels since birth. Plain abdominal radiography reveals
   distended loops of bowel. After appropriate resuscitation and
   management of the child, laboratory analysis of the child's sweat
   reveals increased levels of chloride. What was the most likely cause for
   this patient's presentation?**

   A. Meconium ileus
   B. Volvulus neonatorum
   C. Malrotation of the gut
   D. Intestinal atresia
   E. Hirschsprung's disease

Common surgical conditions and the subspecialties: Endocrine disease

48. **Which among the following statements concerning primary
   hyperaldosteronism is incorrect?**

   A. It results from an adenoma of the adrenal cortex in the majority of cases
   B. It leads to sodium retention
   C. It may result in hypertension
   D. It may suppress plasma renin activity
   E. It leads to metabolic acidosis

Organ and tissue transplantation: Transplant immunology

49. Which of the following statements regarding transplant rejection is incorrect?

A. Hyperacute rejection is a complement mediated response

B. Accelerated rejection may be due to HLA incompatibility

C. Acute rejection commonly occurs between 7–21 days post transplantation

D. Chronic rejection is associated with fibrosis of the internal blood vessels of the transplant

E. Acute rejection is characterized by the presence of leukocytes, macrophages, and T-cells within the interstitium

Professional behaviour and leadership: Evidence and guidelines

50. A researcher plans a study to investigate whether inappropriate steroid prescription is a risk factor for bowel perforation. He decides to perform a case–control study instead of a cohort study. Which of the following best describes an advantage of a case–control study over a cohort study?

A. It provides information on a wide range of outcomes

B. It may be performed with minimal expertise

C. It is able to directly measure the incidence of a disease

D. It is able to analyse exposure to rare factors

E. The chronological sequence of events can be assessed

1. Answer: B

Regional lymph nodes are one of the important means of metastasis for colonic malignancy. Hence it is essential to have a sound understanding of the lymphatic drainage of the colon. The lymphatics draining the colon can be classified into four main groups: (1) epiploic nodes, (2) para-colic nodes, (3) intermediate mesocolic nodes, and (4) principal nodes. The lymph thus drains from the epiploic to paracolic, then to the intermediate mesocolic, and finally to the principal lymph nodes that lie at the root of mesocolon. The pathways of nodal spread of the intermediate mesocolic and the principal lymph nodes follow the course of the arterial supply and the venous drainage of the respective colonic segments. Lymph from the caecum drains primarily to the ileocolic lymph nodes that lie along the ileocolic artery and the efferent lymph nodes from here pass to the superior mesenteric lymph nodes. The lymph from the ascending colon passes to the epiploic and paracolic lymph nodes, to the intermediate nodes that lie along the right colic vessels, and from them to the superior mesenteric lymph nodes (that lie at the root of the superior mesenteric artery). The lymph from the transverse colon passes to the lymph nodes that lie along the middle colic artery (and from them to the superior mesenteric lymph nodes). The lymph from the descending colon passes to the intermediate colic lymph nodes along the left colic artery and thence to the inferior mesenteric lymph nodes (that lie at the root of the inferior mesenteric artery).

2. Answer: E

An ideal urine output in an adult (and in the postoperative period) is greater than 0.5 mL/kg/hour. If the urine output falls below this level, the cause should be investigated immediately and appropriate management instituted. Oliguria in the postoperative period is defined as a urine output of less than 30 mL/hour for 4 consecutive hours. The commonest cause of poor urine output and subsequent renal dysfunction in the postoperative patient is hypovolaemia and thus adequate fluid therapy should be considered first. Intravenous diuretics should not be given during the initial management of oliguria or a suspected renal dysfunction. A fall in urine output is one of the early signs of renal dysfunction; changes in serum creatinine occur later when established renal damage has occurred (e.g. acute tubular necrosis). The commonest causes of postoperative renal dysfunction are hypovolaemia, hypotension, sepsis, nephrotoxic drugs, and pre-existing renal disease.

3. Answer: D

Some of the characteristic histological changes of malignant tumours include:

- Increased mitosis
- Abnormal mitosis (tripolar, tetrapolar, sunburst, or bizarre)
- An increase in the nuclear:cytoplasmic ratio
- Pleomorphism (variance of size and shape of tumour cells)
- Hyperchromatism (increased amounts of DNA leading to dark-stained nuclei).

In addition, there may be focal or extensive areas of haemorrhage and necrosis due to the abnormal vascularity associated with malignant changes. The surrounding tissues may also have infiltrative borders with evidence of vascular or lymphatic spread.

4. Answer: A

Bone cysts are benign fluid containing lesions that occur in the metaphysis of long bones. They mostly occur in children from 4–10 years of age and present as pathological fractures. Bone metastasis can be sclerotic or lytic depending on the primary tumour and usually present as bone pain or pathological fractures. Chondrosarcomas are malignant mesenchymal tumours which produce cartilage, arising from within the bone or from malignant transformation of benign cartilage tumours such as osteochondromas. They usually occur in people over the age of 60. Ewing's sarcomas are round cell tumours of bone or soft tissue, which usually affect young people aged 5–15 years. On radiography they appear as lytic lesions with the periosteal reaction giving rise to an onion-skin appearance. Osteosarcomas are aggressive tumours which arise from the medullary cavity of long bones and present as painful masses in patients aged 10–25. About 25% present later in life in association with Paget's disease.

5. Answer: D

Peptic ulcers (and subsequent perforation) occur more commonly in men than in women, and can be attributed to the regular use of non-steroidal anti-inflammatory drug (NSAID) analgesia for chronic painful conditions (e.g. osteoarthritis). These drugs irritate the gastric mucosa and increase gastric secretion, thus inducing ulcers that may eventually require urgent attention (e.g. due to perforation, obstruction, haemorrhage). The other risk factors include *Helicobacter pylori* infection, smoking, excessive alcohol consumption, and Zollinger–Ellison syndrome. The majority of symptoms include epigastric pain, nausea, and vomiting. The pain may radiate to the back or shoulder tip. After a convincing history, the diagnosis of a perforated peptic ulcer may be suggested by finding free air under the diaphragm on erect chest radiography. There may be elevated serum amylase levels which may not be as significantly raised as in acute pancreatitis. A CT scan of the abdomen may help to support the diagnosis and define the extent of the lesion. The complications of perforated peptic ulcer include peritonitis and upper GI bleeding.

6. Answer: C

The effects of trauma or surgery gives rise to changes in metabolism called the catabolic adrenergic–corticoid phase. This is characterized by a raised basal metabolic rate, which in the absence of adequate calorific intake, will result in proteolysis. Although there is a diabetogenic state, the blood glucose levels usually remain normal unless in states of high glucose consumption such as sepsis or shock. Blood ketone levels remain normal as increased production is balanced with increased metabolism and excretion in the urine. In the proteolytic state, the action of glucocorticoids results in muscle breakdown and a negative nitrogen balance.

7. Answer: D

If blood pressure is unresponsive to noradrenaline or dopamine in critical care situations, adrenaline is the first choice for change of inotropes. The current 'Surviving Sepsis' guidelines recommend the administration of hydrocortisone but do not recommend an adrenocorticotropic hormone (ACTH) stimulation test prior to this. In addition, hydrocortisone is preferable to dexamethasone; fludrocortisone may also be added. Activated protein C was previously used for sepsis-related organ dysfunction with a high risk of death (APACHE II >25) but it has been withdrawn (October 2011) and is no longer in use. At this stage, changing the patient's inotropes again would probably not be effective in relation to other options. Nitric oxide is not of benefit in such cases (i.e. it may exacerbate systemic vasodilatation) but is a non-proven therapy in adult respiratory distress syndrome (ARDS).

8. Answer: D

The posterior (or dorsal) interosseous nerve of the forearm (C7–C8) is the continuation of the deep branch of the radial nerve after the latter crosses the supinator muscle. It provides purely motor innervation and is considerably smaller than the deep branch of the radial nerve. It descends in front of extensor pollicis longus on the interosseous membrane. It forms a gangliform enlargement behind the carpus, from which filaments are distributed to the carpal ligaments and articulations. The nerve supplies all the extensor muscles in the forearm, apart from anconeus, extensor carpi radialis longus, and extensor carpi radialis brevis. Posterior interosseous neuropathy therefore affects only motor function, resulting in finger drop and radial wrist deviation on extension.

9. Answer: D

Insulin is secreted by the beta cells of the pancreatic islets of Langerhans. It increases tissue uptake of glucose, amino acids, and lipids. It stimulates glycogenesis, protein synthesis, and lipid oxidation. Insulin also inhibits gluconeogenesis and promotes intracellular uptake of potassium and phosphate.

Glucagon is secreted by the alpha cells of the pancreas islets; it promotes gluconeogenesis and thereby physiologically opposes the action of insulin.

The other endocrine secretions of the pancreas include somatostatin (from delta cells) and pancreatic polypeptide (from F-cells). Somatostatin inhibits digestion by having an inhibitory effect on GI motility and secretions. Pancreatic polypeptide is also a regulator of the digestive process and its secretion is stimulated by fasting, decreased blood sugar, and protein ingestion.

10. Answer: E

A Pancoast tumour is an apical lung tumour that may involve the brachial plexus, sympathetic ganglia, and vertebral bodies. It can cause pain, upper limb weakness, and Horner's syndrome.

Horner's syndrome is due to ipsilateral cervical sympathetic chain involvement. It is characterized by ptosis, miosis, enophthalmos, decreased sweating of the affected side of the face, and loss of the ciliospinal reflex. The ciliospinal reflex refers to pupillary dilatation caused by a painful stimulus to the head, neck or upper trunk.

Other causes of Horner's syndrome include carotid body tumours, carotid artery dissections or aneurysms, and syringomyelia.

11. Answer: E

Legg–Calvé–Perthes disease represents osteonecrosis of the capital femoral epiphysis of the femoral head in childhood, occurring principally in boys aged between 5–10 years. It may be a result of the changing vascularization of the femoral head at this stage of development. Presentation is with pain and limping, usually affecting just one hip, but occasionally both, developing over a month. Plain radiographs of the hip are useful in establishing the diagnosis but technetium-99 bone scanning is required to delineate the extent of avascular changes before they are evident on plain radiographs.

12. Answer: C

A 'fistula' is defined as an abnormal connection between two epithelial surfaces. A fistula-in-ano involves a fistula track communicating between the skin and the anal canal or rectum. Blockage of deep intramuscular gland ducts is thought to predispose to abscess formation, which then discharge to form the fistula. Goodsall's rule determines the path of the fistula track between openings: if the external opening of a fistula (characterized in this case by the abscess) lies behind a line drawn transversely across the anus the track should curve towards an internal opening in the midline posteriorly (i.e. at 6 o'clock). However, if the external opening lies in front of the transverse anal line, the track is likely to pass radially in a straight line towards the internal opening. Causes of fistula-in-ano include chronic inflammatory conditions (e.g. anorectal abscesses, inflammatory bowel disease, tuberculosis and diverticular disease). The condition is commonly investigated by MRI or endoanal ultrasound scanning. Definitive treatment includes fistulotomy and excision for low trans-sphincteric fistulas; and seton insertion (tight or loose) with staged sphincter repair.

13. Answer: C

Fat-soluble vitamins include vitamins A, D, E, and K. Loss of lipolytic enzymes results in a loss of fat emulsification and digestion resulting malabsorption of these fat-soluble vitamins. Fat malabsorption also exacerbates calorie malnutrition and results in fatty chyme which promote colonic bacterial overgrowth and fatty, floating, offensive stool and flatus. There is also malabsorption of iron, calcium, and phosphate resulting from the loss of alkalinization of chyme rendering these patients at a higher risk of developing iron deficiency and osteoporosis.

14. Answer: D

Patients have a right to information about their condition and the various treatment options available to them, although the amount of information providing to each patient will vary (according to the nature of the condition, the complexity and risks associated with the procedure, etc.) According to the General Medical Council, some of the information which should be provided to the patient includes:

1. Details of the diagnosis (and the likely prognosis if the condition is left untreated)
2. Options for treatment or management of the condition, including the option not to treat
3. Options for further investigation prior to treatment
4. The purpose of a proposed investigation or treatment
5. The likely benefits and the probabilities of success
6. Advice about whether a proposed treatment is experimental
7. Plan to monitor and re-assess the patient's condition and any side effects
8. The name of the doctor who will have overall responsibility for the treatment and, where appropriate, names of the senior members of his or her team
9. A reminder that patients have a right to seek a second opinion and that they can change their minds about a decision at any time.

Although the patient should be informed of the surgeon's own complication rate for the procedure, it is not necessary to provide a comparative figure against the national rate of complications of the procedure.

15. Answer: E

The urinary bladder is situated in the abdomen (i.e. not the pelvic cavity) in infants and children, even when empty. It is embryologically derived from two sources: the cloaca and mesonephric ducts. The primitive cloaca is divided by the urorectal septum into the urogenital sinus and rectum. The bladder develops mostly from the vesicular part of the urogenital sinus, and the bladder trigone is formed from the mesonephric ducts being drawn into the bladder floor. The transitional epithelium of the bladder is derived from the endoderm of the urogenital sinus, whereas the epithelium of the ureters and renal pelvis are derived from mesoderm. The venous drainage of the bladder is to the internal iliac veins, which drain the majority of pelvic viscera.

The vertex of the bladder is directed anteriorly towards the upper part of the symphysis pubis (i.e. fascial separation), and from it the median umbilical ligament (i.e. an unpaired remnant of the embryonic urachus) continues upward on the deep surface of the anterior abdominal wall to the umbilicus. The median umbilical ligament is covered by the median umbilical fold.

16. Answer: C

Antidiuretic hormone (ADH) is synthesized in the hypothalamus and secreted by the posterior pituitary gland. Several factors regulate ADH secretion. These include: (1) Hypothalamic osmoreceptors that secrete ADH in response to raised plasma osmolarity. (2) Stretch receptors (baroreceptors) that are situated in the atria of the heart, which are sensitive to circulating blood volume. The stretch receptors are activated by an increased volume of blood returning to the heart from the venous system, resulting in inhibition of ADH secretion. (3) Stretch receptors that are situated in the aorta and carotid arteries are stimulated when the circulating volume decreases and the blood pressure falls, thereby stimulating ADH secretion. (4) Trauma, such as head injury or burns, or any cause of prolonged hypoxia can also stimulate ADH secretion. An increase in ADH production will lead to water retention, which will result in oliguria and hyponatraemia (dilutional).

17. Answer: E

Benign prostatic hyperplasia (BPH) arises in the transitional zone of the prostate (periurethral glands and stroma). It is a common finding in elderly males, and its incidence increases with age. As the prostate enlarges the patient usually develops lower urinary tract symptoms. Compression of the prostatic urethra leads to a rise in intravesical pressure, which eventually leads to detrusor atony.

Enlargement of the posterior lobes of the prostate is usually seen in prostatic cancer.

Phimosis is not a routine feature of BPH but all patients with lower urinary tract symptoms should have their external genitalia examined to exclude this pathology.

18. Answer: B

Very few medications have to be stopped in a patient undergoing a minor day-case procedure under local anaesthesia. The risk of stopping a long-term medication preoperatively is usually greater than continuing it intraoperatively. Withdrawal of corticosteroids may result in Addisonian crisis (tachycardia, hypotension, oliguria, and confusion). Patients on long-term corticosteroid therapy may develop adrenal dysfunction during the peri- or postoperative period, subsequently requiring an increased dose of steroids (or intravenous steroid treatment). Antiplatelet agents such as aspirin may be stopped at least 5 days prior to surgery to prevent excessive blood loss during surgery. However, if the risks (of stopping aspirin) are greater than the benefits then it is advisable to obtain a medical or anaesthetic opinion. The other important drug that may have to be stopped before surgery (particularly major surgeries) is warfarin (i.e. patients will have to be commenced on intravenous heparin during the pre-, peri-, and postoperative period whilst monitoring the APTT levels). Beta-blockers, antidiabetic agents, and thiazide diuretics do not have to be stopped in patients undergoing a minor day-case procedure under local anaesthesia.

19. Answer: B

Carotid endarterectomy involves the removal of stenotic plaque within the carotid artery, whilst blood flow is shunted to maintain cerebral perfusion. NICE guidance states that patients with stable neurological symptoms from acute non-disabling stroke or TIA, who have symptomatic carotid stenosis of 50–99% according to the NASCET (North American Symptomatic Carotid Endarterectomy Trial) criteria, or 70–99% according to the ECST (European Carotid Surgery

Trial) criteria, should be assessed and referred for carotid endarterectomy within 1 week of symptom onset. They should undergo surgery within a maximum of 2 weeks of symptom onset, whilst receiving best medical treatment (blood pressure control, antiplatelet agents, cholesterol lowering through diet and drugs, lifestyle advice, etc.) The patient in this case has had a transient ischaemic attack affecting the right side of the brain due to a 71% right carotid artery stenosis, and should therefore undergo a carotid endarterectomy on this side. His left internal carotid is completely occluded and therefore no intervention should be considered on this side. The role of endarterectomy for asymptomatic carotid disease is topical, with emerging evidence that it reduces the risk of future stroke.

20. Answer: D

Frey's syndrome is not an immediate complication of parotid surgery. It typically develops after 6 months and the main features are sweating and vasodilation of the skin supplied by the auriculotemporal nerve. The auriculotemporal branch of the trigeminal nerve carries sympathetic fibres to the sweat glands of the scalp and parasympathetic fibres to the parotid gland. Misdirected re-innervation after surgery leads to gustatory sweating and flushing in the skin supplied by the auriculotemporal nerve. Other late complications after parotid surgery include the development of greater auricular nerve neuroma. Facial nerve injury is more an intraoperative/early complication of parotid surgery.

21. Answer: A

Nitric oxide synthase (NOS) acts on L-arginine within endothelial, neuronal, and macrophage cells. It contains an unpaired electron and therefore acts as a highly reactive free radical. Asymmetrical dimethylarginine is an endogenous inhibitor of NOS. Shear stress within vessels induces an increased production of NO from endothelial cells. NO diffuses out into the smooth muscle cells to activate guanylyl cyclase, which in turn converts guanosine triphosphate (GTP) to cyclic guanosine monophosphate (GMP). This subsequently causes smooth muscle relaxation and vasodilatation. NO also prevents platelet aggregation and adhesion as part of the negative feedback mechanism which ensures clot formation at the site of injury. NO also acts as a neurotransmitter in non-adrenergic, non-cholinergic nerves.

22. Answer: D

Urinary tract stones are very common with a peak incidence between 25–50 years of age. Stones obstruct the ureters at natural sites of narrowing, which are the pelviureteric junction, the point at which the iliac vessels cross the ureter and the vesicoureteric junction. The commonest site of stone formation is in the upper urinary tract and most are usually formed within the collecting system. CT urography has superseded IVU as the investigation of choice. Renal ultrasound is not apt for identifying small stones but can effectively identify hydronephrosis.

23. Answer: E

This elderly patient has presented with melaena and evidence of haemodynamic compromise, altogether suggesting a major bleeding episode whilst on warfarin therapy. Under these circumstances, it is advisable to withhold warfarin and administer IV vitamin K, together with either fresh frozen plasma (FFP) or prothrombin complex concentrate (PCC). If in doubt, it is imperative to review local policy or to consult with the duty haematologist. As long as PCC is not contraindicated, it is now used preferentially over FFP as the latter may not completely reverse the effects of warfarin. The rate of fatal haemorrhage in patients who are anticoagulated with warfarin is approximately 1%, thereby emphasizing the need for awareness of warfarin reversal guidelines.

24. Answer: C

Twelve per cent of men and 24% of women will develop gallstones, although only 10–20% of all stones become symptomatic. Asymptomatic gallstones therefore need no intervention. Elective laparoscopic cholecystectomy is considered in the following:

- Symptomatic gallstones failing conservative management (dietary manipulation) or by patient choice
- Episodes of septic gallbladder complications to prevent recurrence (in patients who are fit for surgery)
- Episodes of complications (e.g. pancreatitis) or to prevent recurrence of complications.

25. Answer: B

The portal vein arises from the confluence of the splenic and superior mesenteric veins behind the neck of the pancreas, in front of the IVC between the vertebral levels L1 and L2. It drains the GI tract from the lower oesophagus to the anorectal junction. Porto-systemic anastomoses are seen at the umbilicus, lower oesophagus, retroperitoneum, and anorectal junction. The portal vein lies behind the common bile duct and hepatic artery in the lesser omentum. The common bile duct lies to the right of the hepatic artery. The inferior mesenteric vein lies to the left of the inferior mesenteric artery in the left colonic mesentery and drains into the splenic vein behind the tail of the pancreas.

26. Answer: B

The duration of the cardiac cycle is 0.8 seconds. During exercise each phase shortens but with disproportionate shortening of ventricular relaxation. The cardiac cycle can be divided into seven phases:

- Atrial contraction contributes about 10% of ventricular filling at rest but 40% during exercise.
- Isovolumetric contraction, which is initiated by the QRS complex, leads to a rapid increase in ventricular pressure but not in volume, as ejection has not occurred.
- Rapid ejection occurs when ventricular pressure exceeds those in the pulmonary artery and aorta.
- Reduced ejection occurs as ventricular repolarization occurs (T wave).
- Isovolumetric relaxation leads to a drop in ventricular pressures and abrupt closure of the aortic and pulmonary valves (S2).
- Rapid filling occurs as ventricular pressure falls below that of the atria.
- Reduced filling occurs as the ventricles become less compliant and the intraventricular pressure increases.

27. Answer: D

This patient is most likely to have a basal skull fracture. Trauma, such as that due to falling from heights or road traffic accidents, is the commonest cause of this type of fracture. Basal skull fractures commonly involve the roof of the orbits, the sphenoid bone, and parts of the temporal bone. The classical signs and symptoms of basal skull fracture include periorbital haematoma ('panda' or 'racoon' eyes), subconjunctival haemorrhage (i.e. where the posterior margins of the haemorrhage cannot be seen), Battle's sign (retromastoid bruising; this sign is often the last to develop, from 24–48 hours in some patients), and rhinorrhoea or otorrhoea (blood mixed with CSF and so does not clot; this is consequent to damage to the cribriform plates). Recognized complications of basal skull fracture include meningitis (especially following CSF rhinorrhoea), facial palsy and VIth nerve palsy. CT scanning is the investigation of choice for suspected basal skull fracture (and for other serious head injuries). Specific indications for CT imaging include: a GCS of less than 13; unreliable history or examination due to alcohol and/or drug ingestion; loss of consciousness for more than 5 minutes persisting/progressive headache; persistent vomiting;

ante- and/or retrograde amnesia; clinical suspicion of basal skull fracture; and skull fracture with neurological signs and/or convulsions. Patients with GCS of less than 8 have a risk of airway compromise and will need to be intubated. The Le Fort classification system describes maxillofacial trauma as follows:

- Le Fort I: transverse maxillary fracture with two segments; the floating palate contains the alveolus, palate, and pterygoid bones.
- Le Fort II: pyramidal fracture across nasal bones, the medial orbital wall, and down into the maxilla.
- Le Fort III: craniofacial dysfunction with detachment of the midfacial skeleton from the skull base.

28. Answer: D

There are two drainage patterns to the inguinal lymph nodes. The horizontal group of lymphatics drain along the inguinal ligament; infection and malignant cells from the skin of the lower anterior abdominal wall, retroperitoneum, penis, scrotum, vulva, vagina, gluteal region, lower anal canal, and perineum. The vertical group drains lymph from penis, scrotum, gluteal regions and the lower limbs along the great saphenous vein. Testicular cancer spreads primarily to the para-aortic lymph nodes.

29. Answer: E

Chemoreceptors and stretch receptors are stimulated by neurotransmitters such as serotonin, acetylcholine, histamine, and substance P trigger nausea and vomiting. These stimuli are then conducted via the afferent vagal nerves to the emetic centre in the medulla. The chemoreceptor trigger zone senses potentially toxic substances in blood and initiates emesis. Nausea due to motion sickness, inner ear disease, and disequilibrium produced by alcohol excess is sensed through the vestibular apparatus and mediated largely by acetylcholine and histamine receptors. The central cortex and the limbic systems modulate complex experiences such as taste, smell, memory, and emotion in connection to past experiences and produce anticipatory nausea via neural pathways which are less well understood.

30. Answer: C

Epididymitis most commonly occurs on its own although in 20–40% of the cases it causes concomitant orchitis (epididymo-orchitis). It is as common as testicular torsion in pre- pubertal males. Epididymo-orchitis has a more insidious onset and is less severe than in torsion. Testicular orientation is normal as opposed to torsion, where the testis is usually high lying. Prehn's manoeuvre (elevation of the scrotum above the pubic symphysis) may relieve the pain of epididymitis, whilst exacerbating the pain of testicular torsion. However, it is not usually performed as it is extremely uncomfortable for the patient, and is not an accurate means of excluding torsion. Imaging (e.g. by testicular ultrasound) is a more sensitive means of diagnosis, although scrotal exploration should never be delayed if there is sufficient clinical suspicion of torsion. Idiopathic scrotal oedema is an uncommon condition of unknown aetiology. It is a self-limiting condition, with a peak incidence at 5–7 years of age. It is associated with mild scrotal erythema and oedema, and normal, non-tender testes.

31. Answer: E

Chest drains are commonly inserted to drain air, fluid or both from the pleural cavity. They should ideally be inserted within the 'safe triangle' of the anterior chest wall. The safe triangle is bordered by the anterior border of the latissimus dorsi, the lateral border of the pectoralis major muscle, a line superior to the horizontal level of the nipple, and an apex below the axilla. Within this safe triangle, the chest drain should be inserted by blunt dissection into the fifth intercostal space, just above the superior border of the rib underneath (i.e. in order to avoid the neurovascular bundle travelling along the inferior aspect of the rib above).

The parietal pleura is punctured with an artery forceps and a finger is used to enlarge the hole. The end of the tube is held with a clamp and advanced so that the most proximal hole is in the pleural cavity. The tube is connected to an underwater seal and is secured to the skin with a suture.

32. Answer: A

In the physiological state, the sinoatrial node is under the influence of the sympathetic and parasympathetic nervous systems. Atropine is a muscarinic receptor antagonist (a competitive antagonist for the muscarinic acetylcholine receptor), which works by abolishing the parasympathetic influences (i.e. blocking acetylcholine released from the postganglionic vagus nerve endings in the cardiac tissue) resulting in an increased heart rate. Atropine is a naturally occurring alkaloid; it is absorbed from the GI tract and excreted in the urine. It undergoes hepatic metabolism and has a plasma half-life of about 2–3 hours. When used as premedication for anaesthesia, atropine decreases bronchial and salivary secretions (leading to dry mouth), inhibits the bradycardia associated with some anaesthetic drugs (such as halothane, suxamethonium, and neostigmine), and helps prevent bradycardia from excessive vagal stimulation. Other anticholinergic effects of atropine include dilatation of the pupils, urinary retention, inhibition of sweating (anhidrosis) and constipation.

33. Answer: B

The boundary between the greater (i.e. the general cavity of the abdomen) sac and lesser sac is known as the epiploic foramen (or 'omental foramen'; 'foramen of Winslow'). This passage has the following borders:

- Anterior: the free border of the lesser omentum (i.e. the hepatoduodenal ligament). This has two layers and within these layers are the common bile duct, hepatic artery and hepatic portal vein.
- Posterior: the peritoneum covering the inferior vena cava.
- Superior: the peritoneum covering the caudate lobe of the liver.
- Inferior: the peritoneum covering the first part of the duodenum and the hepatic artery, the latter passing forward below the foramen before ascending between the two layers of the lesser omentum.
- Left lateral: gastrosplenic ligament and splenorenal ligament.

34. Answer: C

Primary biliary cirrhosis (PBC) is a chronic progressive disease of the liver characterized by the destruction of the intrahepatic bile ducts eventually leading to liver cirrhosis. In the presence of characteristic liver function tests, antimitochondrial antibody positivity (found in 96% of all cases), normal bile ducts and the absence of gallstones on the ultrasound scan makes PBC the most likely diagnosis. A liver biopsy maybe performed to confirm the diagnosis, showing characteristic prominent portal inflammatory infiltrate composed of lymphocytes, histiocytes, and macrophages surrounding the bile ducts causing peri-portal fibrosis and moderate biliary stasis. Although the aetiology of PBC is unclear, autoimmunity is thought to play a major role.

35. Answer: C

The second part of the duodenum (D2) lies along the transpyloric plane (of Addison), at the level of the 1st lumbar vertebra (L1). Other key structures at this point include the fundus of the gallbladder, splenic and renal hila, neck of pancreas, origin of the superior mesenteric artery, origin of the hepatic portal vein, gastric pylorus, the attachment of the transverse mesocolon and the tip of the 9th costal cartilage. Posterior to D2 lies the right renal hilum; the other structures mentioned are not directly related to D2. It should be noted that D2 begins at the superior duodenal flexure, passing inferiorly to the level of the lower border of L3, before making a sharp turn medially into the inferior duodenal flexure. The pancreatic and common bile ducts enter the descending duodenum (known as the hepatopancreatic duct) through the major duodenal papilla (ampulla of Vater). The minor duodenal papilla is also located here and serves as the outlet of the accessory pancreatic duct. The junction between the embryological foregut and midgut lies just below the major duodenal papilla.

36. Answer: B

Intussusception is more common in boys and usually occurs under the age of one. It is associated with haemophilia, Henoch–Schönlein purpura, haemangiomas, and GI lymphomas. Although the precise aetiology is not clear, intussusception is known to occur with greater frequency in children who have undergone recent abdominal surgery—either intraperitoneal or retroperitoneal operations. Intussusception is the invagination (or 'telescoping') of a segment of bowel into its adjoining lower segment. The mesentery and associated vessels may also become involved with the intraluminal loop and squeezed within the engulfing segment. Clinical features of this condition include severe colicky abdominal pain (causing intermittent inconsolable cries with the child drawing up their legs) and vomiting. Between attacks, the infant may appear in good health. The infant may pass 'redcurrant jelly' stool. Abdominal examination may reveal a 'sausage-shaped' mass and per rectal examination may reveal blood.

37. Answer: B

The nerves which arise from the posterior cord of the brachial plexus include the upper subscapular nerve (C5 and C6), middle subscapular nerve (i.e. the thoracodorsal nerve, supplying latissimus dorsi; C6, C7, C8), lower subscapular nerve (C5 and C6), axillary nerve (C5 and C6) and radial nerve (C5, C6, C7, C8, T1). The long thoracic nerve (i.e. the nerve of Bell, supplying serratus anterior), has a root value of C5, C6, and C7. It arises from the roots of the brachial plexus; the other nerves arising from the roots include the dorsal scapular nerve (C5) and the branches to scalene muscles (C5–C8).

38. Answer: D

Radiation proctitis refers to inflammation of the rectum caused by radiotherapy, commonly to the prostate or bowel. It is characterized by erythematous friable mucosa with overlying telangiectasia. In the early stages, patients present with tenesmus and diarrhoea. Late symptoms may take up to a year to manifest and consist of tenesmus, peri-anal pain, discharge, and rectal bleeding. Occasionally it may be complicated by low-grade obstruction or fistulation with adjacent structures. Radiation proctitis can be treated with sucralfate, metronidazole, prednisolone enemas or mesalazine enemas. Patients may also benefit from hyperbaric oxygen therapy. Argon plasma coagulation via endoscopy and bipolar electrocoagulation may be used to control refractory bleeding in haemorrhagic proctitis.

39. Answer: B

The fish bone is likely to have been stuck in the piriformis recess, which is a pear-shaped opening bounded by the aryepiglottic folds medially; and the laryngopharynx, thyroid cartilage and hypothyroid membrane laterally. Sharp objects may lodge in this recess and pierce the mucous membrane, injuring the internal laryngeal nerve lying just beneath it. This nerve supplies sensation to the laryngeal mucosa above the vocal folds. Damage to this nerve may therefore result in insensitivity of the mucous membrane of the superior part of the larynx to food, resulting in a loss of cough impulse and increased risk of aspiration.

40. Answer: A

Aortic dissection refers to a tear in the intimal layer of the aorta and propagation by the formation of a subintimal haematoma. This forms a false lumen that occupies much of the circumference of the lumen, resulting in a reduction in blood flow to the major arteries supplied by the aorta. It can be classified by Stanford classification into Type A, which involves the ascending aorta, and Type B, which does not.

An acute myocardial infarction will also present with acute-onset chest pain; however, there is usually no difference in blood pressure between both arms. If aortic dissection is misdiagnosed as myocardial infarction, treatment with thrombolytics or anticoagulants may potentially be catastrophic.

Boerhaave's syndrome refers to oesophageal rupture due to vomiting. It presents with Mackler's triad of chest pain, vomiting and subcutaneous emphysema.

Cardiac tamponade from a pericardial effusion will present with Beck's triad of hypotension, raised jugular venous pressure and muffled heart sounds.

41. Answer: C

When surgical procedures are undertaken, universal precautions are essential and should be practised to minimize the risk to the operator and assistants, as well as to reduce the risk of transmission of blood-borne diseases. The precautions for each procedure may vary according to the risk of contact with the procedure. Appropriate protective clothing in the operating theatre should include double gloving, water-repellent gown and apron, protective headwear, masks, and protective eyewear and footwear. Rubber gloves do not protect against sharps injury although they reduce the risk of disease transmission. Needles should never be re-sheathed, and sharp objects should be transferred in an appropriate container. Fixed retraction devices help in reducing the number of times the assistants' hands pass through or block the operating field inadvertently or inappropriately (thus minimizing the risk of injury due to sharp objects). In addition, fixed retraction devices help in keeping number of assistants required to a minimum.

42. Answer: A

The duodenum is responsible mainly for the absorption of carbohydrates, protein, minerals (e.g. calcium, magnesium, iron, chloride, sodium and zinc); and the jejunum, responsible for the absorption of glucose, protein, folic acid, and vitamins C, B1 (thiamine), B2, and B6. The terminal ileum, however, is the main site of absorption of amino acids, lipids, cholesterol, and the fat-soluble vitamins (e.g. A, D, E and K).

As the terminal ileum is also responsible for 90% of bile salt resorption from the gut, resection of the terminal ileum is likely to result in a significant interruption of the enterohepatic circulation. This stimulates an increase in bile salt synthesis by cholesterol transmetabolism in the liver, thereby increasing the risk of gallstone formation. Furthermore, because the terminal ileum contains intrinsic factor-dependent receptors that are important in vitamin B12 uptake, the resultant vitamin B12 deficiency may lead to macrocytic anaemia and subacute degeneration of the cord.

The increase in intraluminal osmotic content (of substances otherwise absorbed in the terminal ileum) may also result in loosening of the stool after the procedure.

43. Answer: B

Rupture of the extensor pollicis longus tendon is a recognized complication of Colles' fractures. It may occur either acutely, or more commonly, 2 weeks after the injury, when the blood supply to the tendon becomes interrupted by repeated abrasions against the rough fracture edges.

Other of Colles' fractures include:

- Fracture malunion
- Subluxation of the radioulnar joint and fracture displacement
- Impingement on rotation caused by a prominent ulnar head
- Median nerve damage (which presents as pain and paraesthesia over the radial three-and-a-half digits with sparing of sensation over the thenar eminence)
- Sudeck's atrophy: reflex sympathetic dystrophy, which leaves the hand painful, stiff, and hypersensitive

44. Answer: E

Primary hyperparathyroidism may be defined by a circulating level of PTH which is inappropriately high for the prevailing level of calcium. It implies hyperfunction of one or more parathyroid glands with a change in the set point for the control of calcium. It has an incidence of 0.5 per 1000 and is most common between 40–60 years of age, when it is twice as common in women as in men. In other age groups, the gender incidence is roughly equal. In young people of either sex, it is important to investigate the possibility of multiple endocrine neoplasia. The clinical presentation of hyperparathyroidism can involve:

- Renal calculi (i.e. in 10–15% of patients with primary hyperparathyroidism)
- Bone resorption leading to bone pain, pathological fractures, and rarely, osteitis fibrosa cystica
- Rarer features of metastatic calcification (e.g. nephrocalcinosis, corneal calcification, chondrocalcinosis, etc.)
- Polyuria, thirst, weakness and vomiting
- Acute pancreatitis (i.e. a rare presentation of primary hyperparathyroidism).

Features attributable to hypercalcaemia may be evident in primary and tertiary hyperparathyroidism. In secondary hyperparathyroidism, the clinical picture may be complicated by hypocalcaemia. In chronic renal failure, coexistent osteomalacia results in renal osteodystrophy.

45. Answer: D

The Salter–Harris classification is a system used to describe the pattern of fractures involving the epiphysis, and to predict their prognosis. It should be noted that fractures of the epiphysis and growth plate are more common in boys, and are usually seen either in infancy or between the ages of 10–12 years.

It is apparent that this child demonstrates a Salter–Harris type IV fracture, which is one that occurs through the shaft, the epiphyseal plate, the epiphysis, and into the joint. The detached piece of bone therefore consists of fragments of the shaft, epiphyseal plate, and epiphysis. This may interfere with subsequent bone growth, as there is disruption of the growth plate and the articular surface. Type IV fractures therefore usually require open reduction and internal fixation. It is vital to understand the Salter–Harris fracture classification and its applications both clinically and academically, as the management and prognosis of these injuries varies significantly with classification type.

46. Answer: C

Necrotizing enterocolitis is the most common gastrointestinal surgical emergency presenting in neonates. It most commonly presents in premature infants weighing less than 1500 g and has a mortality rate of more than 50%. Initial symptoms include feeding intolerance, high gastric residual, abdominal distension and bloody stool. The infant may later become peritonitic as the bowel perforates, leading to haemodynamic instability. The diagnosis may be facilitated by abdominal radiography, which may reveal distended loops of bowel, pneumatosis intestinalis (i.e. gas within the bowel wall), portal venous gas, and pneumoperitoneum. Management is with supportive intervention involving intermittent gastric decompression, fluid and electrolyte replacement, and total parenteral nutrition. Where medical management has failed or bowel is perforated, surgical excision of dead bowel is required.

47. Answer: A

Meconium ileus is a common and early presentation of neonates with cystic fibrosis. The condition occurs more frequently in boys than girls and presents during the first days of life with gross abdominal distension, bilious vomiting, and failure to pass meconium. Plain radiography of the abdomen may show dilated loops of intestine with thickened bowel walls. Free gas or very large air-fluid levels may suggest bowel perforation. Uncomplicated meconium ileus can be managed with the use of diatrizoate meglumine (Gastrografin) enemas after adequate intravenous fluid administration. If this fails, laparotomy is indicated to evacuate the obstructing meconium. The differential diagnoses for meconium ileus include malrotation of the gut, volvulus neonatorum, and Hirschsprung's disease.

Due to the underlying pathology of cystic fibrosis—a mutated CFTR gene resulting in defective ion transport across epithelial cells of the lungs, pancreas, and other organs—a positive sweat test (i.e. with raised chloride content of sweat) is diagnostic of the condition.

48. Answer: E

Primary hyperaldosteronism results from excessive autonomous secretion of aldosterone by an adenoma of the adrenal cortex (Conn's syndrome; 60–70%) or by bilateral hyperplasia of the zona glomerulosa (in about 30–40% of cases). Aldosterone, by inducing reabsorption of sodium in the distal tubule, enhances secretion of potassium and hydrogen ions, leading to hypernatrae-mia, hypokalaemia, and metabolic alkalosis. Hypertension is due to intravascular fluid retention secondary retention to sodium retention. In essence, Conn's syndrome is characterized by increased aldosterone secretion, suppressed plasma renin activity, hypertension and hypokalae-mia. The hypertension and hypokalaemia may be treated with a potassium-sparing agent such as spironolactone (first line). The second-line agents that are useful in the treatment of primary hyperaldosteronism include thiazides diuretics, angiotensin-converting enzyme (ACE) inhibitors, calcium channel antagonists and angiotensin II blockers. In patients with Conn's syndrome, the preoperative blood pressure response to spironolactone could be used as a valuable predictor of the blood pressure response to unilateral adrenalectomy. Surgery, in the form of an adrenal-ectomy (e.g. laparoscopic), is the mainstay of treatment for Conn's syndrome.

49. Answer: B

Four types of rejection are commonly recognized following transplantation. They are: hypera-cute, accelerated, acute and chronic. Hyperacute rejection occurs within minutes of transplan-tation and is a complement mediated response in recipients with pre-existing antibodies to the donor. This may be due to a HLA class I antibody or an ABO incompatibility. Accelerated rejection is cell-mediated and is seen in sensitized patients 2–4 days following transplantation. A biopsy reveals a florid cellular infiltrate (macrophages and T-lymphocytes). Acute rejection is the outcome of the immune response of the allograft in a non-sensitized patient and most commonly occurs between 7–21 days post transplantation. In acute rejection, graft antigens are recognized by T cells, and the resulting cytokine release eventually leads to tissue distortion, vascular insuf-ficiency, and cell destruction. Histologically, there is a presence of leucocytes, macrophages and T cells within the interstitium. Chronic rejection is the commonest cause of late graft loss and is characterized by an insidious, irreversible deterioration of function associated with fibrosis of the internal blood vessels of the transplant in the months following transplantation.

50. Answer: D

A case–control study is one that compares the characteristics of a group of patients with a particular condition with a 'control' group of patients without that condition. This form of study methodology is advantageous because rare diseases can be studied with relative ease (i.e. as they are independent of disease incidence); a wide range of risk factors can be investigated; there is no loss to follow-up; and they are relatively inexpensive and quick to perform. The results of such studies are usually quoted as an odds ratio (i.e. the ratio of the odds of an event occurring in one group to the odds of it occurring in another group).

Basic sciences: Applied anatomy

1. **Which of the following arteries does not arise from the axillary artery?**
   A. Superior thoracic artery
   B. Lateral thoracic (pectoral) artery
   C. Thoraco-acromial artery
   D. Costo-cervical trunk
   E. Subscapular artery

Basic sciences: Physiology

2. **Which of the following is not a recognized process during angiogenesis in wound healing?**
   A. Proteolytic degradation of the parent vessel basement membrane
   B. Recruitment of fibrocytes to the wound site
   C. Migration of endothelial cells towards the angiogenic stimulus
   D. Proliferation of endothelial cells behind the leading front of migrating cells
   E. Maturation of endothelial cells with organization into capillary tubes

Basic sciences: Pathology

3. **Which among the following is not a feature of Marfan's syndrome?**
   A. Arachnodactyly
   B. Pectus excavatum
   C. Pes cavus
   D. Aortic dissection
   E. Inferonasal dislocation of the ocular lens

Common surgical conditions and the subspecialties:
Trauma and orthopaedics

4. **A 21-year-old professional squash player presents to the Emergency Department with severe, stabbing pain above his right knee joint. He states that the pain was of sudden onset and arose when he took a sharp stride during a match. On examination, he walks with a limp and is unable to extend the leg. There is a swelling over the supra-patellar region with a low-lying patella. Knee jerk is absent on the affected side. What is the most likely disgnosis?**

   A. Fracture of the patella

   B. Tear of the adductor magnus muscle

   C. Injury to the posterior cruciate ligament

   D. Tear of the quadriceps tendon

   E. Tear of the biceps femoris tendon

Common surgical conditions and the subspecialties: General presenting symptoms or syndromes

5. **A 77-year-old woman with a history of atrial fibrillation and ischaemic heart disease is brought to Emergency Department with a 12-hour history of generalized abdominal pain associated with nausea and vomiting. She has also had five episodes of diarrhoea, with semi-altered blood and mucus in the stool. Examination of the abdomen reveals generalized abdominal tenderness with signs of peritonism and absent bowel sounds. However, the patient's pain seems out of proportion to her physical signs. Of the following options, which one is the most likely diagnosis?**

   A. Toxic megacolon

   B. Acute diverticulitis

   C. Ruptured abdominal aortic aneurysm

   D. Perforated peptic ulcer

   E. Mesenteric ischaemia

Perioperative care: Assessing and planning nutritional management

6. **Which of the following is not a metabolic complication of total parenteral nutrition?**

   A. Low phosphate

   B. Low calcium

   C. Deranged liver function tests

   D. Hyperchloraemic acidosis

   E. Low potassium

The assessment and management of the surgical patient:
Clinical decision-making

7. A 35-year-old gentleman presents with a 3-month history of progressive dysphagia for both solids and liquids. He experiences pain on swallowing and regurgitation of food a few hours postprandially. He denies any symptoms of acid reflux but has anorexia and weight loss. After an inconclusive oesophagogastroduodenscopy (OGD), a barium swallow demonstrates proximal dilatation of the oesophagus and failure of relaxation of the lower oesophageal sphincter. Manometric tests reveal incomplete relaxation of the gastro-oesophageal sphincter with a high resting tone that does not fall to gastric fundal pressure. What is the most appropriate first-line management in this patient?

A. Amlodipine
B. Amyl nitrite
C. Intrasphincteric botulinum toxin
D. Oesophageal balloon dilatation
E. Oesophageal myotomy

Basic sciences: Applied anatomy

8. A 75-year-old lady is scheduled for a total hip placement for severe osteoarthritis of her hip. The surgeon's preferred approach to the hip joint is the lateral approach, which involves splitting the tensor fascia lata, followed by the gluteus medius and gluteus minimus, to reach the hip joint. He explains to the patient that during this approach, the nerve supply to the tensor fascia lata and gluteus medius is at risk. What nerve does the surgeon specifically refer to in this case?

A. Femoral nerve
B. Inferior gluteal nerve
C. Lateral femoral cutaneous nerve of the thigh
D. Sciatic nerve
E. Superior gluteal nerve

Basic sciences: Physiology

9. Which of the following is the site of action of the antidiuretic hormone (ADH)?

A. Proximal convoluted tubule
B. Descending limb of loop of Henle
C. Ascending limb of loop of Henle
D. Distal convoluted tubule
E. Proximal collecting duct

Basic sciences: Pathology

10. Which is the commonest type of a tracheo-oesophageal fistula?

    A. No fistula

    B. Proximal fistula

    C. Double fistula

    D. Distal fistula

    E. Cervical 'H' fistula

Common surgical conditions and the subspecialties: Trauma and orthopaedics

11. A 25-year-old lady falls onto her outstretched left hand whilst under the influence of alcohol. She is taken to her local Emergency Department where she complains of severe pain in her left forearm. Anteroposterior and lateral radiographs of the affected forearm reveal a fracture of the proximal ulna with a disruption of the proximal radioulnar joint. What is the eponymous name used to describe such a pattern of injury?

    A. Barton's fracture

    B. Colles' fracture

    C. Galeazzi fracture

    D. Monteggia fracture

    E. Smith's fracture

Common surgical conditions and the subspecialties: Skin, head, and neck

12. A 55-year-old school teacher presents to her new GP for a routine health assessment. Despite having no symptomatic history of note, examination reveals multiple non-tender, soft lumps over her upper and lower limbs. The lumps are 3 cm in diameter on average, non-pulsatile, non-reducible and not tethered to the overlying skin or underlying structures. Which one of the following conditions is the most likely?

    A. Dercum's disease

    B. Dermatofibroma

    C. Hereditary haemorrhagic telangiectasia

    D. Type 1 neurofibromatosis

    E. Type 2 neurofibromatosis

Perioperative care: Coagulation, deep vein thrombosis, and embolism

13. Which of the following statements is true regarding haemostasis?

A. Activated partial thromboplastin time (APTT) measures the haemostatic activity of the extrinsic pathway

B. Prothrombin time measures the haemostatic activity of the intrinsic pathway

C. Thrombin time measures the haemostatic activity of the common pathway

D. Bleeding time measures the haemostatic activity of the platelet phase

E. Heparin acts on the clotting factors II, VII, IX, and X

The assessment and management of the surgical patient: Planning investigations

14. A 32-year-old Middle Eastern man is being investigation for a 2-month history of malaise, lethargy, weight loss, intermittent pyrexia and loose stools. The gastroenterologist believes this to be the result of a malabsorption syndrome and organizes for the patient to undergo a jejunal biopsy. Which of the following options is true of jejunal biopsies?

A. They are contraindicated in elderly patients with an ASA (American Society of Anesthesiologists) grade of III or above

B. The biopsy histology from healthy individuals from tropical regions may have a specimen mucosal structure which would commonly be regarded as abnormal in Europeans

C. The finding of subtotal villous atrophy is exclusive to gluten-sensitive enteropathy

D. The procedure can be diagnostic of Whipple's disease

E. Villous atrophy is evident only on electron microscopy of the biopsy

Basic sciences: Applied anatomy

15. A thoracic surgeon carefully negotiates the axillary region during explorative surgery for multiple gunshot wounds in a soldier. Which of the following statements regarding the anatomy of the axillary region is most accurate?

A. Inadvertent damage to the thoracodorsal nerve during axillary dissection may result in winging of the scapula

B. The lymph nodes lateral to pectoralis minor are considered as level III nodes

C. The third part of the axillary artery is surrounded by cords of the brachial plexus

D. The intercostobrachial nerve is commonly sacrificed during axillary dissection

E. The third part of axillary artery gives off the subscapular artery

Basic sciences: Physiology

16. **Which of the following statements regarding the autonomic nervous system is incorrect?**
    A. A pre-ganglionic sympathectomy would be a reasonable treatment option for Raynaud's disease
    B. Increased parasympathetic stimulation of the salivary glands is likely to result in a greater volume of saliva produced, with reduced potassium and increased sodium content
    C. Post-ganglionic sympathetic neurons release predominantly noradrenaline
    D. A spinal cord lesion at the T10 level is most likely to result in 'dry orgasm'
    E. Increased activity within the parasympathetic innervation of the heart will have a negative chronotropic effect

Common surgical conditions and the subspecialties: Gastrointestinal disease

17. **A 30-year-old male is referred by his GP to the Emergency Department with perianal pain and swelling. He is diagnosed with a perianal abscess and undergoes an incision and drainage procedure. A few months later, he presents to the colorectal clinic with persistent perianal discharge. Rectal examination reveals an opening adjacent to the anus at the 1 o'clock position but no obvious internal opening is felt. A presumed diagnosis of fistula-in-ano is made, and he is listed for examination under anaesthesia (EUA). What is the most likely type of fistula to be seen in this patient?**
    A. Submucosal
    B. Intersphincteric
    C. Trans-sphincteric
    D. Suprasphincteric
    E. Extrasphincteric

Perioperative care: Preoperative assessment and management

18. **Which of the following is not predictive of the risk of a perioperative life-threatening cardiac event in a patient with known ischaemic heart disease?**
    A. Age greater than 70 years
    B. Right pneumonectomy for advanced squamous cell carcinoma of the lung
    C. Mitral regurgitation
    D. Aortic stenosis
    E. Ruptured abdominal aortic aneurysm repair

The assessment and management of the surgical patient: Surgical history and examination (elective and emergency)

19. **A 35-year-old gentleman is referred by his GP to the colorectal clinic for a suspicious perianal lump. On digital rectal examination and subsequent proctoscopy, a firm, irreducible mass is found arising from the lower half of the anal canal. Which additional clinical finding would support a diagnosis of squamous cell carcinoma instead of adenocarcinoma?**

   A. History of pruritis ani associated with the emergence of the lump
   B. History of infective colitis
   C. History of recent blood or mucus in the stool
   D. History of recurrent haemorrhoids
   E. Palpable superficial inguinal lymphadenopathy

Basic sciences: Applied anatomy

20. **What is the main arterial supply to the body of the pancreas?**

   A. Common hepatic artery
   B. Left gastric artery
   C. Superior mesenteric artery
   D. Splenic artery
   E. Right gastric artery

Basic sciences: Physiology

21. **A 45-year-old male suffers a moderate closed head injury and is brought to the resuscitation room with a GCS score of 10. Which of the following measures will not be useful in maintaining cerebral perfusion and oxygen delivery?**

   A. $15°$ head-up tilt
   B. Mechanical ventilation maintaining low to normal levels of CO_2
   C. Mannitol
   D. Steroids
   E. Placement of an intraventricular catheter

Common surgical conditions and the subspecialties:
Gastrointestinal disease

22. **A pregnant 18-year-old girl who has smoked throughout her pregnancy undergoes a vaginal delivery at 36 weeks. The newborn is found to have an abdominal wall defect. The defect is small and to the right of the umbilicus, through which oedematous loops of small bowel are seen protruding. Which of the following conditions best describes this clinical picture?**

    A. Exomphalos major
    B. Prune belly syndrome
    C. Exstrophy
    D. Gastroschisis
    E. Exomphalos minor

Perioperative care: Haemostasis and blood products

23. **A 41-year-old flight attendant presents to her GP with a 2-week history of bleeding gums. She has been taking warfarin for 3 months, after suffering from a below-knee deep vein thrombosis. She has a blood pressure of 130/85 mmHg and a heart rate of 74/min. ECG reveals a normal sinus rhythm, and subsequent blood tests reveal an INR of 8.5. What is the most appropriate treatment for this patient?**

    A. Stop warfarin only
    B. Stop warfarin and administer oral vitamin K 1 mg
    C. Stop warfarin and administer factor VII
    D. Stop warfarin and administer fresh frozen plasma
    E. Stop warfarin and administer prothrombin complex concentrate

The assessment and management of the surgical patient:
Case work-up and evaluation

24. **A 60-year-old man presents to the Emergency Department with sudden-onset, severe, tearing chest pain radiating through to his back. His blood pressure is normal and equal in both arms. ECG, CXR, and troponin levels are normal. A CT aortogram reveals aortic dissection distal to the left subclavian artery and involving the proximal abdominal aorta. How can this pattern of aortic dissection best be classified?**

    A. Stanford type A
    B. DeBakey type I
    C. DeBakey type II
    D. DeBakey type IIIa
    E. DeBakey type IIIb

Basic sciences: Applied anatomy

25. A 30-year-old lady is referred by her GP with a 3-month history of a lump in her neck. Examination reveals a firm lump in the anterior triangle on the right side of the neck, which moves up with deglutition. Which of the following structures is responsible for this upward movement on swallowing?

A. Pyramidal lobe

B. Berry's ligament

C. Ligament of Treitz

D. Thyroglossal duct

E. Cricothyroid membrane

Basic sciences: Physiology

26. A 55-year-old man is found to have microcytic anaemia on a routine blood test, and wishes to know more about the condition from his GP. Which of the following statements regarding the physiology of anaemia is false?

A. Anaemia has no effect on the oxygen dissolved in the blood

B. Anaemia has no effect on the oxygen saturation of haemoglobin

C. Anaemia has no effect on the oxygen carrying capacity of the blood

D. Anaemia reduces the amount of oxygen released from binding, for the same drop in venous PO_2

E. Rapidly deteriorating clinical indices are often noted when Hb levels acutely fall below 7g/dL

Common surgical conditions and the subspecialties: Gastrointestinal disease

27. A 7-year-old boy is brought to the Emergency Department with a 12-hour history of vomiting, severe abdominal pain and lethargy. His parents also describe two episodes of convulsions during this period. Examination reveals a pale and dehydrated child whose abdomen is rigid, with severe generalized tenderness and absent bowel sounds. The child has a temperate of 40.4°C, blood pressure of 82/64 mmHg and pulse rate of 144/min. Which of the following conditions is this child most likely to have?

A. Volvulus neonatorum

B. Acute appendicitis

C. Bacterial peritonitis

D. Necrotizing enterocolitis

E. Meckel's diverticulitis

Basic sciences: Applied anatomy

28. A 24-year-old female has been in labour for more than 20 hours and the crown of the foetal head is now visible through the vaginal orifice. The attending obstetrician decides to perform a mediolateral episiotomy to enlarge the birth orifice and prevent tearing of perineal structures. Which of the following structures is not incised during a mediolateral episiotomy?

   A. Perineal skin
   B. Posterior wall of vagina
   C. Perineal body
   D. Attachment of bulbospongiosus muscle
   E. Fascia around the urinary bladder

Basic sciences: Physiology

29. A 32-year-old female with a hiatus hernia and oesophagitis was commenced on a proton pump inhibitor to control her symptoms of reflux. Which of the following statements is true regarding the physiology of the gastric acid pump?

   A. Gastric acid is produced by G cells in the antrum of the stomach
   B. Gastric acid secretion is stimulated by high hydrogen ion (H^+) concentration
   C. The proton is exchanged with magnesium ions
   D. The proton pump is the final pathway of histamine and acetylcholine stimulated acid production
   E. H^+ secretion occurs by diffusion down a concentration gradient

Common surgical conditions and the subspecialties: Gastrointestinal disease

30. A 60-year-old man presents to his GP with a 2-day history of left iliac fossa pain (LIF) and fresh rectal bleeding. He has no history of weight loss or loss of appetite, but reveals a longstanding history of constipation. Physical examination reveals mild left iliac fossa tenderness with no signs of peritonism. Which of the following statements is not true about the most likely condition that this patient has presented with?

   A. The underlying pathology occurs at sites of vascular entry into the bowel wall
   B. The underlying pathology involves all layers of the bowel wall
   C. The underlying pathology most commonly occurs in the descending and sigmoid colon
   D. The condition is most common in Western populations
   E. The underlying pathology almost never occurs in the rectum

Basic sciences: Applied anatomy

31. A 25-year-old man presents to his GP with a painful swelling in the floor of his mouth that becomes more painful during meals. Bimanual examination of the patient's mouth suggests the presence of a stone in Wharton's duct. Which of the following provides the best anatomical description of the opening of the Wharton's duct?

A. Buccal mucosa opposite the upper second molar

B. Buccal mucosa opposite the lower second molar

C. Either side of the frenulum of the tongue

D. Floor of the mouth

E. None of the above

Basic sciences: Pharmacology

32. A 75-kg male is undergoing an elective inguinal hernia repair under local anaesthetic. From the options chose the correct maximum dose of 0.5% bupivacaine he can be given with adrenaline.

A. 20 mL

B. 30 mL

C. 45 mL

D. 55 mL

E. 75 mL

Basic sciences: Applied anatomy

33. A 34-year-old bowler presents with a gradual onset of right shoulder pain. He specifically describes severe pain when he abducts and laterally rotates his arm. Examination confirms severe pain on arm movement between 70–120 degrees of abduction. Which structure is he not likely to have damaged?

A. Teres major

B. Teres minor

C. Supraspinatus

D. Infraspinatus

E. Subscapularis

Common surgical conditions and the subspecialties: Breast disease

34. **A 45-year-old female is referred to the breast clinic with a smooth, firm and well-circumscribed lump that has grown rapidly in the last 2 weeks. Ultrasound imaging of the lump reveals a smooth, encapsulated 7-cm lump from which core biopsies are taken. The biopsy results confirm a fibroepithelial tumour consisting of epithelial cells and spindle cell stroma. What is the most likely diagnosis?**
    A. Fibrocystic disease of the breast
    B. Ductal carcinoma *in situ*
    C. Fibroadenoma
    D. Lobular carcinoma
    E. Phyllodes tumour

Basic sciences: Applied anatomy

35. **Which of the following is the most superficial structure encountered whilst dissecting into the popliteal fossa?**
    A. Tibial nerve
    B. Posterior tibial artery
    C. Superficial peroneal nerve
    D. Popliteal artery
    E. Sural nerve

Common surgical conditions and the subspecialties: Breast disease

36. **A 21-year-old female is referred by her GP to the rapid access breast clinic with a lump in her right breast. She says that it has been present for the past ten weeks and is painless. There is no bleeding or discharge from her nipples. Examination of the breast reveals a smooth, firm and mobile 2-cm lump in the upper outer quadrant of the right breast. There is no palpable axillary lymphadenopathy. Her paternal aunt died from breast cancer at the age of 62. What is the most likely diagnosis?**
    A. Mondor's disease
    B. Paget's disease
    C. Cystosarcoma phyllodes
    D. Fibroadenoma
    E. Fibrocystic disease

Basic sciences: Applied anatomy

37. **Which among the following statements about the inferior vena cava is correct?**
    A. It lies to the left of the abdominal aorta
    B. It is contained in a groove on the posterior surface of the pancreas
    C. It enters the diaphragm at the vertebral level T10
    D. It is a retroperitoneal structure
    E. It has three valves in the abdominal cavity before it enters the diaphragm

Common surgical conditions and the subspecialties: Gastrointestinal disease

38. **A 75-year-old lady is referred to the surgical assessment unit with progressively worsening abdominal pain. She is a chronic smoker and suffers with hypertension and ischaemic heart disease. The abdominal pain has been ongoing for several months. It occurs an hour after eating, rises steadily, plateaus, and declines after 1–2 hours. It does not radiate to the back and is not associated with nausea or vomiting. Her son is concerned as she seems to have lost her appetite and a significant amount of weight. Blood tests reveal normal LFTs, amylase, Hb, and a WCC of 14 × 10^9 cells/L. What is the most likely diagnosis?**
    A. Chronic gastritis
    B. Chronic cholecystitis
    C. Chronic mesenteric ischaemia
    D. Chronic pancreatitis
    E. Inflammatory bowel disease

Basic sciences: Applied anatomy

39. **A 63-year-old hyperthyroid patient notices a new prominent nodule within the right lobe of her thyroid gland. A biopsy of the lump subsequently confirms malignancy. She then undergoes a total thyroidectomy. During the procedure, the surgeon's field of vision is intermittently obscured by considerable bleeding from the gland. Which of the following statements is correct regarding the vessels of the thyroid gland?**
    A. The inferior thyroid artery is usually the first branch of the external carotid artery and supplies the inferior poles of the gland
    B. The superior thyroid artery is the first branch of the internal carotid artery and descends to supply the superior poles of the gland
    C. The inferior thyroid artery is the largest branch of the thyrocervical trunk arising from the subclavian artery
    D. About 20% of people have an unpaired thyroid ima artery that usually arises directly from the brachiocephalic trunk
    E. The middle thyroid arteries supply the middle of the lobes

Common surgical conditions and the subspecialties: General presenting symptoms or syndromes

40. **A 70-year-old man presents to the Emergency Department with a 4-hour history of haematemesis and melaena. He denies any previous peptic ulcer disease or NSAID use. He is found to be cold and clammy, with a pulse rate of 115/min and blood pressure of 96/50 mmHg. Abdominal examination reveals a midline laparotomy scar from a previous aortic abdominal aneurysm repair, and epigastric tenderness. His past surgical records reveal an aorto-bifemoral graft repair a year ago. What is the most likely diagnosis?**
   A. Acute myocardial infarction resulting from severe anaemia
   B. Aorto-enteric fistula
   C. Bleeding gastric ulcer
   D. Bleeding duodenal ulcer
   E. Bleeding oesophageal varices

Basic surgical skills: Principles of safe surgery

41. **Surgeons are required to possess a good working knowledge of the various types of suture needles and their utility in various surgical procedures. Which one of the following descriptions of needle type is most appropriate for the corresponding surgical procedure?**
   A. Blunt round-point needle for tendon repair
   B. Blunt taperpoint for ligament repair
   C. Reverse cutting needle for mass closure of the abdominal wall
   D. Round-bodied needle for bowel anastomosis
   E. Tapercut needle for suturing of liver

Common surgical conditions and the subspecialties: General presenting symptoms or syndromes

42. A 35-year-old man presents to the Emergency Department with a 2-day history of progressively worsening severe abdominal pain. He denies any previous medical history but admits to consuming large amounts of alcohol daily. Examination reveals pyrexia and tachycardia, together with a diffusely tender, peritonitic abdomen. Initial blood tests reveal: CRP 210 mg/L, WCC 12 × 10⁹ cells/L, mildly deranged LFTs, hyperlipidaemia, and an undetectable amylase level. Erect chest radiography reveals no evidence of pneumoperitoneum. The patient undergoes surgery, revealing a normal appendix but a large volume of free pus in the abdomen (which was later confirmed to be sterile). Which of the following options is the most likely diagnosis?

    A. Acute cholecystitis
    B. Acute pancreatitis
    C. Perforated duodenal ulcer
    D. TB ileitis
    E. Ischaemic colitis

Basic sciences: Applied anatomy

43. A 26-year-old lady undergoes a high tie of the sapheno-femoral junction and stripping of the long saphenous vein by the vascular surgeons. Prior to the operation the surgeon counselled the patient regarding the possible complications of infection, bleeding, bruising, scarring, and numbness along the medial aspect of the lower leg. Which nerve supplies the sensation to the medial aspect of the lower leg?

    A. Common peroneal nerve
    B. Deep peroneal nerve
    C. Superficial peroneal nerve
    D. Saphenous nerve
    E. Sural nerve

Common surgical conditions and the subspecialties: General presenting symptoms or syndromes

44. A 49-year-old gentleman with a longstanding history of Crohn's disease presents to his GP with increased frequency of micturition. Urinalysis demonstrates that he has sterile pyuria. Which of the following is the lesion likely to be?

    A. Colo-vesical fistula
    B. Recto-vesical fistula
    C. Terminal ileitis
    D. Transverse colitis
    E. Vesico-vaginal fistula

Assessment and management of patients with trauma (including the multiply-injured patient): Organ-specific trauma

45. A 30-year-old man is involved in a road traffic accident and is brought to the Emergency Department complaining of abdominal and back pain. He has no other overt injuries but has left loin and left upper quadrant tenderness on abdominal examination. He undergoes a CT scan of his abdomen which shows a normal spleen but a 3-cm renal laceration with a perinephric haematoma. How would you classify this injury on the basis of the American Association for Surgery of trauma classification of renal injuries?

A. Grade 1
B. Grade 2
C. Grade 3
D. Grade 4
E. Grade 5

Common surgical conditions and the subspecialties: Skin, head, and neck

46. A 45-year-old female presents to her GP with a slow-growing, firm, and painless mass in the lateral aspect of her cheek anteroinferior to her right ear. She has no associate lymphadenopathy or facial muscle distortion related to it. What is the most likely diagnosis?

A. Adenoid cystic carcinoma
B. Mumps infection
C. Pleomorphic adenoma
D. Salivary gland calculus
E. Warthin's tumour

Common surgical conditions and the subspecialties: General presenting symptoms or syndromes

47. A 30-year-old woman presents to the Emergency Department with a 48-hour history of severe right-sided abdominal pain, painful micturition, fever, chills, and rigors. Her temperature is 38.3°C. On examination, she is warm with sweaty peripheries and is tender over her left loin region. There are pus cells and casts on examination of her urine. What is the most likely diagnosis?

A. Ruptured ovarian follicle
B. Ascending cholangitis
C. Urinary tract infection
D. Pyelonephritis
E. Uncomplicated retrocaecal appendicitis

Common surgical conditions and the subspecialties:
Gastrointestinal disease

48. **A 21-year-old female is referred by her GP to the colorectal surgeons for a 2-month history of lethargy, weight loss and intermittent blood loss per rectum. The patient subsequently undergoes a flexible sigmoidoscopy and biopsy. Which of the following histological features would favour a diagnosis of Crohn's disease instead of ulcerative colitis?**
   A. Crypt abscesses
   B. Inflammatory infiltration of the lamina propria
   C. Glandular distortion
   D. Goblet cell depletion
   E. Non-caseating granulomata

Organ and tissue transplantation: Transplant immunology

49. **Which of the following statements regarding human leukocyte antigen (HLA) is incorrect?**
   A. They are a group of genes located along chromosome 6 that code for antigen-presenting proteins
   B. Class I HLAs express intracellular antigens and are expressed on all nucleated cells
   C. Class II HLAs includes the subtypes A, B, and C
   D. HLA-B27 is associated with seronegative spondyloarthropathies
   E. Acute transplant rejection is predominantly an immune response against foreign HLA protein

Management of the dying patient: Palliative care

50. **An 82-year-old female with terminal metastatic colorectal cancer is receiving optimal doses of morphine sulphate therapy. Which of the following effects may be expected with the addition of a partial opioid agonist?**
   A. Increased analgesia
   B. Increased respiratory depression
   C. Increased sedation
   D. No change
   E. Reduced analgesia

1. Answer: D

The axillary artery is a large artery supplying the lateral aspect of the thorax, the axilla and the upper limb. Its origin is at the lateral margin of the first rib (before which it is called the subclavian artery); after passing the lower margin of teres major, it is known as the brachial artery. The axillary artery is divided into three parts by the pectoralis minor muscle (the first part is between the outer border of the 1st rib and the pectoralis minor muscle, the second part is behind the pectoralis minor muscle, and the third part is after the pectoralis minor muscle). The first part has one branch—the superior thoracic artery; the second part has two branches—the lateral thoracic (pectoral) artery and the thoraco-acromial artery; and the third part has three branches—the subscapular artery (which divides into the circumflex scapular artery and the thoraco-dorsal artery), the anterior circumflex humeral artery, and the posterior circumflex humeral artery. The costo-cervical trunk arises from the second part of the subclavian artery.

2. Answer: B

Angiogenesis or neovascularization refers to the formation of new blood vessels from pre-existing vessels at the site of injury. Four general steps are recognized during this process: (1) proteolytic degradation of the parent vessel basement membrane, allowing formation of a capillary sprout; (2) migration of endothelial cells towards the angiogenic stimulus; (3) proliferation of endothelial cells behind the leading front of migrating cells; and (4) maturation of endothelial cells with organization into capillary tubes. Several factors induce angiogenesis, including vascular endothelial growth factor, TGFα, platelet-derived growth factor, basic fibroblast growth factor, and TGFβ. Angiogenic capillary sprouts invade the fibrin/fibronectin-rich wound clot and within a few days organize into a microvascular network throughout the granulation tissue. Fibrocytes, which play a role in the formation of extracellular matrix and contribute to the myofibroblast population in the wound, do not play a role in angiogenesis.

3. Answer: E

Marfan's syndrome, estimated to affect approximately 1 in 5000 of the population, is an autosomal dominant connective tissue disorder characterized by skeletal, cardiovascular, ocular and pulmonary system abnormalities. It is caused by mutation of the *FBN1* gene on chromosome 15. This gene normally controls production of fibrillin, a protein which plays an important role in the structural development of the connective tissue. The most readily visible signs are associated with the skeletal system such as long, slender limbs associated with long and slender fingers and toes (arachnodactyly). Other skeletal abnormalities include scoliosis, pectus excavatum or pectus carinatum. Abnormal joint flexibility, a high-arched palate, pes cavus (high-arched feet), stooping of the shoulders, and stretch marks are other associated findings. Cardiac manifestations include dilatation of the aortic root, which may progress to aortic dissection. Ocular manifestations include myopia, astigmatism, superotemporal dislocation of the lens, and glaucoma (note that inferonasal dislocation of the lens is a feature of homocystinuria).

4. Answer: D

A quadriceps tear may occur in both young athletes and older patients. The usual mechanism of injury is from kicking, sprinting or whilst being engaged in a sports activity which exerts sudden strain to the quadriceps tendon. Patients with a tear of the quadriceps tendon typically present with acute knee pain and suprapatellar swelling, and an antalgic gait with inability to extend the knee or perform straight leg raise. There may be a palpable defect in the suprapatellar area and a low-lying patella, but swelling may initially obscure this finding. Neurological examination of the thigh and knee may be normal except for decreased quadriceps motor function and an absent knee jerk.

5. Answer: E

This patient is presenting with the typical history, signs and symptoms of mesenteric ischaemia. Mesenteric ischaemia commonly occurs following embolisation from one of the cardiac chambers, commonly the left ventricle, and, as such, this condition is more common in patients who have atrial fibrillation. The risk factors for this condition include atherosclerosis, hypertension, hypercoagulable states, diabetes mellitus and age. The middle colic artery is commonly affected. The clinical presentation includes sudden-onset severe abdominal pain, with the pain commonly being out of proportion to the clinical findings; nausea and vomiting; and diarrhoea. The stools may be mixed with blood and mucus (due to desloughing of the ischaemic bowel wall). Arterial blood gas analysis is a useful initial investigation and may reveal a metabolic acidosis. Plain abdominal radiography in addition to ruling out other causes for acute abdominal pain, may demonstrate 'thumb printing' (i.e. mucosal oedema) of the affected colon. Angiography, ultrasound scanning, and CT scanning are other investigations that may be indicated to diagnose the condition. The immediate management of patients with bowel ischaemia includes oxygen administration, venous access, appropriate fluid resuscitation, parenteral broad-spectrum antibiotics and adequate analgesia. Surgery (resection of the ischaemic bowel) remains the mainstay of treatment.

6. Answer: B

Metabolic complications occur in approximately 5% of patients having TPN. These include:

- Hypo/hyperglycaemia
- Deranged LFTs
- Hyperchloraemic acidosis
- Hypophosphataemia
- Hypercalcaemia
- Hypo/hyperkalaemia
- Hypo/hypernatraemia
- Deficiency of trace elements such as vitamins, essential fatty acids, folate, zinc, and magnesium.

'Refeeding syndrome' is a rare but well-known complication which results from the rapid shift of potassium and phosphate into the cells. It may manifest itself with cardiac arrest and death.

7. Answer: D

This is a case of achalasia of the cardia: a neuromuscular failure of relaxation at the lower end of the oesophagus with progressive dilatation, tortuosity, incoordination of peristalsis and often hypertrophy of the oesophageal segment above. There is effectively a functional obstruction at the lower end of the oesophagus. The primary neurological defect involves the ganglion cells of Auerbach's myenteric plexus in the lower oesophageal sphincter and oesophageal body.

Abnormalities have also been reported in the vagal dorsal motor nucleus, the nucleus ambiguus and in the smooth muscle of the oesophagus. The management of achalasia usually starts with balloon dilatation (i.e. repeated monthly), with the 10% that fail going on to have surgery (i.e. Heller's cardiomyotomy, involving a longitudinal cut in the distal 3–4 cm of oesophageal muscle; the operation has a success rate of about 90%). Pharmacological treatment (e.g. intrasphincteric injection of botulinum toxin) should be considered as the initial therapy for patients with achalasia who are at high risk for the complications of pneumatic dilatation or surgical myotomy. However, medium- to long-term relief cannot usually be gained by pharmacological treatment alone.

8. Answer: E

There are several different approaches to the hip and different nerves may be damaged depending on which approach is used.

The superior gluteal nerve arises from lumbosacral plexus (i.e. from the dorsal branches of L4, L5, and S1). It exits the pelvis and enters the gluteal region through the upper margin of the greater sciatic notch, just superior to the piriformis muscle. It courses with the superior gluteal artery between gluteus medius and minimus, whilst supplying motor branches to both these muscles, as well as the tensor fascia lata. The nerve is therefore at risk during the lateral approach to the hip.

The posterior approach to the hip joint involves an incision through the deep fascia and gluteus maximus and then division of the external rotators. The sciatic nerve is in danger with this approach. The anterior approach involves the planes between tensor fascia lata and sartorius, followed by the rectus femoris and gluteus medius. The lateral femoral cutaneous nerve of the thigh is in danger with the anterior approach.

9. Answer: E

The collecting ducts account for 4–5% of renal sodium reabsorption and 5% of renal water reabsorption. However, at times of extreme dehydration, over 25% of filtered water may be reabsorbed from the collecting ducts. This occurs under the influence of ADH, which stimulates aquaporin formation to facilitate water reabsorption and inhibit diuresis.

The proximal convoluted tubule is responsible for the reabsorption of the vast majority of ultrafiltrate contents mostly via passive transport and also via some active transport.

The loop of Henle generates the hypertonic medullary osmotic pressure required to allow the collecting ducts to reabsorb water via the countercurrent multiplier system. It is highly dependent on adequate renal perfusion and the provision of adequate quantities of energy (adenosine triphosphate) to power the membrane NA/K pumps.

10. Answer: D

Oesophageal atresia with tracheo-oesophageal fistula occurs in 1 in 3000–5000 live births. Five anatomical variants are described: no fistula, distal fistula, double fistula, proximal fistula, and cervical 'H' fistula. Distal fistula is the commonest and is seen in 87% of all cases. No fistula is seen in about 10% and the other variants are rare.

Presentation may be antenatal with polyhydramnios, or postnatal with frothy oral secretions and feeding difficulty. Pneumonitis and sepsis can occur due to aspiration. Early definitive surgical correction is very successful with survival approaching 100%.

11. Answer: D

The pattern of injury in this case describes a Monteggia fracture-dislocation, which involves a fracture of the upper ulna with dislocation of the radial head. The history is one of a fall, usually with twisting and pronation of the forearm. An adequate lateral radiograph is required to fully demonstrate the fracture-dislocation. The radial head is dislocated forwards and is no longer seen pointing directly to the capitulum, while the ulna is bowed forwards. Closed reduction by manipulation may suffice in children but the fracture is so unstable that internal fixation by plating is usually necessary in adults. The arm should be immobilized in plaster for 6 weeks with the elbow held in flexion to prevent re-dislocation of the radial head. A Galeazzi fracture-dislocation provides almost a 'mirror image' to this, and involves a fracture of the lower radius with subluxation (or dislocation) of the distal radioulnar joint.

A Barton's fracture is a fracture-dislocation of the distal radius, where the fracture line runs across the volar lip of the radius and into the wrist joint; the hand and the fragment of distal radius undergo a proximal and volar displacement. The more common Colles' fracture usually involves a transverse fracture of the distal radius about 2.5 cm from the distal radioulnar joint, presenting with a 'dinner fork' deformity of the wrist. It involves dorsal angulation and dorsal displacement of the distal fragment, radial deviation of the hand, supination and proximal impaction. Finally, a Smith's fracture (i.e. 'reverse Colles' fracture') is a fracture of the distal radius, which occurs if the patient lands with the wrist in flexion. The radial fragment is displaced anteriorly and the fracture does not extend into the joint (i.e. unlike in a Barton's fracture). A lateral radiographic view shows the fragment to be displaced and tilted anteriorly—the opposite of a Colles' fracture.

12. Answer: A

Dercum's disease ('adiposis dolorosa') is a rare condition that mainly affects obese women (female:male ratio = 30:1) and usually manifests after menopause. Although familial tendencies exist, the majority of cases are sporadic. The condition is characterized by the formation of circumscribed adipose tissue deposits, which may be painful, in the subcutaneous tissues of the extremities and other regions (the commonest site being the knees). The lesions vary in diameter from 0.5–5 cm. The disease may be associated with emotional instability, fatigue, weakness, and rarely, dementia. Histological examination reveals no abnormalities of the adipose tissue (i.e. no fat necrosis as seen in panniculitis, although giant cell formations may be seen). No definitive treatment currently exists. In contrast, a dermatofibroma is a benign neoplasm of dermal fibroblasts and would therefore be tethered to the skin. Hereditary haemorrhagic telangiectasia (Osler–Weber–Rendu syndrome) is a dominantly inherited genetic condition in which there are haemangiomata scattered over the mucous membranes, predisposing to gastrointestinal bleeding.

Type I neurofibromatosis (von Recklinghausen's disease) is an autosomal dominant condition involving two or more of the following: six café-au-lait macules (>5 mm prepubertally or >15 mm postpubertally), two neurofibromas of any type (or one plexiform neurofibroma), axillary or inguinal freckling, optic gliomas, Lisch nodules, distinctive osseous lesions (e.g. sphenoid dysplasia), or a 1st-degree relative with type 1 neurofibromatosis. Type 2 neurofibromatosis implies the presence of either bilateral vestibular schwannomas (as seen on CT or MRI) or a 1st-degree relative with type 2 neurofibromatosis and an unilateral vestibular schwannoma or neurofibroma/meningioma/glioma/schwannoma/juvenile cataract.

13. Answer: C

APTT is a measure of the intrinsic pathway and is often a useful measure when patients are on heparin therapy (it is useful to note that heparin affects the intrinsic pathway mainly but its effect on factor Xa). PT is a measure of the extrinsic pathway and is prolonged with the use of warfarin, which reduces the production of vitamin K-dependent clotting factors II, VII, IX, and X. Thrombin time is a measure of the common pathway, while the bleeding time is a measure of platelet function.

14. Answer: D

In order to obtain jejunal biopsies, a Crosby–Watson capsule is swallowed and guided through the pylorus, duodenum and jejunum with screening. When in position, a small sample of mucosa is obtained by suction, the capsule immediately retrieved, and the sample placed in 10% formalin. Complications of this procedure include transient sore throat and, very rarely, haemorrhage, perforation, and capsule retention. Option A is incorrect as these circumstances alone should not preclude jejunal biopsy, which is warranted in elderly patients presenting with features of late-onset coeliac disease such as iron-deficiency anaemia, osteoporosis and weight loss. Option B alludes to the abnormal histology seen in tropical sprue (i.e. featuring villous atrophy and malabsorption occurring in the Far and Middle East and Caribbean); however, these individuals are not likely to be considered 'healthy' at presentation. Option C is incorrect as subtotal villous atrophy is seen in various conditions other than coeliac disease, including severe tropical sprue, cows' milk (or soya) insensitivity in children, Whipple's disease, hypogammaglobulinaemia, neomycin therapy, laxative abuse, etc. Option E is incorrect as the villous atrophy may be evident under a simple magnifying glass. Option D is correct; jejunal biopsy in Whipple's disease reveals stunted villi, with macrophage deposition in the lamina propria containing periodic acid–Schiff (PAS)-positive granules. The bacteria (*Tropheryma whippelii*) may be seen within macrophages on electron microscopy.

15. Answer: E

The axillary artery originates at the lateral margin of the 1st rib (before which it is called the subclavian artery) and ends at the lower margin of teres major (after which it is called the brachial artery). The first, second, and third parts of the axillary artery lie medial, behind and lateral to pectoralis minor respectively. These parts of the axillary artery give off one, two and three branches respectively:

- First part:
  - Superior thoracic artery
- Second part:
  - Thoraco-acromial artery
  - Lateral thoracic artery
- Third part:
  - Subscapular artery
  - Anterior humeral circumflex artery
  - Posterior humeral circumflex artery.

Within the axillary region, level I lymph nodes lie lateral to pectoralis minor, level II lie behind, and level III lie medial to the pectoralis minor. If the intercostobrachial nerve is divided during axillary dissection, paraesthesia over the medial aspect of the inner upper arm may result. If the long thoracic nerve is divided, a winged scapula will result from denervation of serratus anterior. However, if the thoracodorsal nerve is divided there will be weakness of arm adduction, extension, and internal rotation from denervation of latissimus dorsi. The cords of the brachial plexus are anatomically related to the second part of the axillary artery: the lateral, posterior, and medial cords lie laterally, posteriorly, and medially to this part of the artery, respectively.

16. Answer: D

Raynaud's disease is characterized by excess arterial and arteriolar constriction within the peripheral circulation. Therefore, a reduction in the sympathetic-mediated tone of these vessels via a pre-ganglionic sympathectomy is a reasonable option to treat this disorder.

The salivary glands are influenced to a much greater extent by the parasympathetic rather than the sympathetic division of the autonomic nervous system. Increased parasympathetic activity increases the flow rate in the salivary glands but less time is allowed for the duct cell secretion of potassium into the salivary fluid. Consequently, the potassium content of the saliva is reduced. Noradrenaline is the neurotransmitter released by the majority of post-ganglionic sympathetic neurons. Genital erection and ejaculation requires coordinated activity from both divisions of the autonomic nervous system. The sympathetic fibres from T11 to L2 govern ejaculation whereas genital erection is mediated by parasympathetic innervation arising from the sacral region of the spinal cord. A lesion at the T10 level would therefore affect both erection and ejaculation. 'Dry orgasm', where the patient can generate and maintain an erection but is unable to ejaculate, can be a side effect of drugs such as beta-blockers. The parasympathetic innervation of the heart is almost exclusively restricted to the atria and structures therein, including the sinoatrial node (SAN). Increased parasympathetic activity reduces the slope of the pacemaker potential in the SAN, resulting in a reduced heart rate—a negative chronotropic action.

17. Answer: B

An intersphincteric fistula is the commonest type of fistula-in-ano. The anatomical (Parks') classification of fistulas depends on the precise track a given fistula takes and can be:

- Submucosal (5%): superficial to all sphinteric structures.
- Intersphincteric (60%): passes deep to part of, or all of, the internal sphincter.
- Trans-sphincteric (25%): passes through the external sphincter to lie deep to part of it (or all of it). Divided into low (<1/2) or high (>1/2) according to the amount of sphincter encircled.
- Suprasphincteric (5%): passes above the external anal sphincter below the levator ani.
- Extrasphincteric (5%): passes above the levator ani. May originate in the rectum rather than in the anal canal.

18. Answer: C

Patients with a history of ischaemic heart disease are at an increased risk of developing perioperative and postoperative cardiac events such as myocardial infarction and cardiac failure. The Goldman's Cardiac Risk Index is a prognostic indicator for predicting the likelihood of developing a perioperative life-threatening cardiac event in a patient with ischaemic heart disease. The risk factors include: age greater than 70 years, raised jugular venous pressure, presence of a 3rd heart sound, significant myocardial ischaemic event in the preceding 6 months (i.e. not simply angina pectoris), surgery on the abdomen or thorax, symptomatic aortic stenosis, poor general condition, and emergency surgery. Cardiopulmonary exercise testing (which measures metabolic parameters while the patient exercises on a bicycle ergometer) is an objective method of assessing cardiac risk and provides more information than a treadmill test. Serum brain natriuretic peptide (BNP) is another laboratory marker that is being evaluated as a test to predict cardiac events.

19. Answer: E

The upper two-thirds of the anal canal are divided from the lower third by the dentate (or pectinate) line. In embryological terms, this line represents the hindgut–proctoderm junction (i.e. the 'squamo-columnar' junction). The lymphatic drainage between the two areas is different; the region above the dentate line drains along the superior rectal vessels to the abdominal nodes, whereas lymphatic drainage from under the dentate line is to the inguinal nodes. The several distinctions that can be made based upon the location of a structure relative to the dentate line are shown in Table 3.1.

Table 3.1 Features of the anal canal in relation to the dentate line

Distinctive feature	Below dentate line	Above dentate line
Arterial supply	Middle and inferior rectal arteries (from internal iliac artery)	Superior rectal artery (from inferior mesenteric artery)
Venous drainage	Middle and inferior rectal veins (to internal iliac vein)	Superior rectal vein (to inferior mesenteric vein)
Innervation	Inferior rectal nerves	Inferior hypogastric plexus
Embryological origin	Ectoderm	Endoderm
Epithelium	Stratified squamous	Columnar
Lymphatic drainage	Superficial inguinal nodes	Internal iliac nodes and inferior mesenteric nodes
Haemorrhoid classification	External (i.e. painful)	Internal (i.e. not painful)

None of the other options particular favour a diagnosis of squamous cell carcinoma over adenocarcinoma or vice versa.

20. Answer: D

The blood supply to the pancreas is from the superior and inferior pancreaticoduodenal arteries and the splenic artery. The superior pancreaticoduodenal artery is a branch of the gastroduodenal artery, which is a branch of the common hepatic artery of the coeliac axis. The inferior pancreaticoduodenal artery is a branch of the superior mesenteric artery. The pancreaticoduodenal arteries supply the head of the pancreas. The body and tail are supplied by the pancreatic branches from the splenic artery.

21. Answer: D

The Munro–Kelly doctrine highlights that the cranium is a fixed volume vault, which contains 85% brain, 10% CSF fluid and 5% blood. An increase in the intracranial volume therefore causes a rapid rise in the intracranial pressure (ICP), such that the increase in volume of one component is forced to be compensated for by the decrease in volume of another. A slight head-up tilt reduces venous congestion, potentially improving cerebral perfusion. Patients should be intubated and ventilated to maintain good oxygenation; and also to ensure adequate elimination of carbon dioxide, thereby minimizing its vasodilatory effect and thus controlling intracranial blood volume and ICP. Mannitol is an osmotic diuretic and a potent free radical scavenger. It decreases CSF production and causes a reduction in blood viscosity, thereby increasing cerebral blood flow. Steroids are not indicated in head injury. They are only useful in reducing the inflammatory reaction that is associated with organized masses such as tumours. An intraventricular catheter can be placed to measure the ICP and to allow therapeutic drainage.

22. Answer: D

There are two main types of congenital abdominal wall defects: gastroschisis and exomphalos (or 'omphalocele'). Gastroschisis is more common than exomphalos. It has a male preponderance and is seen in 1 in 3000 live births. The defect is typically to the right of the umbilicus, from which it is separated by a narrow skin bridge. Exposed midgut protrudes through a small open defect in the abdominal wall. The intestinal contents are not contained within a sac. In contrast, exomphalos is where organs herniate through an abdominal wall defect and are contained within a sac. Exomphalos minor has a small defect (<4 cm) and the umbilical cord inserts to the left of the hernial sac rather than the apex. Exomphalos major has a large abdominal wall defect (>4 cm) and the umbilical cord inserts into the apex of the sac.

The sac is trilaminar, comprising amnion, Wharton's jelly and peritoneum. Prune belly syndrome (abdominal wall dysplasia) refers to failure of development of the anterior abdominal wall musculature and is associated with urinary tract dilatation and testicular maldescent.

23. Answer: B

For patients on warfarin with evidence of minor bleeds (i.e. as in this case), is it advisable to withhold warfarin for at least a day, and to consider giving either vitamin K 0.5–2 mg orally or 5 mg by slow intravenous injection or infusion. This should be repeated in 24 hours if the INR remains high and bleeding persists. Warfarin should then be restarted a lower dose. It is nonetheless imperative to consider the risks and benefits of reversing the anticoagulation. The patient described is at low risk from warfarin reversal. In addition, there is no suggestion of haemodynamic compromise or any evidence of pulmonary embolism. In contrast to such 'minor' bleeding, 'major' bleeding is defined as being intraorbital, intracranial, retroperitoneal, or muscular (i.e. risking compartment syndrome). Any evidence of haemodynamic instability should also raise the suggestion of major bleeding. In such cases, an urgent coagulation screen must be performed, with urgent advice sought from the duty haematologist regarding aggressive reversal of the coagulopathy with vitamin K, stopping warfarin and administering prothrombin complex concentrate or fresh frozen plasma.

24. Answer: E

Aortic dissection can be classified using the Stanford or the DeBakey classification. The Stanford classification is more commonly used in clinical practice.

- Stanford classification:
  - ◆ Type A: ascending aorta involved
  - ◆ Type B: ascending aorta not involved.

Reprinted from *The Annals of Thoracic Surgery*, 10, 3, Daily PO, Trueblood HW, Stinson EB, Wuerflein RD, Shumway NE, 'Management of acute aortic dissections', pp. 237–47. Copyright 1970, with permission from The Society of Thoracic Surgeons.

- DeBakey classification:
  - ◆ Type I: ascending aorta extending into descending aorta
  - ◆ Type II: ascending aorta only
  - ◆ Type III: descending aorta distal to left subclavian artery
  - ◆ Type IIIa: Type III extending proximally and distally, mostly above the diaphragm
  - ◆ Type IIIb: Type III extending only distally, potentially extending below the diaphragm

This classification was published in *Journal of Thoracic Cardiovascular Surgery*, 49, DeBakey ME *et al.*, 'Surgical management of dissecting aneurysms of the aorta', pp. 130–49. Copyright Elsevier 1965.

25. Answer: B

In adults, the thyroid gland is a bilobed structure lying in the anterior neck. The two lateral lobes are connected by the isthmus, which may have an associated pyramidal lobe extending cephalad towards the base of the tongue

The pretracheal fascia splits to enclose the thyroid gland. The posteromedial aspect of the gland is attached to the side of the cricoid cartilage, and the first and second tracheal rings, by a condensation of the pretracheal fascia called the posterior suspensory ligament of Berry. This is responsible for the upward movement of the thyroid gland on swallowing.

The ligament of Treitz is the suspensory ligament of the duodenum, which arises from the right crus of the diaphragm and inserts into the third and fourth parts of the duodenum (and frequently into the duodenojejunal flexure).

26. Answer: C

Anaemia decreases the oxygen carrying capacity of blood by virtue of the fact that there is less haemoglobin to bind with oxygen. However, anaemia does not affect the amount of oxygen dissolved in the blood, or the haemoglobin oxygen saturation (i.e. since it is the 'quantity' and not the 'quality' of the oxygen-binding haemoglobin that is reduced in anaemia.) Because the overall oxygen carrying capacity of the blood is reduced in anaemia (i.e. the blood carries less oxygen overall), a smaller oxygen gradient exists between the blood and tissues, resulting in less oxygen being released from binding, for the same drop in venous PO_2. Such hypoxic states may predispose to tissue hypoxia in the long term. In acute-onset anaemia (i.e. from rapid blood loss), a drop in haemoglobin levels to between 8 g/dL and 10 g/dL may cause minimal to moderate symptoms, depending on the patient's constitution and comorbidities. However, an acute drop in haemoglobin to under 7 g/dL would rapidly manifest with symptoms of anaemia (e.g. shortness of breath, faintness, lethargy).

27. Answer: C

The signs and symptoms in this child are suggestive of spreading/established infection in the peritoneal cavity. Bacterial peritonitis in children may occur as a result of a ruptured viscus (e.g. ruptured appendicitis or ruptured Meckel's diverticulitis), or as a complication of abdominal surgery. The child may present with classical signs of peritonitis such as abdominal pain, pyrexia, nausea, vomiting, tachycardia, low blood pressure and decreased urine output. High pyrexia may result in febrile convulsions. Abdominal examination may reveal a board-like rigidity, guarding and rebound tenderness. Bowel sounds are commonly absent in established peritonitis. Erect chest radiography may demonstrate free gas under the diaphragm, alluding to a perforated viscus. The organisms frequently responsible for bacterial peritonitis in children include *Escherichia coli, Klebsiella pneumoniae*, and *Pseudomonas* species.

28. Answer: E

An episiotomy is performed when a perineal laceration seems to be inevitable, in order to protect the fascia supporting the urinary bladder, urethra, external anal sphincter, levator ani and rectum. An uncontrolled tear of these structures will result in poor perineal support of pelvic organs, resulting in prolapse of the urinary bladder (cystocoele) and incontinence in later life. An episiotomy therefore entails a clean cut that is made away from these important structures.

29. Answer: D

Gastric acid is secreted by oxyntic (parietal) cells that are located in the body of the stomach. They secrete H^+ by active pump-mediated membrane transport. The H^+- K^+-ATPase proton pump is found embedded on the apical membrane and is the final common pathway of histamine and acetylcholine stimulated gastric acid production. Gastric acid secretion is inhibited by increased concentrations of intraluminal H^+, secretin, and gastric inhibitory peptide. In contrast to parietal cells, gastric chief cells, which are located mainly in the gastric fundus, secrete pepsinogen, gastric lipase, and chymosin. Another key cell in the stomach is the G cell, which is located mainly in the gastric antrum, and secretes gastrin.

30. Answer: B

The most likely diagnosis in this scenario is diverticular disease. Diverticular disease most commonly occurs in Western populations. Inherent weaknesses of the bowel wall at points of vascular entry, colonic hypersegmentation, and low fibre intake (which is believed to cause raised intraluminal pressures) are possible contributing factors to the development of such diverticulae. These diverticulae are usually acquired, although they can rarely be congenital. Acquired diverticulae are out-pouchings of the bowel wall involving only mucosa, submucosa and serosa.

These occur mostly in the descending and sigmoid colon, and almost never occur in the rectum. In contrast, congenital diverticulae (e.g. Meckel's diverticulum) occur anywhere in the colon and involve all layers of the bowel wall (i.e. they are 'true' diverticulae.).

31. Answer: C

The duct of the submandibular gland is also known as Wharton's duct. It runs along the floor of the mouth and opens onto either side of the frenulum of the tongue. In contrast, the parotid duct (Stenson's duct) opens into the buccal mucosa opposite the second upper molar tooth. The sublingual gland has about 8–20 ducts. The smaller sublingual ducts (ducts of Rivinus) either join the submandibular duct or open separately into the mouth on the elevated crest of mucous membrane (plica sublingualis). One or more of these join to form the major sublingual duct (duct of Bartholin), which opens into the submandibular duct. Eighty per cent of the calculi in salivary glands are found in the submandibular gland and the Wharton's duct because of the primarily mucoid secretions of the submandibular gland, and the upward drainage angle of Wharton's duct.

32. Answer: C

Bupivacaine is a long-acting anaesthetic agent that is used for local and epidural anaesthesia. The maximum dose without adrenaline is 2 mg/kg, and with adrenaline, is 3 mg/kg. Adrenaline is a vaso-constrictor and decreases plasma clearance of the local anaesthetic, therefore allow a higher dose to be administered safely without reaching the systemic circulation. The maximum dose for a 75 kg man = 3 × 75 = 225 mg.

As 1 mL of 0.5% bupivacaine contains 5 mg, for a 75-kg man: 225/5 = 45 mL is the maximum volume.

It is important to remember that bupivacaine is more cardiotoxic than other commonly used local anaesthetic agents, and its toxicity does not produce any neurological 'warning signs' prior to myocardial depression and cardiovascular collapse.

33. Answer: A

The rotator cuff is a musculotendinous cuff formed by the tendons and insertions of the rotator cuff muscles to reinforce the articular capsule of the glenohumeral joint. It holds the head of the humerus in the glenoid cavity and stabilizes the joint through tonic contractions of the mus-cles. Frequent microtrauma to the shoulder joint through activities such as bowling or throw-ing, which require abduction of the arm, results in injuries and tears of the rotator cuff. As the supratendinous part of the rotator cuff is relatively avascular, this tears initially, resulting in severe pain and weakness when abducting the arm from 70 to 120 degrees. The reason that pain is not felt before and after this range of abduction is because the tendons of the rotator cuff are not anatomically 'impinged' by the head of the humerus during this time. Of the options listed, only teres major does not form part of the rotator cuff and cannot be implicated in the pain of such tendon impingement.

34. Answer: E

Phyllodes tumours are fibroepithelial tumours composed of epithelial and stromal components. They are usually benign but about 25% are malignant and metastasize. As even the benign forms have malig-nant potential, all phyllodes tumours are considered to be breast cancer. They usually present between the ages of 40–50 years (premenopausal) as fast-growing, discrete, firm masses that may be difficult to distinguish from fibroadenomas. In patients under the age of 25 years, FNA may be relied upon; if over 25 years or if doubt remains, core biopsy or excision biopsy may be used to confirm the diagnosis.

35. Answer: A

The popliteal fossa is the shallow depression posterior to the knee joint, the boundaries of which are: superomedial—semitendinosus; superolateral—biceps femoris; inferomedial—medial head of gastrocnemius; and inferolateral—lateral head of gastrocnemius. Its roof is formed by the skin, superficial fascia (containing the short saphenous vein), three cutaneous nerves (terminal branch of posterior cutaneous nerve of thigh, posterior division of medial cutaneous nerve, and peroneal or sural communicating nerve), and the deep (or popliteal) fascia. The floor is formed by the popliteal surface of the femur, knee joint capsule, oblique popliteal ligament and the strong fascia covering the popliteus muscle. During dissection within this fossa, the tibial nerve is the most superficial structure encountered, followed by the popliteal vein, and lastly, the popliteal artery. Other contents of the popliteal fossa include the common peroneal nerve and six or seven popliteal lymph nodes.

36. Answer: D

Fibroadenoma is the most commonly diagnosed breast tumour in women under 30 years of age. They are benign tumours originating from the breast lobule. They show proliferation of both epithelium and connective tissue elements, and are considered an 'aberration of normal development and involution' (ANDI). Most fibroadenomas measure 2–3 cm in diameter and are common between the ages of 16–24; the incidence decreases towards menopause. Fibroadenomas are usually mobile, firm and smooth lumps but are sometimes lobulated. They may be multiple in approximately 10% of cases. The diagnosis is confirmed by triple assessment: (1) clinical examination, (2) radiological assessment (mammography or ultrasound scan), and (3) cytological (FNA) or histological (core biopsy) confirmation. Over a 5-year period, 50% increase in size, 25% remain stable, and 25% decrease in size. The risk of malignant transformation is approximately 1 in 1000.

37. Answer: D

The inferior vena cava (IVC) conveys blood to the right atrium from all structures below the level of the diaphragm. It is formed by the union of the common iliac veins anterior to the L5 vertebral body to the right of the midline (note that the abdominal aorta bifurcates at the level of L4, just left of the IVC). It ascends anterior to the vertebral column, lying to the right of the abdominal aorta. Both the abdominal aorta and the IVC are retroperitoneal structures. The IVC is contained in a deep groove on the posterior surface of the liver. It crosses the diaphragm at the level of T8, between its median and right leaves, and inclines slightly anteromedially. It then passes through the fibrous pericardium and opens into the inferoposterior aspect of the right atrium. The abdominal part of the inferior vena cava is devoid of any valves.

38. Answer: C

Mesenteric ischaemia can be classified as follows:

Acute mesenteric ischaemia is caused by sudden intestinal hypoperfusion due to trauma, emboli, etc. It commonly results from thromboembolic arterial occlusion, usually of the superior mesenteric artery. Acute mesenteric ischaemia may also result from mesenteric venous occlusion, systemic vasculitis, sudden episodes of reduced cardiac output or sudden drops in systemic vascular resistance. Rarely, acute mesenteric ischaemia may be secondary to intestinal obstruction (e.g. strangulated hernia, intussusception or volvulus). The typical presentation involves sudden, severe, colicky abdominal pain associated with vomiting or diarrhoea (both of which may be bloody due to haemorrhage into the bowel lumen), in an elderly patient with a history of cardiac or arterial disease.

In contrast to this, chronic mesenteric ischaemia ('intestinal angina') refers to longstanding hypoperfusion of the gut due to atherosclerotic occlusive disease of the mesenteric arteries, resulting in inability to meet the metabolic demands of post-prandial gut function.

A high level of clinic suspicion is required in diagnosing a patient with the given presentation. Patients typically present with colicky, epigastric pain occurring 30–60 minutes after eating, which may be relieved by defecation. They tend to develop profound food fear from this, resulting in progressive weight loss and malnourishment. Diagnosis is by angiography (CT/MR or standard), which should include a lateral view of the aorta and the origins of the coeliac axis, and the superior and inferior mesenteric arteries. Duplex ultrasound is an alternative imaging tool. Treatment is by surgical (open or endovascular) reconstruction of one or more of the mesenteric arteries. Three vessel reconstructions provide the best results, albeit with a 40% recurrence rate.

39. Answer: C

The thyroid gland is a highly vascular structure supplied by paired superior and inferior thyroid arteries. The first branch of the external carotid artery is usually the superior thyroid artery, which descends downwards to supply the superior pole. It then divides into anterior and poste-rior branches, which anastomose in the midline. The inferior thyroid artery is the largest branch of the thyrocervical trunk arising from the subclavian artery, supplying the inferior poles of the gland. Around 10% of the population have a small unpaired thyroid ima artery that usually arises directly from the brachiocephalic trunk. However, its origin may vary. Although there is a middle thyroid vein, there is no middle thyroid artery.

The superior and middle thyroid veins drain into the internal jugular vein and the inferior thyroid veins drain into the brachiocephalic veins.

40. Answer: B

Aorto-enteric fistula should be excluded in any patient presenting with gastrointestinal bleed-ing following an AAA repair, as it is a serious and life-threatening complication of aortic graft surgery. It may present several months to years after the initial operation. The graft will most commonly erode and ulcerate into the duodenum to cause significant haemetemeis and sub-sequently, melaena. If the patient is stable, the diagnosis may be confirmed with a contrast CT scan. However, any unstable patient providing a high enough degree of clinical suspicion should undergo emergency laparotomy without further delay.

41. Answer: D

It is vital for surgeons to understand the principles behind the various types of suture needles and their applications in surgery. Round-bodied needles tend to separate tissue fibres (i.e. instead of cutting them). They are therefore used in bowel and vascular anastomoses, as they encourage tissues to close tightly around the suture material, forming a leak-proof suture line.

Blunt round-point needles literally 'dissect' rather than cut, and are useful when suturing extremely friable vascular tissue (e.g. liver, kidney, and spleen) and mass closure of the abdominal wall. For tough tissues like skin, ligament and tendon, reverse cutting needles are beneficial as their triangular cross section (with the apex on the outer convex curvature of the needle) offers the most effective tissue penetration with minimal collateral trauma. Reverse cutting needles are especially useful in ophthalmic and cosmetic procedures, where minimal trauma, early tissue regeneration, and minimal scar formation are the primary aims.

Blunt taperpoint needles are employed when needlestick injury is a major concern (i.e. in high-risk patients). In contrast, tapercut needles combine the initial penetration of a cutting needle with the minimized trauma of the round-bodied needle, making this needle appropriate for use on fascia, ligament, or scar tissue.

42. Answer: B

In the presence of generalized tenderness and sterile pus from the abdomen, cholecystitis is unlikely. In the case of a perforated peptic ulcer, pneumoperitoneum is usually visible on erect

CXR. Such perforations would also be apparent intraoperatively, with gastric or duodenal contents within the abdomen.

The diagnosis of pancreatitis would be most appropriate for this scenario as this would be in keeping with the severe generalized abdominal pain and normal intra-abdominal viscera visualized during laparotomy. In acute pancreatitis, acinar necrosis will result in the amylase rising to a level as high as 2000 units/dL. This begins to decrease within 3–4 days. The urinary amylase rises initially but remains steady for 4–7 days. In the presence of hyperlipidaemia, the serum amylase will often be masked. The urinary amylase is therefore highly useful in such patients. In the acute stages of pancreatitis, the inflammatory fluid or pus is often sterile due to sterile necrosis of the pancreas gland.

43. Answer: D

The saphenous nerve is the largest cutaneous branch of the femoral nerve. It is associated closely with the long saphenous vein and can be damaged easily during varicose vein surgery.

The sural nerve runs on the posterolateral aspect of the leg along with the short saphenous vein to supply sensation to the lateral aspect of the ankle, foot and 5th toe. It is easily damaged during stripping of the short saphenous vein.

The superficial peroneal nerve supplies sensation to the dorsum of the foot except for the 1st dorsal web space and innervates the peroneus longus and brevis muscles.

The deep peroneal nerve supplies sensation to the 1st dorsal web space and innervates tibialis anterior, extensor hallucis longus and extensor digitorum longus muscles.

The common peroneal nerve supplies the biceps femoris and gastrocnemius muscles. Damage to this nerve will result in failure to dorsiflex and evert the foot and hence, foot drop.

44. Answer: C

Sterile pyuria is defined as the presence of increased numbers of white cells ($>10/mm^3$) in urine that appears sterile using standard culture techniques. Its usual causes include:

- A treated urinary tract infection, within 2 weeks of treatment
- An inadequately treated urinary tract infection, or one with a fastidious culture requirement
- Renal stones
- Prostatitis
- Chlamydia urethritis
- Renal papillary necrosis (e.g. from analgesic excess)
- Tubulo-interstitial nephritis
- Genitourinary tuberculosis (always consider doing three early morning urine samples)
- Interstitial cystitis
- Urinary tract neoplasm
- Polycystic kidney.

In rarer instances, Crohn's disease of the terminal ileum may induce an inflammatory response to the right ureter and result in sterile pyuria.

45. Answer: C

Approximately 5–10% of abdominal injuries affect the kidneys. They usually present with back/loin pain with macroscopic haematuria; features of shock are rare. The diagnosis is usually made by CT scanning.

The American Society for Surgery trauma classification of renal injuries is as follows:

- Grade 1: contusion
- Grade 2: <1 cm laceration not affecting medulla/collecting system
- Grade 3: >1 cm laceration not affecting medulla or collecting system
- Grade 4: laceration involving medulla or collecting system
- Grade 5: shattered kidney or avulsed renal artery or vein

Reproduced from E. Moore et al., Organ injury scaling: spleen, liver and kidney. 29, 12, pp. 1664, with permission from Wolters Kluwer.

Treatment is usually conservative for grades 1–3. Grades 4 and 5 may require exploration/nephrectomy.

46. Answer: C

Eighty per cent of the salivary gland tumours occur in the parotid gland. Of the parotid gland tumours, 80% are benign, and of these, 80% are pleomorphic adenomas. They usually occur in the fifth decade and should be treated by superficial parotidectomy. Warthin's tumours or papillary cystadenomas are also benign tumours of the parotid which are more common in men in their 70s. Adenoid cystic carcinoma is the commonest malignant tumour of salivary glands and is more common in smaller glands than the parotid. It presents with facial pain and facial paresis. Salivary gland calculi occur most commonly in the submandibular glands due to its dependent position and higher concentration of mucous; they usually present with pain and swelling whilst eating. Finally, parotitis secondary to mumps is usually bilateral and affects young patients.

47. Answer: D

Pyelonephritis usually presents with severe loin pain, chills, rigors, pyrexia, painful micturition, and increased urinary frequency and urgency. There may be renal angle tenderness and tenderness over the iliac fossa on the affected side. Pyelonephritis may present with associated constitutional symptoms such as headache, lassitude and nausea. The risk factors for pyelonephritis include the use of urinary catheters, cystoscopy, surgeries on the urinary tract, renal stones and an enlarged prostate in males. Urine microscopy reveals pus cells and cast cells. Ultrasound is a very useful investigation towards diagnosis. Plain abdominal radiography may reveal a renal calculus, which may be the aetiology of pyelonephritis. In pyelonephritis caused by underlying anatomical disorders or a pathological obstruction, an intravenous pyelogram (IVP) or CT scan of the abdomen (i.e. CT of the kidneys, ureters and bladder) are valuable investigations, and may demonstrate enlarged kidneys with poor contrast flow through the kidneys. Some recognized complications of pyelonephritis include chronic pyelonephritis, renal scarring and renal failure, perinephric abscess and sepsis. Of the other options, it is important to note that uncomplicated retrocaecal appendicitis is unlikely to present such a severe clinical picture, although it may do so if ruptured.

48. Answer: E

Ulcerative colitis is a relapsing and remitting inflammatory disorder of the colonic mucosa. It may present solely with proctitis (about 50%) or extend proximally to involve part of the colon (left-sided colitis, about 30%) or the entire colon (pancolitis, in ~20%). It is histologically characterized by mucosal inflammation with general inflammatory cell infiltration, goblet-cell mucus depletion, glandular distortion, mucosal ulceration and crypt abscesses. In contrast, Crohn's disease is a chronic inflammatory gastrointestinal disease characterized by transmural granulomatous inflammation. It may affect any part of the gut but favours the terminal ileum (in 50%) and proximal colon. Unlike ulcerative colitis, there is unaffected bowel between areas of active disease (i.e. skip lesions). Histologically, Crohn's is characterized by neutrophil infiltrates and lymphoid aggregates, non-caseating granulomata and preservation of crypt architecture. Patchy inflammation may exist anywhere along the gastrointestinal tract in Crohn's disease.

49. Answer: C

Human leucocyte antigen (HLA), the human form of major histocompatibility complex (MHC), is a large group of genes located along chromosome 6 that code for the proteins expressed on cell surfaces that present antigens. Class I HLA expresses intracellular antigens and is expressed on all nucleated cells, whilst Class II HLA is expressed only by antigen presenting cells (which express phagocytosed material to CD8+ cells). The subtypes of Class I HLA are A, B, and C and those of Class II are DR, DP, DQ. The significance of these subtypes is that specific forms are associated with an increased likelihood of developing certain diseases/conditions. For example, the presence of HLA-B27 is associated with conditions such as ankylosing spondylitis, enteropathic spondyloarthropathies (associated with inflammatory bowel disease), psoriatic arthritis, and reactive arthritis—grouped as 'sero-negative spondyloarthropathies. Acute transplant rejection occurs within hours and days, and is predominantly an immune response against foreign HLA protein. Hyperacute transplant rejection, which begins within minutes of transplant, is complement-mediated immunity driven by pre-existing antibodies, such as in ABO-mismatch.

50. Answer: E

Partial opioid agonists, when used in association with morphine, may produce a reduction in the overall analgesic effect due to partial antagonism. A commonly used partial agonist is buprenorphine, which works as an agonist at the µ opioid receptor, and an antagonist at the κ receptor. It has very high affinity and low intrinsic activity at the mu receptor and will displace morphine, methadone and other full opioid agonists from this receptor. Its partial agonist effects give buprenorphine several clinically desirable pharmacological properties: lower abuse potential, lower level of physical dependence (and less withdrawal discomfort), a ceiling effect at higher doses, and greater safety in overdose compared with full opioid agonists.

Basic sciences: Applied anatomy

1. Which of the following structures is unlikely to be damaged during a carotid endarterectomy procedure?

A. Hypoglossal nerve

B. Buccal branch of the facial nerve

C. External laryngeal nerve

D. Ansa cervicalis

E. Pharyngeal branch of the vagus nerve

Basic sciences: Physiology

2. Which among the following statements concerning myofibroblasts is incorrect?

A. They are characterized by the presence of stress fibres that contain α-smooth muscle actin and indented nuclei

B. They have structural properties between those of fibroblasts and smooth muscle cells

C. They are present in the healing wound for up to 48 hours from the time of injury

D. They help to contract the granulation tissue and deposit new extracellular matrix

E. They are responsible for wound contracture and scarring

Basic sciences: Pathology

3. Which of the following tumour markers is not paired with the appropriate malignancy?

A. CA19–9: pancreatic cancer

B. ACTH: small-cell lung cancer

C. Calcitonin: papillary thyroid carcinoma

D. CA 15–3: breast cancer (occasionally)

E. Alpha-fetoprotein: hepatocellular cancer.

Common surgical conditions and the subspecialties:
Trauma and orthopaedics

4. An 18-year-old rugby player is brought to the Emergency Department
    with a painful right shoulder after falling awkwardly during a tackle. On
    examination, there is fullness in the deltopectoral groove and lowering
    of the anterior axillary fold. The acromion appears to be more
    prominent than on the contralateral side. The affected arm is slightly
    abducted and externally rotated. What is the most likely diagnosis?

    A. Acromioclavicular joint subluxation
    B. Fracture of the greater tuberosity of the humerus
    C. Anterior dislocation of the shoulder
    D. Fracture of the acromion process
    E. Posterior dislocation of the shoulder

Common surgical conditions and the subspecialties:
Trauma and orthopaedics

5. Which among the following statements regarding the Salter–Harris
    classification of bone injuries in children is correct?

    A. It is a classification for fractures involving the metaphysis and the diaphysis
    B. Growth arrest is common in Salter–Harris type II injury
    C. In Salter–Harris type III injuries, growth disturbance is very unlikely
    D. Salter–Harris type V is described as a comminuted fracture of the metaphysis
    E. Salter-Harris fractures account for <5% of all fractures in children

Perioperative care: Coagulation, deep vein thrombosis, and embolism

6. A 30-year-old woman with a previous history of deep vein
    thrombosis and end-stage renal failure undergoes a cadaveric kidney
    transplantation. Postoperatively she develops severe generalized
    abdominal and pelvic pain. Ultrasound imaging reveals an occluded
    transplant renal vein, necessitating a transplant nephrectomy. The
    patient then undergoes extensive investigations and is diagnosed with
    protein C deficiency. Which of the following options best describes the
    pathophysiological process responsible for her symptoms?

    A. Failed inactivation of Factors VIIIa and Va
    B. Failed synthesis of antithrombin
    C. Reduced activity of tissue factor pathway inhibitor
    D. Failed inactivation of factor IXa
    E. Reduced protein S synthesis

Assessment and management of patients with trauma (including the multiply injured patient): Fractures

7. **A 12-year-old boy falls from the carousel of his playschool, injuring his left forearm. Examination reveals tenderness over his distal radius. Two-view radiography demonstrates a displaced fracture through the distal epiphysis also involving a fragment of metaphyseal bone. Which of the following categories of fracture does this injury best describe?**
   A. Salter–Harris type I
   B. Salter–Harris type II
   C. Salter–Harris type III
   D. Salter–Harris type IV
   E. Salter–Harris type V

Basic sciences: Applied anatomy

8. **A 55-year-old hypertensive man with a 60-pack-year smoking history is referred by his GP to the vascular surgeon for the incidental finding of an expansile, pulsatile mass in his left popliteal fossa. Further imaging confirms the presence of a popliteal artery aneurysm. Whilst in clinic, the surgeon asks his surgical trainee to describe the anatomy of the popliteal fossa. Which of the following structures is most likely to lie immediately superficial to the popliteal artery aneurysm?**
   A. Common peroneal nerve
   B. Small saphenous vein
   C. Popliteal fascia
   D. Popliteal vein
   E. Sural nerve

Basic sciences: Physiology

9. **Which of the following is not true about the control of respiration?**
   A. The medullary respiratory centre controls the rhythm of breathing
   B. The pneumotaxic centre controls the duration of inspiration
   C. The apneustic centre is located in the lower pons
   D. Chemoreceptors respond to a rise in pH
   E. Peripheral chemoreceptors are located in the carotid bodies

Basic sciences: Pathology

10. **A 40-year-old man presents to the neck lump clinic with a prominent solitary thyroid nodule. The fine-needle aspirate cytology performed shows features similar to benign adenomatous hyperplasia. He subsequently undergoes a thyroid lobectomy and the histology of the surgical specimen confirms a diagnosis of follicular carcinoma. Which of the following is a characteristic of follicular carcinoma?**

A. It arises from the parafollicular cells of the thyroid gland

B. Fine-needle aspiration cytology can sufficiently differentiate it from benign adenomatous hyperplasia

C. The majority of such cases are multifocal

D. Metastasis tends to occur via the bloodstream to the bone and other remote sites

E. Its peak incidence is between the ages of 30–45 years

Common surgical conditions and the subspecialties:
Trauma and orthopaedics

11. **A 28-year-old professional footballer is injured during a training session, sustaining a closed fracture of his left tibia with no fibular involvement. The nurses in the Emergency Department apply an above-knee backslab, with which the patient remains comfortable. What is the next most appropriate step in managing this patient?**

A. Admit for observation on the ward

B. Advise to weight bear as tolerated, and discharge with fracture clinic follow-up

C. Advise not to weight bear, and discharge with fracture clinic follow-up

D. Arrange for operative intervention at the next available opportunity

E. Request a CT scan of the injured region from the Emergency Department

Common surgical conditions and the subspecialties: General presenting symptoms or syndromes

12. **A 24-year-old medical student presents to the Emergency Department after vomiting 100 mL of fresh blood following a 6-hour stretch of binge drinking. He is otherwise fit and healthy, and denies regular alcohol abuse. Examination reveals a heart rate of 85/min and a blood pressure of 125/85 mmHg. What is the most likely diagnosis?**

A. Acute gastritis

B. Aorto-oesophageal fistula

C. Mallory–Weiss tear

D. Peptic ulcer disease

E. Ruptured oesophageal varices

Perioperative care: Assessing and planning nutritional management

13. A 65-year-old male with Crohn's disease presents with a high output enterocutaneous fistula. He is started on total parenteral nutrition (TPN) to decrease the fistula output and improve his general nutritional status. Which of the following statements are false regarding TPN?

A. It may cause fatty liver when used over a long period

B. It increases the risk of acalculous cholecystitis

C. It may result in metabolic complications such a refeeding syndrome, resulting in hyperkalaemia, hypermagnesaemia, and hyperphosphataemia

D. Sepsis due to fungal infections is especially common in patients receiving TPN

E. Volume overload, hyperglycaemia, and hyperchloraemic acidosis are early complications of TPN

The assessment and management of the surgical patient: Planning investigations

14. A 35-year-old female with a BMI of 36 experiences persistent gastro-oesophageal reflux symptoms despite lifestyle and dietary modification, and maximum antisecretory therapy. Which of the following tests should first be performed before considering antireflux surgery in this patient?

A. Cardiac sphincter manometry

B. Gastric emptying study

C. Oesophageal motility study

D. Oesophageal pH monitoring off therapy

E. Oesophageal pH monitoring on therapy

Basic sciences: Applied anatomy

15. An orthopaedic surgeon performs an arthroscopic subacromial decompression on a 45-year-old woman suffering from supraspinatus tendinopathy. Which of the following statements regarding the anatomy of the shoulder joint is most accurate?

A. The shoulder joint most commonly dislocates in a posterior fashion

B. Weakness of teres major will result from trauma to the nerve related to the surgical neck of the humerus

C. The shoulder joint capsule receives most support from its inferior aspect

D. The subacromial bursa usually communicates with the shoulder joint cavity

E. The origin of triceps lies within the shoulder joint capsule

Basic sciences: Physiology

16. Which of the following statements concerning foetal and adult red blood cells is incorrect?

A. Each foetal haemoglobin molecule comprises two alpha chains and two gamma chains

B. Gamma haemoglobin chains have a greater affinity for 2,3 DPG than beta haemoglobin chains

C. The Bohr shift is a significant factor in ensuring sufficient oxygen delivery to foetal tissues

D. The life span of red blood cells in a term infant is nearly half that of the maternal red blood cells

E. By the end of a healthy term pregnancy, foetal haematocrit would be expected to be approximately 50% higher than the maternal haematocrit

Common surgical conditions and the subspecialties: Skin, head, and neck

17. A 60-year-old man undergoes a neck dissection involving excision of level II–IV lymph nodes with preservation of the jugular vein, accessory nerve, and sternomastoid. What is the name of this operation?

A. Modified radical neck dissection type 1

B. Supraomohyoid selective neck dissection

C. Posterolateral selective neck dissection

D. Lateral selective neck dissection

E. Modified radical neck dissection type 2

Perioperative care: Haemostasis and blood products

18. An adolescent boy with mild von Willebrand's disease is due to see his dentist for a tooth extraction. A similar extraction 2 years ago resulted in bleeding that had required a two-unit blood transfusion. What is the best form of bleeding prophylaxis for this boy prior to surgery?

A. Cryoprecipitate

B. Desmopressin

C. Fresh frozen plasma

D. Factor VIII concentrate

E. Platelet transfusion

The assessment and management of the surgical patient:
Planning investigations

19. **A 65-year-old retired army officer presents to the Emergency Department describing a 3-day history of progressively worsening colicky hypogastric pain, abdominal distension and absolute constipation. Examination reveals a soft but grossly distended abdomen, with no evidence of shifting dullness but with high-pitched bowel sounds. Plain abdominal radiography reveals a single distended (5-cm) loop of peripherally placed bowel. At this point, the patient's blood results return as normal and the patient is placed nil by mouth. What is the next most appropriate step in the management of this patient?**

   A. Computed tomography scan with contrast enema (barium)
   B. Computed tomography scan with contrast enema (gastrografin)
   C. Contrast small bowel follow-through
   D. Laparotomy
   E. Magnetic resonance imaging

Basic sciences: Applied anatomy

20. **Which of the following is not true about the jejunum?**

   A. It is bright pink in appearance and is thin walled
   B. It only has a sparse amount of lymphoid tissue
   C. The mesentery of the jejunum has fat deposited near the root and is scanty at the intestinal end
   D. The jejunal mesenteric vessels form only single or double arcades with long vasa recta
   E. The jejunal mesentery is attached to the posterior abdominal wall to the left of the aorta

Basic sciences: Physiology

21. **Which of the following hormones is not produced by the anterior pituitary gland?**

   A. Adrenocorticotrophic hormone
   B. Antidiuretic hormone
   C. Growth hormone
   D. Thyroid stimulating hormone
   E. Prolactin

Common surgical conditions and the subspecialties:
Neurology and Neurosurgery

22. **A 45-year-old woman presents with a 2-week history of left arm weakness. The problem began with severe pain in the neck radiating into the left shoulder, followed by weakness in that arm. Examination reveals winging of the left scapula with weakness of left shoulder abduction and elbow extension. Sensory loss was noted over the lateral aspect of the left shoulder, with an absent left triceps reflex. Which of the following options represents the most accurate diagnosis in this patient?**

    A. C7 entrapment radiculopathy
    B. Central C5/6 disc prolapse
    C. Neuralgic amyotrophy
    D. Suprascapular nerve entrapment
    E. Traction of the lateral cord of the brachial plexus

Perioperative care: Assessing and planning nutritional management

23. **A 7-year-old girl presents to the Emergency Department with a 12-hour history of profuse diarrhoea and vomiting. The provisional diagnosis is of viral gastroenteritis and the patient is admitted for intravenous fluid resuscitation. Once her diarrhoea and vomiting resolves, the doctors encourage oral fluid intake but she refuses this, so intravenous crystalloids are prescribed. Assuming a body weight of 25 kg, which of the following is the most appropriate rate of infusion of maintenance fluids for this patient?**

    A. 49 mL/hour
    B. 58 mL/hour
    C. 67 mL/hour
    D. 790 mL/day
    E. 1800 mL/day

The assessment and management of the surgical patient:
Differential diagnosis

24. **A 37-year-old cyclist is brought to the Emergency Department after he was hit from behind by a car travelling at about 50 mph. On examination, he has severe bruising over his left anterolateral chest wall. A puncture wound is noticed at the level of the left 6th intercostal space and decreased air entry is noted over the base of the left lung. A CXR reveals fractures of the lower four ribs on the left side and a raised left hemidiaphragm. What is the most likely diagnosis?**

    A. Cardiac tamponade
    B. Traumatic haemothorax
    C. Left basal pneumonia
    D. Tension pneumothorax
    E. Rupture of the diaphragm

Basic sciences: Applied anatomy

25. A 30-year-old-man sustains a fall and presents with bleeding from his right nostril. On examination, he looks well and is haemodynamically stable. Anterior rhinoscopy reveals bleeding from the anterior part of the nasal septum corresponding to Little's area. Which of the following arteries is not responsible for the epistaxis?

A. Sphenopalatine artery
B. Greater palatine artery
C. Anterior ethmoidal artery
D. Superior septal perforator artery
E. Superior labial artery

Basic sciences: Physiology

26. A 73-year-old male is brought into hospital obtunded and tachypnoeic. Apart from complaining of a headache, he is unable to give a coherent history. On examination, he is found to be tachycardic, with a blood pressure of 100/80 mmHg. An arterial blood gas (ABG) sample reveals metabolic acidosis with a high anion gap. Which of the following is not a cause of metabolic acidosis with a high anion gap?

A. Salicylate overdose
B. Starvation
C. Diabetic ketoacidosis
D. Uraemic acidosis
E. Renal tubular acidosis

Common surgical conditions and the subspecialties: Gastrointestinal disease

27. A 54-year-old lady presents to the Surgical Emergency Assessment Unit with a 12-hour history of central colicky abdominal pain and vomiting. She underwent a subtotal colectomy and formation of an end ileostomy for ulcerative colitis 8 years previously. Her ileostomy has not functioned for nearly 72 hours. Examination reveals mild abdominal distension and diffuse central abdominal tenderness. Plain abdominal radiography reveals multiple distended loops in the centre of the abdomen. What is the most likely diagnosis?

A. Sigmoid volvulus
B. Small bowel obstruction secondary to adhesions
C. Acute colonic pseudo-obstruction
D. Incarcerated femoral hernia
E. Bacterial peritonitis

Basic sciences: Applied anatomy

28. **A 12-year-old boy presents with a 3-day history of migratory abdominal pain and vomiting. He is found to have localized peritonism in his right iliac fossa warranting an appendicectomy. During the operation the appendix is felt to be retrocaecal and very adherent to the surrounding structures. The surgeon extends the wound laterally to get better access. Which structure needs to be identified and preserved when making this transverse incision?**

   A. Iliohypogastric nerve

   B. Ilioinginal nerve

   C. Intercostobrachial nerve

   D. Inferior epigastric artery

   E. Superficial epigastric artery

Basic sciences: Physiology

29. **Which of the following statements regarding the renin–angiotensin system is not true?**

   A. Angiotensin-converting enzyme (ACE) is found mainly in pulmonary and vascular endothelium

   B. Aldosterone causes salt and water retention and increases potassium excretion

   C. Low perfusion pressure is the sole stimulus for renin release from the juxtaglomerular cells

   D. Angiotensin II is a powerful vasoconstrictor

   E. Renin catalyses the cleavage of angiotensin I from angiotensinogen

Common surgical conditions and the subspecialties: Endocrine disease

30. **A 29-year-old woman is referred by her GP with a 3-month history of a painless lump in the anterior aspect of the neck. She does not describe any hoarseness of voice. Examination reveals a lump in the left anterior triangle, which moves up and down with swallowing. FNA cytology of the lump reveals nuclear grooves and intranuclear inclusions. What is the most likely diagnosis?**

   A. Follicular adenoma

   B. Follicular carcinoma

   C. Papillary carcinoma

   D. Medullary carcinoma

   E. Anaplastic carcinoma

Basic sciences: Applied anatomy

31. Which of the following is not a remnant of the Wolffian duct?

    A. Hydatid cyst of Morgagni
    B. Appendix epididymis
    C. Tunica vaginalis
    D. Organ of Giraldes
    E. Ductulus aberrans

Common surgical conditions and the subspecialties: Endocrine disease

32. A 40-year-old lady with intermittent headaches, palpitations and excessive sweating has recently been diagnosed with a phaeochromocytoma. Which one of the following is the ideal initial management of her condition?

    A. Alpha blockade initially, followed by beta blockade (i.e. once alpha blockade is sufficiently established)
    B. Alpha and beta blockade simultaneously
    C. Beta blockade initially, followed by alpha blockade (i.e. once beta blockade is sufficiently established)
    D. Alpha blockade alone
    E. Beta blockade alone

Basic sciences: Applied anatomy

33. A 14-year-old boy falls from a tree onto his right shoulder, in such a manner that his shoulder is depressed, and his head and neck are forcefully flexed to the other side of the body. Examination in the Emergency Department reveals paralysis of his right upper limb as it hangs limply by his side. It is found to be abducted and medially rotated with an extension of the elbow and pronation of the forearm so that the palmar surface of the hand is facing posteriorly. What is/are the most likely nerve root/s to have been injured?

    A. C5 only
    B. C5 and C6
    C. C6 and C7
    D. C7 and C8
    E. C8 and T1

Common surgical conditions and the subspecialties: Breast disease

34. **A 45-year-old woman presents to the breast clinic with four episodes of spontaneous blood-stained nipple discharge. Examination reveals no skin or nipple changes, masses or lymphadenopathy. On expression, a serosanguinous secretion is discharged from the opening of a duct. What is the most likely diagnosis?**

    A. Breast abscess
    B. Duct ectasia
    C. Duct papilloma
    D. Galactorrhoea
    E. Prolactinoma

Basic sciences: Applied anatomy

35. **A 31-year-old motorcyclist is brought to the Emergency Department following a high-speed road traffic accident. On examination, he is noticed to have bruising on his right arm. He is unable to actively extend his wrist or the fingers of this hand. Plain radiography of the arm reveals a mid-shaft fracture of the humerus. Which of the following nerves is most likely to be damaged following a mid-humeral fracture?**

    A. Anterior interosseous nerve
    B. Axillary nerve
    C. Radial nerve
    D. Median nerve
    E. Musculocutaneous nerve

Common surgical conditions and the subspecialties: General presenting symptoms or syndromes

36. **Which of the following is not a recognized feature of Pancoast's syndrome?**

    A. Pain in the shoulder region radiating toward the axilla and scapula
    B. Facial nerve palsy
    C. Wasting of the intrinsic muscles of the hand
    D. Compression of major vessels in the thoracic inlet
    E. Horner's syndrome

Basic sciences: Applied anatomy

37. Which of the following nerves does not pass through the superior orbital fissure?

A. Ophthalmic branch of the trigeminal nerve

B. Trochlear nerve

C. Optic nerve

D. Abducens nerve

E. Oculomotor nerve

Common surgical conditions and the subspecialties: General presenting symptoms or syndromes

38. A 5-month-old boy is brought into the Paediatric Emergency Assessment Unit with abdominal pain. His mother describes 'abdominal colic' that occurs every few minutes, causing the child to 'curl up in a ball'. The pain is associated with two episodes of bilious vomiting. He is prone to constipation and has not opened his bowels for 2 days. On examination he is apyrexial, pale and lethargic. The abdomen is distended and a tender sausage-shaped lump is palpable in the right flank. Blood tests showed a WCC of 12 × 10⁹ and a urea of 9 mmol/L. An urgent ultrasound scan revealed a 'target sign'. What is the most likely diagnosis?

A. Appendix abscess

B. Intussusception

C. Pyloric stenosis

D. Strangulated inguinal hernia

E. Meckel's diverticulum

Basic sciences: Applied anatomy

39. A 22-year-old brick layer presents to his GP with altered sensation over the medial aspect of his right hand and reduced hand function. He had sustained a fracture of the medial epicondyle of the right humerus about 10 weeks ago. On examination, there is wasting of the hypothenar eminence with loss of abduction and adduction of the fingers. Which nerve do you think is most likely to have been injured in this patient?

A. Axillary nerve

B. Radial nerve

C. Ulnar nerve

D. Median nerve

E. Musculocutaneous nerve

Common surgical conditions and the subspecialties:
Gastrointestinal disease

40. **A 37-year-old male presents with a 2-day history of central abdominal pain which gradually localizes to his right groin. He also complains of a lump in his right groin. Clinical examination is highly suggestive of an incarcerated inguinal hernia. The patient undergoes emergency surgery; intraoperatively, the appendix is found to lie within a mass of incarcerated, inflamed and oedematous tissue within the inguinal canal. As the appendix does not appear to be inflamed, an appendicectomy is performed through the same scar. Part of the indirect sac is excised, and a mesh repair is undertaken. Which type of hernia does this describe?**
    A. Amyand's hernia
    B. Littre's hernia
    C. Maydl's hernia
    D. Pantaloon hernia
    E. Richter's hernia

Basic surgical skills: Wounds, scars, and contractures

41. **Which of the following is a common characteristic of both keloid and hypertrophic scars?**
    A. They occur most commonly in young patients
    B. They occur late in the wound healing process
    C. They extend beyond the boundaries of the original wound
    D. Wound tension increases the risk of keloid formation
    E. There is often a familial tendency to both of these pathologies

Common surgical conditions and the subspecialties: Cardiovascular and pulmonary disease

42. **Which of the following is not a feature of acute respiratory distress syndrome?**
    A. Bilateral pulmonary infiltrates
    B. Radiological evidence of bilateral pleural effusions, upper lobe diversion of pulmonary vessels and an enlarged heart
    C. Refractory hypoxaemia (PaO$_2$ <8 kPa)
    D. Pulmonary arterial wedge pressure <19 mmHg
    E. PaO$_2$/FiO$_2$ <200 mmHg

Basic sciences: Applied anatomy

43. **A 45-year-old-male undergoes an elective inguinal hernia repair. Intraoperatively, the junior surgical trainee is asked to identify if the hernia is a direct or an indirect hernia. Which anatomical landmark is most likely to help her answer this question?**
    A. Mid-inguinal point
    B. Midpoint of the inguinal ligament
    C. Pubic tubercle
    D. Spermatic cord
    E. Inferior epigastric artery

Common surgical conditions and the subspecialties: Neurology and neurosurgery

44. **A 42-year-old male presents to the Emergency Department with an acute onset of severe occipital headache, described as 'a kick in the back of the head'. He is disoriented and drowsy whilst his history is obtained. A focused examination reveals neck stiffness and fundoscopy reveals subhyaloid haemorrhages. Of the most likely diagnosis that this patient has, what grade of pathology does he demonstrate, according to the Hunter and Hess scale?**
    A. Grade 1
    B. Grade 2
    C. Grade 3
    D. Grade 4
    E. Grade 5

Assessment and management of patients with trauma (including the multiply injured patient): Fractures

45. **A 40-year-old biker is brought to the Emergency Department after being involved in a low-speed road traffic accident. Primary and secondary surveys reveal injuries only to his left leg. Closer examination of his left leg reveals a 5 cm laceration over the medial aspect of the leg with an associated comminuted fracture of the tibia. The wound is moderately contaminated but without any obvious soft tissue loss. Neurovascular status of the leg is intact. How might this injury be classified on the basis of the Gustilo–Anderson classification of open fractures?**
    A. Type I
    B. Type II
    C. Type III A
    D. Type III B
    E. Type III C

Common surgical conditions and the subspecialties: Cardiovascular and pulmonary disease

46. A 1-year-old baby boy is brought into hospital looking cyanotic, short of breath, and failing to thrive. He is admitted and investigated for congenital cyanotic heart disease. Which of the following congenital heart conditions does not typically cause cyanosis?

    A. Atrial septal defect
    B. Right ventricular outflow tract obstruction
    C. Tetralogy of Fallot
    D. Transposition of the great arteries
    E. Total anomalous pulmonary venous drainage

Common surgical conditions and the subspecialties: Gastrointestinal disease

47. A 74-year-old gentleman is referred urgently by his GP to the gastroenterologists for a 2-month history of intermittent rectal bleeding and change in bowel habit. He admits to a recent loss of appetite and weight loss of over 10 kg over the preceding three months. Examination reveals mild jaundice of the sclerae, an enlarged liver (to 6 cm below the costal margin) and shifting dullness within the abdomen. Subsequent imaging of the abdomen confirms ascites, multiple non-specific hepatic deposits, and evidence of tumour-cell implantation on the omental surface. What is the most likely diagnosis?

    A. Desmoplastic small round cell tumour
    B. Malignant peritoneal mesothelioma
    C. Gastrointestinal stromal tumour
    D. Peritoneal carcinomatosis
    E. Budd–Chiari syndrome

Common surgical conditions and the subspecialties: Peripheral vascular disease

48. A 62-year-old retired gentleman with poorly controlled diabetes mellitus presents to the diabetic clinic for annual review. He is found to have a new, early-stage ulcer under the left first metatarsal head. The nurse also notes a slight bony deformity of his left ankle. Of the following options, which is true regarding diabetic foot ulceration?

A. An important predictor of ulceration is the formation of callous at pressure points

B. Lower limb perfusion is poor due to atherosclerosis but improved by autonomic neuropathy

C. Osteomyelitis and Charcot arthropathy are commonly differentiated by plain radiographs of the foot and ankle

D. The main predisposing factor to ulceration is skin infection in the immunocompromised diabetic patient

E. Ulceration of pressure areas on the plantar surface is usually due to atherosclerosis

Organ and tissue transplantation: Transplant immunology

49. A 60-year-old man has end-stage renal failure secondary to type 2 diabetes mellitus. He has had two previous failed kidney transplants and has recently had two blood transfusions for anaemia. He is currently on haemodialysis three times a week. During the operation, just as the ureter is being anastomosed to the bladder, the transplant kidney changes colour from pink to black. Which of the following is not true about the cause of the this condition?

A. It is mediated by T cells

B. It is not as significant in liver grafts

C. It warrants removal of transplanted kidney

D. It is now a rare occurrence

E. Cytotoxic crossmatch has helped to reduce its incidence

Basic sciences: Microbiology

50. A 50-year-old man sustains a dog bite to his right hand, presenting to the Emergency Department 72 hours later with right hand swelling. Examination reveals a puncture wound over the dorsum of the hand, cellulitis, ascending lymphangitis and tender axillary lymphadenopathy. Which antibiotic therapy is most appropriate this case, assuming that the patient has no known drug allergies?

A. Benzylpenicillin and flucloxacillin

B. Ceftriaxone

C. Ciprofloxacin

D. Co-amoxiclav

E. Erythromycin

1. Answer: B

Many vital structures can be damaged during a carotid endarterectomy procedure. The hypoglossal nerve crosses the external carotid artery just above its bifurcation. Damage to this nerve results in loss of normal motor function of the tongue (on protrusion, the tongue is pulled towards the affected side). The buccal branch of the facial nerve does not run close to the field of surgery and, as such, is unlikely to be damaged during a carotid endarterectomy procedure. However, the marginal mandibular branch of the facial nerve can be damaged due to retraction of the nerve during the procedure. The external laryngeal nerve runs close to the superior thyroid artery and supplies the cricothyroid muscle. Damage to this nerve causes loss of phonation over prolonged periods of time. The ansa cervicalis lies within the carotid sheath and supplies the infrahyoid strap muscles. The pharyngeal branch of the vagus nerve is also at risk of injury at a higher level and paralysis of this nerve causes difficulty in swallowing.

2. Answer: C

One of the best characterized subtypes of fibroblasts is the myofibroblast, which plays an important role in scar formation. Myofibroblasts are characterized by the presence of stress fibres that contain α-smooth muscle actin and indented nuclei, thus having structural properties between those of a fibroblast and a smooth muscle cell. Although their precise origin is unclear, the consensus is that fibroblasts (i.e. once migrated into the wound) differentiate into myofibroblasts under the influence of growth factors such as transforming growth factor-beta1 and mechanical stress. In addition to fibroblasts, some smooth muscle cells and pericytes are also thought to be capable of differentiating into myofibroblasts. Myofibroblasts appear in the wound approximately 3 days after wounding and increase in number to a maximal level between days 10–21. Their main function is to contract the granulation tissue and deposit new extracellular matrix. Although they promote wound closure, myofibroblasts are also responsible for subsequent wound contracture and scarring; therefore, a delicate balance of fibroblasts and myofibroblasts is essential for optimum wound healing.

3. Answer: C

Tumour markers are specific products released by some tumours that can be measured by sensitive assays. Some tumour markers can be elevated in benign conditions as well, and therefore cannot be used to diagnose cancer. Changes in concentration are generally used to assess response to treatment or to detect recurrence or progression of the tumour. Thyroglobulin is associated with thyroid cancer and calcitonin is the tumour marker for medullary thyroid cancer. Alpha-fetoprotein is elevated in hepatocellular carcinoma and germ cell tumours. CA-125 is associated with non-mucinous ovarian carcinomas, while CA 15-3 is associated with breast cancer. Carcinoembryonic antigen is mostly elevated in colorectal cancer but may also occasionally be elevated in pancreatic, breast, ovarian, or lung cancer.

4. Answer: C

Anterior (subcoracoid) dislocation is the commonest type of shoulder dislocation (this is in contrast to the hip, where posterior dislocation is most common). The usual mechanism of injury is a fall onto the outstretched arm when the arm is abducted and externally rotated. It can also result from various sporting injuries, commonly, basketball and rugby. The pain is usually severe, and the patient is unwilling to attempt movements of the shoulder. A swelling may be noticed in the delto-pectoral groove (i.e. the displaced humeral head) with an undue prominence of the acromion process. The arm is held in slight abduction and external rotation. There may be flattening and loss of contour of the shoulder just below the acromion process, and lowering of the anterior axillary fold. If the axillary nerve is damaged, patients may present with loss of sensation over the upper, outer aspect of the arm (i.e. the 'regimental badge' area). Posterior dislocation of the shoulder, although uncommon, may occur as a result of a direct blow to the shoulder joint causing the humeral head to be displaced from the glenoid cavity. It may also result from violent muscular contractions induced by an electric shock or an epileptic convulsion. The arm is usually held (or fixed) in internal rotation (compared to external rotation in anterior dislocation), which cannot be rotated outwards even as far as the neutral position. The normal shoulder contour is lost and the anterior aspect of the shoulder appears flat (in contrast to the fullness observed in anterior dislocation).

5. Answer: E

The Salter–Harris classification applies to fractures through the growth plate or the epiphysis (in Salter–Harris types II and IV, the metaphyseal fragment is also involved but the diaphysis is never affected). Salter–Harris types I and II do not involve the germinal layer and therefore growth disturbance is uncommon following these fractures. In Salter–Harris types III and IV, the germinal layer is breached so growth disturbance is likely, although its incidence can be minimized by adequate fracture reduction. Although not originally described, Salter–Harris type V fractures are recognized as a crush injury of the epiphysis, following which, growth arrest is common. This fracture is often diagnosed retrospectively, when disturbance of physeal growth becomes apparent as a limb deformity. Because of the weakness of the growth plate, these injuries are relatively common. Salter–Harris injuries account for less than 5% of all fractures in children. Within the Salter-Harris classification system, types I, II, III, and IV fractures have an incidence of 5%, 75%, 10%, and 10% respectively; while type V fractures are rare.

6. Answer: A

Protein C and protein S are activated by thrombin bound to thrombomodulin on endothelial cells. Together they inactivate factors VIIIa and Va by proteolysis. Protein C is vitamin K-dependant, similar to coagulation factors II, VII, IX, and X.

Coagulation factors are inactivated by various serum protease inhibitors, including antithrombin, tissue factor pathway inhibitor, and heparin.

7. Answer: B

The Salter–Harris classification system is used to describe the pattern of fractures involving the epiphyses, and to predict their prognosis. It was first described by Salter and Harris in 1963. Fractures of the epiphysis and growth plate are more common in boys, and are usually seen either in infancy or between the ages of 10–12 years.

- Type I: A slipped epiphysis, usually occurring in infants but also seen at puberty as a slipped femoral epiphysis; it seldom results in any serious complications.
- Type II: Occurs along the epiphyseal plate but branches into the shaft. The detached fragment of bone consists of the epiphysis plus a triangular fragment of the shaft. This is the most common type of epiphyseal injury, usually occurring in older children and seldom resulting in abnormal growth.

- Type III: Occurs along part of the epiphyseal plate and then cuts into the epiphysis. This results in detachment of part of the epiphysis from the shaft, with the fracture extending into the joint. In order to prevent abnormal growth, accurate reduction is required to restore the joint surface.
- Type IV: Occurs through the shaft, the epiphyseal plate, the epiphysis, and into the joint. The detached pieces of bone comprise fragments of the shaft, epiphyseal plate and epiphysis. There is disruption of the growth plate and of the articular surface.
- Type V: Compression damage to a portion of the growth plate. The crushed epiphysis stops growing; this is not easily detected in the acute setting, often resulting in severe deformity in the long term. This carries the worst prognosis of the epiphyseal injuries, usually involving partial or complete cessation of growth.

8. Answer: D

The structures of the popliteal fossa (from superficial to deep) include the common peroneal nerve, popliteal vein, popliteal artery (i.e. as a continuation of the femoral artery), tibial nerve, and the popliteal lymph nodes. Such anatomy is especially useful when performing local anaesthetic blockade of the common peroneal nerve, as the vein and artery are relatively protected from the needle.

The boundaries of the popliteal fossa are:

- Superolaterally: biceps femoris tendon
- Superomedially: semitendinosus and semimembranosus tendons
- Inferolaterally: plantaris muscle and lateral head of gastrocnemius
- Inferomedially: medial head of gastrocnemius.

The roof of the popliteal fossa (from superficial to deep) is comprised of skin; the superficial fascia (which contains the small saphenous vein, the terminal branch of the posterior cutaneous nerve of the thigh, the posterior division of the medial cutaneous nerve, the lateral sural cutaneous nerve and the medial sural cutaneous nerve); and the deep (popliteal) fascia.

The floor of the popliteal fossa is formed by the popliteal surface of the femur, the knee joint capsule with the oblique popliteal ligament, and the strong popliteus muscle fascia.

9. Answer: D

The medullary respiratory centre has inspiratory and expiratory centres, which control the rhythm of breathing. The pneumotaxic centre is located in the upper pons and controls the duration of inspiration. The apneustic centre is present in the lower pons and prolongs the inspiratory phase.

Central chemoreceptors are located on the ventral surface of the medulla surrounded by cerebral extracellular fluid. Carbon dioxide readily crosses the blood–brain barrier and as $PaCO_2$ rises, so does the pCO_2 of CSF, thus liberating hydrogen ions. This drop in pH stimulates the central chemoreceptors and causes an increase in ventilation.

Peripheral chemoreceptors are located in the carotid body at the carotid bifurcation. They respond to decreased PaO_2, decreased pH and increased $PaCO_2$.

10. Answer: D

Follicular carcinoma of the thyroid is a well-differentiated cancer arising from thyroid follicular cells, and most commonly occurs between the ages of 40–50 years. Like papillary carcinoma, it is three times more common in women than men. On FNA cytology it is impossible to distinguish it from benign adenomatous hyperplasia. A firm diagnosis can only be made on the histology of a surgical specimen. Follicular carcinomas grow slowly and unlike papillary carcinoma, which metastasizes via the lymphatics, it spreads via the bloodstream to the lung, bones and remote sites. In contrast to papillary carcinoma, it is rarely multifocal and the management depends on the extent of capsular invasion, which is also a strong prognostic indicator. Medullary carcinomas of the thyroid arise from the parafollicular C cells and secrete abnormal amounts of calcitonin, but do not share this feature with follicular carcinoma.

11. Answer: A

The patient's closed fracture, together with his history of recent cardiovascular exertion, should alert the clinician to the possibility of compartment syndrome (i.e. increased pressure within the osteofascial compartment with resultant microcirculatory compromise.) Apart from fractures, compartment syndrome may also result from infection, prolonged immobilization in a tight plaster cast, or from muscle hypertrophy in athletes; arterial damage is not necessary for this to occur. If untreated (e.g. by urgent fasciotomy), a vicious circle arises in which tissue swelling results in reduced tissue perfusion and, in turn, tissue ischaemia. This results in further swelling, a further increase in pressure, and a further reduction in microcirculatory perfusion. Necrosis develops within 12 hours; nerve function may be recoverable in time but infarcted muscle is damaged permanently. Eventually, the dead muscle fibroses and shortens, and an ischaemic contracture results. Compartment syndrome may also complicate up to 15% of open fractures. In this case, this patient should not be sent home but admitted to the ward for elevation of his leg and closed monitoring for compartment syndrome. The fracture may be treated conservatively and may not require any surgical fixation.

12. Answer: C

In view of the patient's presentation, previously insignificant medical history and haemodynamically stable state, a Mallory–Weiss tear is the most likely diagnosis. Such tears occur near the gastro-oesophageal junction after forceful or prolonged coughing or vomiting, and often after excessive alcohol intake (or less frequently, from the recurrent morning sickness of pregnancy). They may also result from epileptic convulsions. The tears result in vomiting bright red blood and sometimes passing melaena thereafter. Although bleeding can be profuse, it usually stops spontaneously.

Aorto-duodenal fistula results from erosion of the duodenum into the aorta, due to tumour or previous repair of the aorta with a synthetic graft.

Meckel's diverticulum occasionally occurs in the ileum and may contain ectopic gastric mucosa, which may result in rectal bleeding.

Oesophageal varices represent dilated venous collaterals and result from portal hypertension in patients with liver cirrhosis.

Bleeding from peptic ulcers is the commonest cause of upper GI bleeds. Mucosal erosions develop, commonly due to NSAIDs, steroids, or prolonged alcohol abuse.

13. Answer: C

Refeeding syndrome is a condition in which there are severe electrolyte and fluid shifts associated with metabolic abnormalities in malnourished patients undergoing refeeding, weather orally, enterally, or parenterally. It is thought to arise as a result of rapid hormonal changes which occur in response to a regime rich in carbohydrate and amino acids and as a consequence of depletion of the substrates required for glucose metabolism. The cardinal features include hypophosphatae-mia, hypomagnesaemia, hypokalaemia, hyponatraemia, fluid shifts, and change in glucose, fat, and protein metabolism. Patients with refeeding syndrome may present with symptoms such as ataxia, paralysis, coma, cardiac dysrhythmias, anaemia, respiratory and cardiac failure, acute tubular necrosis, rhabdomyolysis, ileus and confusion. Therefore it is important to identify susceptible patients early, monitor electrolytes daily, and correct deficiencies by oral or parenteral routes.

14. Answer: D

Antireflux surgery is indicated in patients with symptoms of gastro-oesophageal reflux disease (GORD) that are resistant to conservative and medical (i.e. high-dose proton pump inhibitors) management. It is also believed to prevent certain complications of GORD, such as Barrett's oesophagus, oesophageal strictures, ulcer formation, and bleeding. In addition, patients in whom medical therapy cannot be continued (i.e. for undesirable side effects, poor compliance, or unwillingness/inability to pay for long-term medical therapy) and those who simply prefer surgery to indefinite drug therapy are potential candidates for surgery. Laparoscopic (e.g. Nissen) fundoplication is the treatment of choice in most centres. It is common practice for patients to have had undergone upper GI endoscopy at least 6 months prior to surgery to exclude any unsuspected pathology, Barrett's oesophagus, or adenocarcinoma. In addition, oesophageal pH monitoring is performed whilst the patient is off antisecretory therapy to establish the presence of reflux (i.e. when oesophageal pH <4). Oesophageal transit studies may be conducted to exclude primary motor disorders if suspected (e.g. achalasia, scleroderma-related oesophageal dysmotility), and to exclude aperistalsis, which may result in postoperative dysphagia after fundoplication.

15. Answer: B

The axillary nerve (C5, C6) arises from the posterior cord of the brachial plexus and passes through the quadrilateral space just below the shoulder joint. This space is bound superiorly by subscapularis and teres minor; inferiorly by teres major; medially by the long head of triceps brachii; and laterally by the surgical neck of the humerus. It is important to note that the axillary nerve and the posterior circumflex humeral artery, both of which pass through the quadrilateral space, may be damaged by trauma or space-occupying lesions in this region.

The axillary nerve then curves around the posterolateral surface of the humerus deep to the deltoid, dividing into anterior and posterior branches, both of which supply the deltoid muscle. The posterior branch also forms the upper lateral cutaneous nerve of the arm, which supplies the skin overlying the deltoid. The axillary nerve also gives off a branch supplying the teres minor.

The subacromial bursa is the synovial membrane located just below the acromion; it does not usually communicate with the shoulder joint capsule, and is often the site of pathology in shoulder impingement.

The long head of triceps brachii originates at the infraglenoid tubercle of the scapula, while the medial and lateral heads originate from the posterior aspect of the humerus. Therefore, no part of the triceps is considered to lie within the shoulder joint capsule (unlike the biceps brachii, which has a long head that extends inside the capsule to attach to the supraglenoid tubercle of the scapula).

The shoulder or 'glenohumeral' joint has a loose capsule that is lax inferiorly and is therefore at risk of dislocation in an anteroinferior direction (>95%), potentially damaging the axillary artery. Posterior dislocations are rarer and are usually due to electrocution or seizure activity (i.e. causing unbalanced contractions of the rotator cuff muscles, resulting in the humeral head dislocating posteriorly).

16. Answer: B

In foetal haemoglobin (HbF) two gamma chains replace the two beta chains found in HbA (adult haemoglobin). These gamma chains exhibit a *lower* affinity for 2,3 diphosphoglycerate (DPG) than beta chains. This ensures that HbF has a greater affinity for oxygen than HbA does, and is an important factor in ensuring oxygen delivery to the developing foetus. Oxygen transfer is further facilitated by the binding of hydrogen ions by foetal Hb molecules (the Bohr effect), as the pH of foetal blood is lower than that of maternal blood. The lifespan of neonatal red blood cells is approximately 70 days compared with approximately 120 days for maternal red blood cells. However, foetal haematocrit and consequently HbF levels increase throughout pregnancy to a peak value around term, which is about 50% higher than those of the mother.

17. Answer: D

The lymph nodes in the neck are classified into seven levels:

I: submental and submandibular
II: upper jugular (above the level of carotid bifurcation)
III: middle jugular (from the carotid bifurcation to the upper part of cricoid)
IV: lower jugular (from the cricoid to the clavicle)
V: posterior triangle
VI: anterior compartment (from the hyoid to the sternum, pretracheal, and paratracheal)
VII: upper anterior mediastinum

Levels I–V lymph nodes are often involved in the lymphatic regional spread of laryngeal and pharyngeal cancer. Levels VI and VII are mainly involved with thyroid cancer.

Radical neck dissection consists of excision of levels I–V lymphatic structures as well as three non-lymphatic structures: spinal accessory nerve, sternomastoid muscle and internal jugular vein.

Modified radical neck dissection comprises the removal of all level I–V lymph nodes with preservation of one or more non-lymphatic structures:

• Type 1: accessory nerve preserved
• Type 2: accessory nerve and jugular vein preserved
• Type 3: accessory nerve, sternomastoid and jugular vein preserved

Selective neck dissection: one or more lymphatic structures and all three non-lymphatic structures are preserved. It can be subdivided into:

• Supraomohyoid: excision of levels I–III nodes
• Posterolateral: excision of levels II–V nodes
• Lateral: excision of levels II–IV nodes

18. Answer: B

Desmopressin is the treatment of choice for mild von Willebrand's disease, including the type I and the majority of the type II variants (although it is believed to exacerbate thrombocytopenia that can accompany the type IIB variant of the disease). It is of no use in type III (i.e. severe) von Willebrand's disease. Cryoprecipitate or fresh frozen plasma are usually used in cases of bleeding (and not usually for prophylaxis), and would not be used in such patients due to the potential risk of viral transmission from blood products. For severe disease, von Willebrand's factor concentrate, and not factor VIII concentrate, would be used.

19. Answer: B

This patient's history, examination, and radiological findings are highly suggestive of large-bowel obstruction. The patient's relatively stable clinical state (i.e. with no evidence of peritonitis or other signs of bowel or mesenteric ischaemia) and the degree of colonic dilatation observed on radiography (i.e. under 6 cm) are not severe enough to warrant an immediately laparotomy without further investigation. In such cases, a CT scan with water soluble contrast (e.g. gastrografin) enema should be obtained to differentiate between a mechanical cause and pseudo-obstruction. Barium, which carries the risk of causing chemical peritonitis, should be avoided as a contrast agent as the patient may require urgent surgery.

20. Answer: A

Beyond the duodenojejunal flexure the small bowel is divided into the jejunum (proximal one-third) and ileum (distal two-thirds). There are no defining features but the jejunum can be distinguished from the ileum by the following features:

- The jejunum is of larger calibre, thick walled, and redder than the ileum, which is more purplish in appearance. The jejunal wall feels thicker because of the permanent infoldings of the mucous membrane, the plicae semilunaris are larger, more numerous, and closely set in the jejunum, whereas in the upper part of the ileum they are smaller and more widely separated, and in the lower part they are absent.
- The jejunal mesenteric vessels form single or double arterial arcades with long vasa recta while the ileal vessels form multiple arcades with short vasa recta.
- Lymphoid tissue is sparse in the jejunum but numerous in the ileum in the form of Peyer's patches.
- The fat on the jejunal mesentery is abundant near the root and scant near the intestinal end while it is deposited evenly throughout the ileal mesentery. The root of the mesentery extends 15 cm from duodenojejunal flexure at the level of L2, inferomedially to the ileocecal junction in the right iliac fossa.

21. Answer: B

The anterior pituitary or the adenohypophysis is derived from Rathke's pouch. The posterior pituitary/neurohypophysis is a downward projection of the hypothalamus. The hypothalamus is connected to the anterior pituitary gland via the pituitary portal system of blood vessels which carries inhibitory factors from the hypothalamus. In contrast, the posterior pituitary is connected to the hypothalamus by neurons, which transport hormones down to it. The anterior pituitary secretes six hormones: growth hormone, adrenocorticotrophic hormone, thyroid stimulating hormone, follicle stimulating hormone, prolactin and luteinizing hormone. The posterior pituitary secretes antidiuretic hormone and oxytocin.

22. Answer: C

Neuralgic amyotrophy (also known as Parsonage–Turner syndrome, brachial neuritis, and brachial plexitis) refers to the inflammation of branches of the brachial plexus, or other nerves in the upper extremity. It is idiopathic and usually occurs in response to bodily stress (e.g. surgery, influenza, excessive exercise, post-vaccination). It presents with severe pain for days to weeks, followed by weakness and sensory loss over the corresponding territory of the brachial plexus (most commonly C5–C7, as in this case). The diagnosis is obtained by history and physical examination, and by excluding all other possible causes. Neuromuscular studies are useful for both diagnosis as well as determining prognosis. A more diffuse process is usually revealed by such investigations than is present clinically, including bilateral involvement. Scapular winging is a common feature. Treatment is mostly symptomatic, with analgesia in the acute phase, and progressive physical therapy thereafter, to improve ranges of motion and aid subsequent recovery. Surgery is rarely indicated but in rare cases with severe deficits lacking any clinical or electrical recovery by 6 months, neurolysis with or without nerve transfer may be considered. Complete recovery may take weeks to years; 5–10% of patients never fully recover. If another immediate family member has had a similar episode, hereditary neuralgic amyotrophy may be present (5% of cases).

23. Answer: C

Fluid replacement in children follows the same general principles as that in adults (i.e. volume replacement = deficit + maintenance + ongoing losses). In the scenario, the patient's deficit and ongoing losses (e.g. through diarrhoea and vomiting) are assumed to have resolved. The calculation of daily maintenance fluid requirements for children may be performed according to their body weight in kilograms:

- 100 mL/kg for the first 10 kg
- 50 mL/kg for the next 10 kg
- 20 mL/kg for any weight after 20 kg.

Therefore, the child in this case requires (100 mL × 10 kg) + (50 mL × 10 kg) + (20 mL × 5 kg) = 1600 mL per day, for her 25 kg body weight. This equates to approximately 67 mL per hour. More accurate estimations of the maintenance requirements can be made if the surface area is known; 1500 mL of fluids is required for each square metre of surface area. However, this is obviously less practical than calculation by weight in most clinical situations.

24. Answer: E

The clinical signs and symptoms in this patient are most likely to be due to a ruptured diaphragm. Direct penetrating injury to the thoraco-abdominal region is a common cause for diaphragmatic rupture. The injury could be at any level between the 4th and the 10th intercostal space, depending on the patient's respiratory pattern. The other causes include rib fractures and a sudden increase in thoraco-abdominal pressure, as occurs when the patient with a closed glottis is hit in the abdomen. Patients with rupture of the diaphragm may present with hypotension, tachycardia, tachypnoea, chest pain and decreased air entry in the lung base of the affected side. However, diaphragmatic rupture may be difficult to detect clinically, and thus may result in significant morbidity or even mortality. The displacement of abdominal wall contents into the thorax will correlate to the degree of rupture, and bowel sounds may be auscultated in the chest. Rupture may be seen on plain chest radiograph especially with the abnormal location of the nasogastric tube; however, this method is of modest accuracy. Fracture(s) of the lower ribs on the affected side may or may not be present. The differential diagnoses for a raised left hemidiaphragm, both clinically and on plain radiography, include phrenic nerve palsy, atelectasis, diaphragmatic hernia and distended abdominal viscera.

25. Answer: D

Little's area is present in the anteroinferior part of the nasal septum and most bleeds (90%) originate here. It is marked by the convergence of the anterior ethmoidal, superior labial, sphenopalatine and greater palatine arteries. This is also known as Kiesselbach's plexus. In general, epistaxis is very common and has a bimodal age distribution (i.e. 2-10 years and 50-80 years). In children, epistaxis is usually due to nose picking and foreign bodies. Adult epistaxis is more likely to be idiopathic or traumatic in aetiology. In contrast, posterior epistaxis is more common in the elderly and usually arises from the branches of the sphenopalatine artery.

26. Answer: E

Metabolic acidosis results when the body forms more acid than the kidneys can excrete. The diagnosis is made with the use of arterial blood gas sampling. The numerous causes of metabolic acidosis can be classified depending on the anion gap (i.e. a normal anion gap or a raised anion gap).

$$\text{Anion gap} = ([Na^+] + [K^+]) - ([Cl^-] + [HCO_3^-])$$

The normal anion gap ranges from 8–16 mmol/L. The causes of metabolic acidosis with a normal anion gap includes GI tract losses of bicarbonate ions, such as diarrhoea and pancreatic fistula losses, renal tubular acidosis, dilutional causes, drugs (e.g. acetazolamide), Addison's disease, and TPN infusions of amino acids.

An elevated anion gap (>16 mmol/L) may indicate acidosis due to lactic acidosis (e.g. shock, hypoxia, sepsis), uraemia (e.g. renal failure), ketosis (e.g. diabetes mellitus, alcohol), and drugs (e.g. salicylates, biguanides, ethylene glycol, methanol). The diagnosis may require further investigations including toxicology.

Renal tubular acidosis is characterized by the failure to acidify urine correctly and results in the loss of sulphate and phosphate anions. Electrical neutrality is maintained by renal reabsorption of chloride anions, resulting in a hyperchloraemic metabolic acidosis with a normal anion gap. Of the three types of renal tubular acidosis, the proximal and distal types are associated with potassium loss.

27. Answer: B

Small bowel obstructions make up 80–85% of all intestinal obstructions. Of these, adhesional obstructions account for nearly 90% of all cases. Adhesions usually develop following laparotomy and/or 'major' surgery such as resection of large lengths of the bowel. However, it can also arise as a sequela of 'minor' abdominal surgery such as appendicectomy. In females, gynaecological procedures are predisposing factors for adhesion formation. In addition, pelvic inflammatory disease can also lead to adhesions even in the absence of prior surgical intervention to the abdomen. The cardinal features of small bowel obstruction are pain, vomiting and abdominal distension; untreated, this may lead to constipation with reduction in flatus, which then becomes absolute. The pain is usually colicky due to excessive peristalsis, but may become continuous if strangulation or perforation occurs. Vomiting is early in high small bowel obstruction, late in low small bowel obstruction, and delayed or absent in large-bowel obstruction. The management involves appropriate resuscitation of the patient, including nasogastric tube insertion (i.e. attempting to proximally decompress the bowel) and intravenous fluid rehydration—'drip and suck'. Small bowel obstruction secondary to adhesions should rarely lead to surgery (adhesiolysis).

28. Answer: A

The iliohypogastric nerve perforates the posterior part of the transversus abdominis muscle and divides between this and the internal oblique muscle into lateral and anterior cutaneous branches, and muscular branches to both these muscles. This nerve may be cut during a transverse incision for appendicectomy, resulting in muscle weakness and a subsequent predisposition to developing direct inguinal hernias. Like the iliohypogastric nerve, the ilioinguinal nerve also arises from the L1 nerve root, but passes through the 2nd and 3rd layers of abdominal wall musculature and passes through the inguinal canal. It lies inferior to McBurney's point and is therefore less likely to be damaged.

29. Answer: C

Renin is released from the juxtaglomerular cells in response to three main stimuli: reduced renal perfusion, sympathetic stimulation and reduced sodium delivery to the distal tubules.

Renin catalyses the cleavage of angiotensin I from angiotensinogen. Angiotensin I is then converted to angiotensin II, being catalysed by angiotensin-converting enzyme (ACE). ACE is found mainly in the pulmonary and vascular endothelium. Angiotensin II causes powerful and rapid vasoconstriction and also the release of aldosterone from the adrenal gland. Aldosterone causes sodium retention from urine, sweat, saliva and gastric juice, and increased potassium excretion by increasing the exchange between Na and K/H in the renal tubules. Both vasoconstriction and salt and water retention increase renal perfusion, which reduces renin release.

30. Answer: C

Papillary carcinomas of the thyroid are most commonly seen in children and young adults. FNA cytology demonstrates characteristic nuclear grooves, intranuclear inclusions or optically clear nuclei, Orphan Annie cells, and psammoma bodies. They are often multifocal and slow growing with good prognosis. Spread is usually lymphatic (i.e. to cervical lymph nodes). Follicular adenomas are benign tumours that are well encapsulated. Capsular invasion is seen in follicular carcinomas, which tend to exhibit haematogenous spread. Medullary carcinomas are rare, arising from the parafollicular C cells, which secrete calcitonin. Anaplastic carcinomas are rare and aggressive cancers presenting usually in older women as a hard, woody goitre.

31. Answer: A

There are four types of testicular appendages:

- Appendix testis (Hydatid cyst of Morgagni)
- Appendix epididymis
- Paradidymis (organ of Giraldes)
- Ductulus aberrans (vas aberrans of Haller)

The commonest testicular appendage is the appendix testis, which is a remnant of the para-mesonephric (Mullerian) duct. The rest are remnants of the mesonephric duct (Wolffian duct).

Torsion of the testicular appendage is the commonest cause of an acute scrotum in pre-pubertal boys. Testicular appendages are present in 85–90% of testes but only a minority will develop torsion.

The tunica vaginalis (i.e. the serous covering of the testis) is a pouch of serous membrane derived from the processus vaginalis.

32. Answer: A

Phaeochromocytomas are rare neuroendocrine tumours of the adrenal medulla. They normally follow the *rule of tens*—10% are malignant, 10% are familial, 10% are bilateral, and 10% are extra-adrenal. These tumours secrete excessive amounts of catecholamines and related products, leading to their symptoms of headache, sweating, palpitations and paroxysmal hypertension. Management involves alpha blockade (phenoxybenzamine or doxazosin) upon diagnosis. Once alpha-blockers are well established, a beta-blocker (e.g. propranolol) can be added to control tachycardia. Beta-blockers are avoided prior to alpha-blockade as they can enhance the vasopressor effects of noradrenaline.

Laparoscopic adrenalectomy is the treatment of choice for small benign tumours. Open adrenalectomy is reserved for large or malignant tumours.

33. Answer: B

This type of trauma classically injures the upper brachial plexus, particularly the ventral rami of C5 and C6, the consequences of which are in keeping with the clinical findings described. The muscles supplied by the nerves arising from these rami and the superior trunk are paralysed. These muscles are the deltoid, biceps brachii, brachialis, brachioradialis, supraspinatus, infraspinatus, teres minor and supinator. Paralysis of teres minor and infraspinatus (lateral rotators) results in medial rotation of the arm. Paralysis of biceps (a secondary supinator), results in pronation of the forearm. Paralysis of brachialis and biceps brachii results in weakness of elbow flexion. Inability of the patient to flex his upper arm results from paralysis of the deltoid, coracobrachialis and the clavicular head of pectoralis major. Paralysis of the supraspinatus and deltoid muscles results in the loss of abduction at the shoulder joint.

34. Answer: C

There are many different types of nipple discharge. Clear or cloudy white nipple discharge is invariably physiological due to galactorrhoea whereas milky white nipple discharge is often seen in pregnancy and rarely with hyperprolactinaemia. Green or grey nipple discharge may indicate an infection, duct ectasia, fibrocystic disease, or even perimenopausal change. Blood-stained nipple discharge can be caused by duct papillomas, intraductal carcinoma, or infiltrating carcinoma. Duct papillomas are localized areas of epithelial proliferation within large lactiferous ducts. They are hyperplastic rather than neoplastic, and therefore are not premalignant.

Duct ectasia is the dilatation of the larger mammary ducts as they fill up with green fluid and sterile pus. This usually occurs around the menopause and presents with tender lumpy breasts and green nipple discharge. The ducts may rupture to produce periductal mastitis and even breast abscesses.

35. Answer: C

The clinical signs and the type of bony injury are consistent with an injury to the radial nerve. The radial nerve (C5–T1) is the largest branch of the posterior cord of the brachial plexus and is most frequently injured following a mid-shaft fracture of the humerus. The course of this nerve is as follows: after leaving the axilla, the radial nerve gives three sensory branches and innervates the three heads of the triceps muscle and the anconeus. It then winds down the humerus in the spiral groove, after which it gives muscular branches to the brachioradialis, the extensor carpi radialis longus, and the supinator muscles, before bifurcating into sensory and motor branches. The sensory branch, the superficial radial nerve, travels along the radial aspect of the forearm and provides sensation to the 1st web-space region. At the elbow, the motor branch of the radial nerve becomes the posterior interosseous nerve and enters the extensor compartment through the supinator muscle under the arcade of Frohse. There it supplies the remaining extensors of the wrist, thumb and fingers. If the nerve is injured in the region of the spiral groove, all the long extensors of the wrist and fingers are affected, resulting in wrist drop.

36. Answer: B

The most important aetiology of Pancoast's syndrome involves tumours located at the apex or superior sulcus of the lungs (predominantly non-small-cell lung carcinoma) growing by local extension, and involving the brachial plexus (most commonly the lower roots) and cervical sympathetic nerves (stellate ganglion). This results in: (1) pain in the shoulder region radiating toward the axilla and scapula, (2) pain and atrophy of small muscles of the hand due to ulnar nerve involvement, (3) paraesthesia in the medial side of the arm, (4) Horner's syndrome (ptosis, miosis, hemianhidrosis and enophthalmos), and (5) oedema of the arms due to compression of the major vessels in the thoracic inlet. Tumour invasion into the 1st or 2nd thoracic vertebral bodies or intervertebral foramina can result in spinal cord compression. In rare instances, there may also be unilateral recurrent laryngeal nerve palsy producing unilateral vocal cord paralysis and/or phrenic nerve involvement. Facial nerve involvement is not seen in Pancoast's syndrome. Although until recently, lung tumours involving the brachial plexus were generally considered to be inoperable, recent studies have shown that induction chemotherapy (e.g. three courses of split-dose cisplatin and etoposide or paclitaxel) followed by concurrent chemoradiotherapy (e.g. a course of cisplatin/etoposide combined with 45 Gy hyperfractionated accelerated radiotherapy) and surgery may improve the survival of such patients. Nevertheless, multidisciplinary team discussions are imperative when exploring such treatment options.

37. Answer: C

The middle cranial fossa communicates with the orbit via the superior orbital fissure. The orbital fissure is bounded superiorly by the lesser wing of the sphenoid, inferiorly by the greater wing, and medially by the body of the sphenoid. The fissure is wider on its medial aspect. The superior orbital fissure transmits a number of structures including: the oculomotor, trochlear, and abducens nerves; the frontal, lacrimal, and nasociliary branches of the trigeminal nerve; the internal carotid sympathetic plexus; the ophthalmic vein; the orbital branch of the middle meningeal artery; and the recurrent branch of the lacrimal artery. The optic nerve, along with ophthalmic artery, passes through the optic canal which lies lateral to the pituitary fossa.

38. Answer: B

Intussusception refers to the invagination of a segment of bowel within the lumen of an adjacent loop. It usually occurs from 5–12 months of age and is the commonest cause of intestinal obstruction in infants. Causes of intussusception include:

- Idiopathic (possibly due to enlarged Peyer's patches)
- Meckel's diverticulum
- Polyp
- Lymphoma.

In addition to the scenario described, children may also present with redcurrant jelly-like stool and peritonism. The most common type of intussusception is ileocolic.

In contrast, with an appendix abscess, the abdominal pain would have been ongoing for longer, and the child would be pyrexic with significantly raised inflammatory markers. Vomiting in pyloric stenosis is projectile and strictly non-bilious. An inguinal hernia would not present with a palpable mass in the right flank. Meckel's diverticulum is a true (i.e. involving all layers of bowel wall) congenital diverticulum resulting from the incomplete obliteration of the vitello-intestinal duct. The rule of 2's dictates that it occurs in 2% of the population, it lies 2 feet away from the ileo-caecal junction and is 2 inches long. Although it can cause intussusception, it is not individually palpable or visible as a 'target sign' on ultrasound scan.

39. Answer: C

The ulnar nerve (C8, T1) arises from the medial cord of the brachial plexus or, more specifically, the anterior division of the lower trunk. This nerve is commonly damaged following injury to the medial epicondyle of the humerus. It can also be injured in other types of humeral fractures. Ulnar nerve injury may lead to paralysis of the small muscles of the hand; paralysis of the interossei results in loss of adduction and abduction of the fingers. Thumb adduction may be lost due to loss of innervation of adductor pollicis brevis (the other thenar muscles are supplied by the median nerve). Clawing of the little and ring fingers, known as the 'ulnar claw hand', is seen in low ulnar nerve injuries where the extension of the fingers is lost due to paralysis of the medial two lumbricals but the fingers become flexed due to the unopposed action of the long flexors (flexor digitorum superficialis and flexor digitorum profundus). High ulnar nerve lesions cause loss of action of the above flexors to the little and ring fingers and hence there is no clawing of the hand.

40. Answer: A

An Amyand's hernia is an inguinal hernia which contains an appendix within it. It may or may not be inflamed. A Littre's hernia refers to an inguinal hernia containing a Meckel's diverticulum. Maydl's hernia is an inguinal hernia with two adjacent loops of small intestine lying within the hernia sac with a tight neck, whereas the intervening loop of bowel lies within the abdomen and becomes deprived of its blood supply and eventually becomes necrotic. A Pantaloon hernia is an inguinal hernia with a direct and indirect component protruding on either side of the inferior epigastric artery. A Richter's hernia is an inguinal hernia which only contains one side of the bowel wall. This can result in bowel strangulation and ischaemic perforation without necessarily manifesting with obstructive symptoms.

41. Answer: A

Most scars take over a year to fully mature. Wound healing resulting in problematic scarring is more common in younger people.

Keloid scars have a higher incidence in younger people and in those with pigmented skin. There is often a familial tendency. They extend beyond the boundaries of the original wound and occur late in wound healing (>3 months). They do not regress and usually recur following excision. Their incidence is unrelated to wound tension, and is regarded by some to be an autoimmune phenomenon.

Hypertrophic scars also have a higher incidence in younger people. They generally occur early in wound healing and are limited to the boundaries of the original wound. They spontaneously regress but not entirely back to normal, and are more likely to form scar contractures. Wound tension and delayed healing increase the risk of hypertrophic scarring.

42. Answer: B

ARDS is characterized by all of the options listed except B. It is thought to occur following a recognized precipitating cause such as severe sepsis (50%), trauma (30%), gastric aspiration (10%), acute pancreatitis, etc. On plain chest radiography, bilateral pulmonary infiltrate are visible with no evidence of heart failure. An enlarged heart, pleural effusions, upper lobe diversion, alveolar 'bat wing' oedema and 'Kerley B lines' are all radiological signs of heart failure.

43. Answer: E

An inguinal hernia is the abnormal protrusion of the contents of the abdominal cavity through the inguinal canal. The inguinal canal runs from the midpoint of the inguinal ligament (the deep inguinal ring) to a point above and medial to the pubic tubercle (superficial inguinal ring). The anterior wall of the canal is formed by the external oblique aponeurosis. The posterior wall is formed by the conjoint tendon and transversalis fascia. The floor is formed by the inguinal and lacunar ligaments and the roof is formed by the internal oblique and transversus abdominis.

An indirect inguinal hernia protrudes through the deep ring due to a patent processus vaginalis. It is therefore covered by the internal spermatic fascia and lies lateral to the inferior epigastric artery.

In contrast, a direct inguinal hernia occurs as a result of weakening of the transversalis fascia. It is therefore not covered in spermatic fascia and lie medial to the inferior epigastric artery.

44. Answer: C

The nature of this patient's presentation and the findings on examination are suggestive of subarachnoid haemorrhage (SAH). SAH accounts for about 6% of cerebrovascular disease with an annual incidence of about 1 per 10,000. It is the result of bleeding from intracranial vessels into the subarachnoid space. Occasionally, the arachnoid layer gives way and a subdural haematoma develops. Eighty per cent of cases are due to congenital berry aneurysms (with a peak incidence of presentation between 40–50 years of age).

SAH can be graded according to the Hunt and Hess scale, which classifies the severity of disease based on the patient's clinical status (i.e. from an asymptomatic presentation to the other extreme of coma with decerebrate posturing). It is recognized as a predictor of outcome, with a higher grade correlating to lower survival rate. The patient in this scenario demonstrates grade 3 disease, which involves drowsiness with confusion or mild focal neurology (but not yet involving stupor or significant hemiparesis). Other scales which describe the clinical presentation of SAH include the World Federation of Neurosurgical Societies classification, which combines consciousness level and motor deficit in its scoring system.

45. Answer: C

The Gustilo–Anderson classification of open fractures considers the amount of energy, the extent of soft tissue damage and the degree of wound contamination, to determine fracture severity. Type I fractures result from low-energy trauma and involve a wound less than 1 cm in length. Type II fractures also result from low-energy trauma but these comprise wounds greater than 1 cm in length, with more extensive soft tissue damage. The most severe grade is type III, which results from high-energy trauma and involves extensive soft tissue damage and contamination. Type III injuries are subdivided into three categories: type IIIA, comprising a segmental or severely comminuted open fracture but with adequate soft tissue to cover the bone; type IIIB, involving periosteal stripping and bone exposure (thus needing soft tissue cover); and type IIIC, which involves vascular injury requiring repair (regardless of soft tissue injury). Therefore, the progression from grade I to IIIC involves a higher degree of energy towards the injury, greater soft tissue and bone damage, and a higher potential for complications.

46. Answer: A

Atrial septal defect results in a left-to-right shunt and volume overload of the chambers receiving excess blood flow, eventually causing right ventricular failure. As the blood in the left atrium is already oxygenated, mixing with venous blood within the right side of the heart merely decreases cardiac efficiency. In contrast, right-to-left shunts are more dangerous as they allow poorly oxygenated blood into the peripheral vascular system, causing cyanosis.

Right ventricular tract outflow obstruction results in reduced pulmonary blood flow and cyanosis. However, these patients are not typically breathless, and their chest radiographs demonstrate oligaemic lung fields. Tetralogy of Fallot is characterized by four heart malformations which include pulmonary stenosis, overriding aorta, ventricular septal effect and right ventricular hypertrophy. Cyanosis in this pathology is also due to a right-to-left shunt. In infants with transposition of the great arteries, the pulmonary and systemic circuits occur in parallel rather than in series, resulting in the mixing of oxygenated and deoxygenated blood. Total anomalous pulmonary venous drainage is a rare cyanotic congenital defect in which all four pulmonary veins are malpositioned and make anomalous connections with the systemic venous circulation. Due to the lack of systemic blood flow resulting from this condition, these patients may survive only in the presence of a patent foramen ovale or atrial septal defect.

47. Answer: D

This patient's signs and symptoms are suggestive of peritoneal carcinomatosis and malignant ascites probably secondary to colorectal carcinoma and liver metastases. Peritoneal carcinomatosis refers to the presence of malignant cells within the peritoneal cavity. It can lead to the development of ascites. Other recognized causes of peritoneal carcinomatosis (and malignant ascites) include carcinoma of the ovary, endometrium, breast, stomach and pancreas. Tumour cell implantation on the omental surface leads to the classic finding of 'omental caking'. This is followed by serosal invasion and proliferation in the omental fat. Eventually, the omental fat becomes entirely replaced by tumour, resulting in a thick, confluent, soft tissue mass. Desmoplastic small round cell tumour is a highly aggressive malignancy that most often affects young adults. This malignancy rapidly invades the peritoneal surfaces with haematogenous metastasis to the liver, lungs and lymph nodes. Malignant peritoneal mesothelioma is a rare but aggressive tumour derived from the peritoneal mesothelium. Twenty to 30% of mesotheliomas arise from the peritoneum and are associated with asbestos exposure and therapeutic irradiation of the abdomen. There is no history of either of such exposure in this patient. The clinical presentations of gastrointestinal stromal tumours and Budd–Chiari syndrome (occlusion of the hepatic vein or inferior vena cava) are largely different to this presentation.

48. Answer: A

Apart from excluding overt ulceration, it is vital to check for callous formation at pressure areas (e.g. under the first metatarsal head or 'ball of the foot') as this is an important predictor of skin ulceration in diabetic patients with a compromised microcirculation. Progressive, unnoticed trauma secondary to diabetic neuropathy is usually the cause of plantar ulceration in these patients, and is usually initiated by minor skin trauma (i.e. not infection in itself). As lower limb perfusion is often limited by the associated autonomic neuropathy, performing a sympathectomy may help to improve skin perfusion. It is challenging to distinguish Charcot arthropathy and osteomyelitis based on plain radiographic evidence alone.

49. Answer: A

This sequence of events is characteristic of hyperacute rejection. Hyperacute rejection is caused by prior sensitization, which results in the development of preformed antibodies against human leucocyte antigens. Sensitization is mainly due to blood transfusion. This is a type of humoral vascular rejection occurring within minutes to hours following transplantation. This is now a rare event due to preoperative ABO matching and histocompatibility testing. Liver grafts are more tolerant of hyperacute rejection but the reason behind this is not fully understood. The graft must be removed to prevent a systemic inflammatory response in these patients.

50. Answer: D

Antibiotic prophylaxis is not required for the majority of dog bite wounds, as long as the wounds are appropriately cleaned and not at high risk of further complications (e.g. deep wounds or those associated with crush injuries). The patient in this case demonstrates clinical evidence of wound infection, which, in the context of the primary injury, may involve organisms like *Pasteurella* species, *Staphylococcus aureus,* and anaerobes such as *Corynebacterium*. Such a range of pathogens would respond most effectively to a broad-spectrum antibiotic such as co-amoxiclav, than to the other options in the question. In cases of penicillin allergy, doxycycline, and metronidazole, or (if pregnant) ceftriaxone alone, may be used. It is important to note that bites from humans, cats, and rats carry a higher risk of infection than those from dogs, and must therefore be treated more seriously.

Basic sciences: Applied anatomy

1. **A 65-year-old presents to his GP with weakness along the right side of his mouth and lower lip. He states that he has difficulty in closing his mouth and is unable to move his lower lip. On examination, there is loss of sensation over the mandible and the chin on the right side. The patient states that he has noticed these symptoms since he underwent excision of his right submandibular gland for a malignant tumour 2 weeks previously. Which nerve is most likely to have been injured in this patient to cause these symptoms?**
   - A. Mandibular branch of the trigeminal nerve
   - B. Glossopharyngeal nerve
   - C. Lingual nerve
   - D. Marginal mandibular branch of the facial nerve
   - E. Hypoglossal nerve

Basic sciences: Physiology

2. **Which of the following is not a criterion for diagnosing systemic inflammatory response syndrome (SIRS)?**
   - A. Temperature >38°C or <36°C
   - B. Systolic blood pressure <90 mmHg
   - C. Heart rate >90/min
   - D. Respiratory rate >20 or $PaCO_2 < 4.3$ kPa
   - E. WCC > 12,000 or < 4000 × 10^9/L

Basic sciences: Pathology

3. **Which of the following cells are implicated in foam cell formation?**
   - A. Monocytes
   - B. Macrophages
   - C. Endothelial cells
   - D. Platelets
   - E. T cells

Common surgical conditions and the subspecialties:
Trauma and orthopaedics

4. **Which of the following statements concerning fractures of the cervical spine is correct?**
   A. A Jefferson fracture leads to sudden death
   B. Acute fractures of the axis represent about 70% of all cervical spine injuries
   C. Type I axis fractures involve the junction of the odontoid peg with the body
   D. In type II axis fractures, the posterior elements of the axis may be fractured by a hyperextension injury
   E. Odontoid fractures may be visualized using open-mouth odontoid views

Common surgical conditions and the subspecialties: Skin, head, and neck

5. **Which among the following is not a feature of Pierre Robin syndrome?**
   A) Cleft palate
   B) Micrognathia
   C) Severe respiratory and feeding difficulties
   D) Otitis media
   E) Delayed eruption of teeth

Perioperative care: Assessing and planning nutritional management

6. **A 45-year-old man with no significant medical history is currently being kept nil-by-mouth for an elective bilateral inguinal hernia repair. Which of the following describes the best fluid regimen for this patient over the following 24 hours?**
   A. 3 L normal saline with 20 mmol potassium in each bag
   B. 2 L Hartmann's solution and 1 L 5% dextrose with 20 mmol potassium
   C. 1 L normal saline with 20 mmol potassium and 2 L 5% dextrose with 20 mmol potassium in each bag
   D. 1 L dextrose saline and 2L 5% dextrose with 20 mmol potassium in each bag
   E. 3 L dextrose saline

The assessment and management of the surgical patient:
Clinical decision-making

7. **A 35-year-old race car driver is seen in the Emergency Department after being involved in a collision on the track, during which his protective harness failed to restrain him. On examination, he is unable to walk and complains of severe left hip pain. His left leg appears shortened and lies adducted. Plain radiography reveals a posterior dislocation of the hip. Which is the next most appropriate step in managing this patient?**
   A. Admit to the orthopaedic ward and await space on theatre list
   B. Attempt closed reduction in the Emergency Department under local nerve block
   C. Attempt closed reduction in the Emergency Department under sedation
   D. Send the patient to theatre immediately
   E. Urgent CT to exclude an acetabular fracture

Basic sciences: Applied anatomy

8. In view of the possible operative damage to the recurrent laryngeal nerve during thyroid surgery, a patient is requested to undergo laryngoscopy as part of his preoperative assessment to determine the baseline function of his vocal cords. Which muscle is primarily responsible for the abduction of the vocal cords?

   A. Cricothyroid muscle
   B. Lateral cricoarytenoid muscle
   C. Posterior cricoarytenoid muscle
   D. Thyroarytenoid muscle
   E. Transverse arytenoid muscle

Basic sciences: Physiology

9. Which of the following is least responsible for maintaining anal continence towards fluid and gas?

   A. Anorectal angle
   B. Internal anal sphincter
   C. Endoanal cushions
   D. External anal sphincter
   E. N/A—all the above are equally responsible

Basic sciences: Pathology

10. A 71-year-old gentleman is referred by his GP to the urology outpatient clinic with a 3–4 month history of painless haematuria, increased frequency, difficulty in initiating micturition, and loss of weight. He also complains of generalized tiredness and occasional palpitations. He smokes 16–20 cigarettes a day. Prior to his retirement, he worked in a petrochemical industry. On examination, he appears pale and anaemic. Abdominal examination is unremarkable. Per rectal examination reveals a normal prostate gland. What is the most likely diagnosis?

    A. Renal cell carcinoma
    B. Squamous cell carcinoma of the renal pelvis
    C. Angiomyolipoma
    D. Renal tuberculosis
    E. Carcinoma of the bladder

Common surgical conditions and the subspecialties:
Trauma and orthopaedics

11. **A 5-year-old boy is brought to the Emergency Department by his parents after falling off a carousel. Examination reveals an angulated right elbow and a cold distal right hand with no palpable brachial, radial or ulnar pulses. Anteroposterior and lateral radiographs of the elbow reveal a displaced supracondylar fracture of the right humerus. Which of the following options describes the most appropriate initial management?**

A. Applying a plaster cast and arranging urgent outpatient review
B. Initiating thrombolysis to prevent further ischaemia of the upper limb
C. Manipulation of the fracture under general anaesthetic
D. Open reduction and internal fixation of the fracture
E. Surgical exploration of the right antecubital fossa

Common surgical conditions and the subspecialties:
Gastrointestinal disease

12. **A newborn infant is noted to have a protrusion of his bowel from the abdomen, within a semitranslucent sac at the umbilicus. What is the most likely diagnosis?**

A. Duodenal atresia
B. Exomphalos
C. Gastroschisis
D. Hirschsprung's disease
E. Imperforate anus

Perioperative care: Assessing and planning nutritional management

13. **A 70-year-old female on enteral feeding complains of diarrhoea. Which of the following conditions is the least likely cause of her symptoms?**

A. Bacterial contamination
B. Low feed temperature
C. Hyperosmolar feed
D. Reduced fluid replacement
E. Reduced intestinal absorptive capacity

The assessment and management of the surgical patient:
Clinical decision-making

14. **A 52-year-old man with a longstanding history of liver disease secondary to alcoholism presents to the Emergency Department after an episode of profuse haematemesis. Which of the following procedures would be most appropriate for the immediate management of this patient?**
    A. Endoscopic sclerotherapy
    B. High-dose proton pump inhibitors
    C. Intravenous octreotide
    D. Sengstaken–Blakemore tube insertion
    E. Transjugular intrahepatic portosystemic shunting (TIPS)

Basic sciences: Applied anatomy

15. **An obstetrician performs a pudendal nerve block to anaesthetize the perineum of a pregnant woman in labour. Which of the following statements accurately describes the pudendal nerve?**
    A. It arises from the posterior rami of nerve roots S2, S3, and S4
    B. It crosses the ischial spine on the lateral side of the internal pudendal artery
    C. It exists the pelvis through the lesser sciatic foramen
    D. It supplies the levator ani
    E. It supplies the testes

Basic sciences: Physiology

16. **Which among the following statements regarding the autonomic nervous system is correct?**
    A. Accommodation of the lens is achieved via parasympathetic innervation of the ciliary muscle
    B. The pupillary light reflex is an example of 'push–pull' innervation by both the sympathetic and parasympathetic divisions
    C. Spinal cord damage below T10 level is unlikely to affect the micturition reflex
    D. Sweat production is increased in response to the release of noradrenaline from postganglionic sympathetic fibres
    E. Tidal volume is increased during the fight or flight response due to an increased respiratory frequency caused by elevated circulatory levels of adrenaline

Common surgical conditions and the subspecialties: Skin, head, and neck

17. **Prolonged exposure to which of the following types of ultraviolet (UV) light increases the risk of development of skin cancer?**
    A. UVA
    B. NUV
    C. UVB
    D. FUV
    E. UVC

Perioperative care: Haemostasis and blood products

18. **A 30-year-old patient with type 1 von Willebrand's disease attends the Day Surgery Unit for incision and drainage of an abscess on her forehead. She has a past history of menorrhagia and had two uncomplicated dental extractions as an adolescent. What is the most useful test to assess her bleeding tendency?**
    A. Activated partial thromboplastin time
    B. Bleeding time
    C. Plasma factor VIII activity
    D. Platelet aggregation
    E. Prothrombin time

The assessment and management of the surgical patient: Planning investigations

19. **A 19-year-old medical student discovers a fluctuant swelling in the midline of her neck and asks her GP about the potential benefits of undergoing fine needle aspiration cytology (FNAC). The GP reassures her and explains the common indications for FNAC. Which of the following is true regarding FNAC?**
    A. A follicular adenoma may be distinguished from a follicular carcinoma by FNAC
    B. FNAC for suspected breast malignancy provides more information than core biopsy
    C. FNAC is not a part of the triple assessment of a breast lump
    D. FNAC is preferred to radionuclide scanning for evaluating thyroid nodules
    E. FNAC of branchial cysts usually yields serous fluid

Basic sciences: Applied anatomy

20. **Which of the following is not true about coronary blood supply?**
    A. The sinoatrial (SA) node is usually supplied by the right coronary artery
    B. 90% of human hearts are right dominant
    C. The left coronary artery is usually smaller than the right coronary artery
    D. The coronary arteries arise from the sinus of Valsalva
    E. 3% of hearts are codominant

Basic sciences: Physiology

21. **In the action potential of non-nodal cardiac cells, phase 2 corresponds to:**
    A. Rapid influx of calcium
    B. Rapid efflux of calcium
    C. Slow influx of calcium
    D. Slow influx of potassium
    E. Rapid influx of sodium

Common surgical conditions and the subspecialties:
Neurology and Neurosurgery

22. **A 65-year-old painter complains of weakness in his right leg after falling 3 metres from a ladder. His GP performs a full neurological examination and discovers a diminished Achilles tendon reflex on the right. Which nerve is involved in the Achilles tendon reflex and what are its nerve roots?**
    A. Deep peroneal nerve L5, S1
    B. Deep peroneal nerve S1, S2
    C. Tibial nerve L5, S1
    D. Tibial nerve S1, S2
    E. Tibial nerve S2, S3

Perioperative care: Assessing and planning nutritional management

23. **A 21-year-old woman is admitted under the Mental Capacity Act for severe anorexia nervosa. She receives nasogastric feeding, which she initially tolerates well. However, she becomes acutely agitated and confused 3 days later. Examination reveals a heart rate of 120/min (and regular rhythm) and a blood pressure of 95/65 mmHg. She is apyrexial and appears adequately hydrated. Which one of the following investigations would be most immediately appropriate for this patient?**
    A. Serum calcium
    B. Serum sodium
    C. Serum phosphate
    D. Serum urea and electrolytes
    E. Serum vitamin B

The assessment and management of the surgical patient:
Differential diagnosis

24. **A 43-year-old gentleman presents to the Emergency Department with a 2-hour history of sudden-onset, severe epigastric pain, which increases on swallowing. He describes a heavy alcohol intake for the past 10 years but no other serious medical concerns. Examination reveals a regular, thready pulse of 95 per minute and a blood pressure of 100/90 mmHg. Chest radiography reveals gas in the mediastinum and in the subcutaneous tissues. What is the most likely cause of this patient's signs and symptoms?**
    A. Oesophageal perforation
    B. Diaphragmatic rupture
    C. Myocardial contusion
    D. Fracture of the sternum
    E. Traumatic haemothorax

Basic sciences: Applied anatomy

25. **A 28-year-old woman undergoes a wide local excision of a right-sided breast lump along with right axillary clearance. Postoperatively, she complains of numbness in her inner arm and axilla. Which nerve injury has likely caused the patient's symptoms?**
    A. Medial cutaneous nerve of arm
    B. Long thoracic nerve
    C. Thoracodorsal nerve
    D. Intercostobrachial nerve
    E. Axillary nerve

Basic sciences: Physiology

26. **Which of the following statements is true regarding gut hormones?**
    A. Gastrin increases pyloric sphincter pressure to retain food in the stomach while it is acted upon by gastric acid and pepsinogen
    B. Secretin produced by the S cells in the small intestine inhibits gastric acid and pepsin secretion
    C. Somatostatin increases hepatic and splanchnic blood flow
    D. Cholecystokinin is produced by the gallbladder and stimulates gallbladder contraction in response to fat and amino acids
    E. Vasoactive intestinal peptide is secreted by the small intestine in response to food entry

Common surgical conditions and the subspecialties:
Gastrointestinal disease

27. **A 42-year-old female presents to the Surgical Emergency Assessment Unit with a 48-hour history of abdominal pain, vomiting, and feeling generally unwell. She says that she has also noticed her stools to become pale and her urine to darken in colour. On examination, she is jaundiced and is tender over the right upper quadrant. An ultrasound examination reveals a dilated proximal common bile duct with intrahepatic duct dilatation. A MRCP demonstrates a fistula between the gallbladder and the common bile duct, and a large calculus is found in the common bile duct just distal to the fistula. What is the most likely diagnosis?**
    A. Primary biliary cirrhosis
    B. Primary sclerosing cholangitis
    C. Carcinoma of the gallbladder
    D. Mirizzi syndrome
    E. Cholangiocarcinoma

Basic sciences: Applied anatomy

28. **A 65-year-old male is admitted to hospital with abdominal pain, back pain and collapse. Physical examination reveals an expansile, pulsatile mass in his abdomen and weak femoral pulses. As he is haemodynamically stable, he undergoes a CT scan to confirm the suggestion of a ruptured abdominal aortic aneurysm. After a decision to operate is made, emergency repair of his 10 cm aneurysm with a Dacron graft requires extensive mobilization of the aorta and ligation of several segmental vessels. After the operation, he is found to be paraplegic, impotent, and incontinent of urine and faeces. What is the single most likely structure to have been damaged during surgery?**
    A. Inferior intercostal artery
    B. Lumbar artery
    C. Posterior spinal artery
    D. Great anterior segmental medullary artery
    E. Spinal cord

Basic sciences: Physiology

29. **Gastric acid secretion is increased by all the following except:**
    A. Gastrin
    B. Short gastric reflex
    C. Secretin
    D. Histamine
    E. Acetylcholine

Common surgical conditions and the subspecialties: Gastrointestinal disease

30. **Which of the following conditions is most commonly associated with meconium ileus in the newborn?**
    A. Duodenal stenosis
    B. Hirschsprung's disease
    C. Midgut volvulus
    D. Cystic fibrosis
    E. Imperforate anus

Basic sciences: Applied anatomy

31. **A surgeon wishes to obtain access into the popliteal fossa. Of the options listed, which is the first structure to be encountered whilst operating in this region?**
    A. Common peroneal nerve
    B. Popliteal artery
    C. Popliteal vein
    D. Posterior femoral cutaneous nerve
    E. Sural nerve

Common surgical conditions and the subspecialties: Endocrine disease

32. **A 70-year-old woman is recently diagnosed with primary hyperparathyroidism. Which of the following symptoms are not attributable to her hypercalcaemia?**

   A. Bone pain
   B. Abdominal pain
   C. Fatigue
   D. Constipation
   E. Confusion

Basic sciences: Applied anatomy

33. **A 60-year-old man is referred to the head and neck clinic with a lump in his cheek 2 cm anterior to the tragus of his right ear. He describes rapid growth of the swelling over the previous 2 months, associated with right-sided facial droop. Assuming that the lump is a parotid tumour, the surgeon proceeds to examine for regional lymphadenopathy. Which of the following nodes are lymphatic metastases from the parotid most likely to reach?**

   A. Submandibular nodes
   B. Superficial cervical nodes
   C. Deep cervical nodes
   D. Posterior cervical nodes
   E. Supraclavicular nodes

Common surgical conditions and the subspecialties: Skin, head and neck

34. **A 45-year-old male presents to his GP with a dark brown, irregularly pigmented skin lesion on his chest. He complains that it is extremely itchy and bleeds on contact. He is referred to a dermatologist, who informs him that it is malignant with a risk of regional and distant metastasis if left untreated. Which of the following features of this lesion would most accurately correlate with the likelihood of regional and distant metastasis?**

   A. Depth of the lesion
   B. Presence of satellite lesions
   C. Presence of ulceration
   D. Site of the primary lesion
   E. Surface area of the lesion

Basic sciences: Applied anatomy

35. Which of the following groups of lymph nodes is not involved in the lymphatic drainage of the thyroid gland?

A. Brachiocephalic lymph nodes
B. Thoracic duct (directly)
C. Deep cervical lymph nodes
D. Paratracheal lymph nodes
E. Pectoral lymph nodes

Common surgical conditions and the subspecialties: General presenting symptoms or syndromes

36. A 58-year-old gentleman with a history of alcohol abuse is brought to the Emergency Department after being found collapsed outside a pub. He remembers consuming about 15 pints of lager in the morning before developing severe epigastric pain. He then vomited five times prior to his collapse, with the last two episodes being mixed with blood. On examination, he appears pale and in significant discomfort. His blood pressure is 94/78 mmHg, pulse rate is 110/min, and his respiratory rate is 20/min. Abdominal examination reveals upper abdominal guarding and the presence of subcutaneous emphysema over the epigastric region extending to the chest. A plain erect CXR reveals air under the diaphragm and in the mediastinum. What is the most likely diagnosis?

A. Thoracic aortic rupture
B. Boerhaave's syndrome
C. Acute inferior myocardial infarction
D. Ruptured abdominal aorta
E. Perforated peptic ulcer

Basic sciences: Applied anatomy

37. A 63-year-old lady undergoes a parathyroidectomy for the treatment of primary hyperparathyroidism under the care of the endocrine surgeons. Intraoperatively, she is found to have a right inferior parathyroid adenoma, which is excised. On the ward round the following morning, she complains of hoarseness in her voice which she did not experience prior to the operation. What is the most likely cause for her symptoms?

A. Intubation
B. Unilateral damage to the external laryngeal nerve
C. Unilateral damage to the recurrent laryngeal nerve
D. Bilateral damage to the recurrent laryngeal nerve
E. Haematoma of the neck

Common surgical conditions and the subspecialties: General presenting symptoms or syndromes

38. **A 65-year-old diabetic man presents to the Emergency Department with excruciating genital pain 36 hours after undergoing incision and drainage of a perianal abscess. Examination reveals a temperature of 38°C and a pulse rate of 120/min. Purulent discharge is noted from the perianal wound, and his scrotum is found to be oedematous, red, and tender. His perianal skin appears dusky, and subcutaneous crepitations are noted on palpation. Which of the following options is the most likely diagnosis?**

    A. Testicular torsion and scrotal ischaemia
    B. Cellulitis
    C. Fournier's gangrene
    D. Epididymo-orchitis
    E. Isolated scrotal abscess

Basic sciences: Applied anatomy

39. **A 69-year-old gentleman presents to his GP with weakness of his right shoulder. Three months previously, he underwent a right cervical lymph node sampling for suspected metastasis of a squamous cell carcinoma of the floor of his mouth. Examination reveals muscle wasting in his right shoulder and neck, with associated right shoulder droop. The patient is unable to shrug the shoulder and his scapula appears prominently when he attempts to externally rotate his shoulder against resistance. Which of the following nerves is most likely to have been injured in this patient?**

    A. Long thoracic nerve
    B. Median pectoral nerve
    C. Transverse cervical nerve
    D. Supraclavicular nerve
    E. Spinal accessory nerve

Common surgical conditions and the subspecialties:
Gastrointestinal disease

40. **A 75-year-old lady from a residential home presents to clinic with jaundice and weight loss. She also complains of pale, buoyant stools and dark urine. She denies any pain or vomiting. Clinical examination reveals conjunctival pallor, yellow sclera and a non-tender, palpable mass in the right upper quadrant. Routine laboratory investigations reveal grossly elevated bilirubin and ALP levels, and mildly elevated GGT levels. What is the most likely diagnosis?**
    A. Common bile duct stone
    B. Stone in Hartmann's pouch
    C. Empyema
    D. Mucocoele
    E. Carcinoma of the head of the pancreas

Basic sciences: Applied anatomy

41. **A 25-year-old diabetic man presents to his GP with a 48-hour history of neck swelling and dysphagia. He also describes a longstanding history of dental pain originating from his left lower second molar. Examination reveals bilateral, tense neck swellings with overlying erythema, and an elevated and protruding tongue. Which of the following fascial compartments is most likely to be infected?**
    A. Prevertebral space
    B. Retropharyngeal space
    C. Parapharyngeal space
    D. Submandibular space
    E. Carotid sheath

Common surgical conditions and the subspecialties: Breast disease

42. **Which of the following statements is true about the risk factors for breast cancer?**
    A. A woman having her first child in her mid-thirties is at lower risk of breast cancer than a girl attaining menarche at 10 years of age
    B. In the UK, the female lifetime risk of breast cancer is 1 in 9
    C. Nulliparity lowers the risk of breast cancer
    D. Low socioeconomic status increases the risk of breast cancer
    E. Alcohol intake is not a risk factor in the development of breast cancer

Basic sciences: Applied anatomy

43. **A male patient undergoes an elective open inguinal hernia repair. The surgeon opens the spermatic cord to identify the hernia sac. Which structure is is unlikely to be found within the spermatic cord?**

A. Artery to the vas deferens

B. Genital branch of the genitofemoral nerve

C. Ilioinguinal nerve

D. Testicular artery

E. Vas deferens

Common surgical conditions and the subspecialties:
Neurology and neurosurgery

44. **A 32-year-old woman presents to the Emergency Department with an acute, severe occipital headache. Subsequent lumbar puncture and CT imaging demonstrate a subarachnoid haemorrhage. Despite an apparently early recovery, the patient's level of consciousness begins to deteriorate 4 days after the onset of her headache. Which of the following options describes the most likely cause of this sudden deterioration?**

A. Hydrocephalus

B. Intracerebral abscess

C. Medullary coning

D. Meningitis complicated the lumbar puncture

E. Sagittal sinus thrombosis

Assessment and management of patients with trauma (including the multiply injured patient): Assessment, scoring, and triage of adults and children

45. **A 17-year-old cricketer is struck on the outside of his right cheek by a cricket ball travelling at high speed. When he is examined at the scene by the attending medic, his cheek appears to be flat and depressed. He soon develops swelling and ecchymosis around his right eye and complains of dizziness, diplopia of the right eye and numbness over his cheek. What is the most likely injury described in this scenario?**

A. Retinal detachment

B. Intracranial haemorrhage

C. Blunt trauma to parotid gland

D. Maxillary fracture

E. Zygomatic fracture

Common surgical conditions and the subspecialties: Endocrine disease

46. **Which of the following statements is false regarding the renin–angiotensin–aldosterone system (RAAS)?**

    A. Renal artery stenosis accounts for 1% of hypertension and results from the overproduction of renin

    B. ACE inhibitors are contraindicated in renal artery stenosis

    C. The action of angiotensin I on cardiac receptors results in increased contractility and ventricular hypertrophy

    D. The action of angiotensin I on the kidneys results in a reduction of glomerular filtration rate and inhibition of renin release

    E. In the adrenal cortex angiotensin II stimulates the release of antidiuretic hormone

Common surgical conditions and the subspecialties: General presenting symptoms or syndromes

47. **A 63-year-old lady presents to her GP with a 3-month history of upper abdominal pain, lethargy, anorexia, weight loss, and night sweats. There is no recent history of trauma or travel. She appears pale and cachectic on inspection. Further examination reveals a temperature of 37.8°C, epigastric and left hypochondrial tenderness, and painless lymphadenopathy in the neck, axillae, and groins. Liver function tests reveal an elevated lactate dehydrogenase level. An ultrasound scan of the abdomen reveals gross splenomegaly with free fluid in the abdomen and pelvis. At laparotomy, an enlarged spleen is seen with several capsular tears and imminent rupture, so a splenectomy is performed. What is the most likely diagnosis?**

    A. Carcinoid tumour

    B. Kaposi's sarcoma

    C. Non-Hodgkin's lymphoma

    D. Infectious mononucleosis

    E. Multiple myeloma

Common surgical conditions and the subspecialties: Genitourinary disease

48. **An 8-month-old boy is taken to see the GP by his anxious mother, who is worried that his right testicle does not always seem to be present within his scrotum. Which of the following statements is true of undescended testes?**

    A. Inability to palpate the testes is an indication for laparoscopy

    B. One-quarter of undescended testes complete their descent in the first year of life

    C. Surgical exploration and fixation should be performed in the neonatal period to allow for easier repair of the defect

    D. Undescended testes are associated with a reduced risk of testicular malignancy

    E. Undescended testes are associated with normal fertility

Organ and tissue transplantation: Transplant immunology

49. The senior registrar on call for the transplant surgical team receives the HLA tissue typing and mismatch list from a donor, for a number of prospective renal transplant patients. Of the following combinations, which is the best mismatch for receiving the donor kidney?

   A. 1–0–1
   B. 0–1–1
   C. 1–1–0
   D. 0–0–1
   E. 1–1–1

Management of the dying patient: Palliative care

50. An 81-year-old gentleman undergoes endoscopic insertion of a self-expanding metallic stent, as a palliative treatment for inoperable oesophageal adenocarcinoma. Despite good initial symptom control, the patient presents 4 weeks later with intermittent dysphagia to both solids and liquids during meal times. Which of the following options is the most appropriate initial management for this patient?

   A. Carbonated drink ingestion
   B. Endoscopic laser ablation
   C. Endoscopic removal of stent
   D. Nasojejunal tube insertion
   E. Percutaneous endoscopic gastrostomy formation

1. Answer: D

It is most likely that this patient has sustained an injury to the marginal mandibular branch of the facial nerve during surgical removal of the submandibular gland. The submandibular gland occupies most of the submandibular or the digastric triangle. The marginal mandibular branch of the facial nerve courses between the deep surface of the platysma and the superficial aspect of the fascia that overlies the submandibular gland. The nerve supplies muscles of the lower lip and the chin. Injury to the nerve may thus result in difficulty in closing the mouth and loss of sensation over the chin and mandible. The facial artery and vein are located just deep to this nerve. The lingual nerve and submandibular duct (Wharton's duct) lie along the posterior border of the mylohyoid muscle. The hypoglossal nerve courses deep to the tendon of the digastric muscle and then lies medial to the deep cervical fascia.

2. Answer: B

SIRS is a generalized inflammatory response produced by the body in response to a variety of clinical insults such as infection (bacterial, viral, fungal), shock, trauma, burns, pancreatitis and tissue ischaemia. A clinical diagnosis of SIRS can be made when at least two of the following criteria are present: (1) temperature >38°C or <36°C; (2) heart rate >90/min; (iii) respiratory rate >20 or $PaCO_2$ <4.3 kPa; and WCC >12,000 or < 4000 × 10^9/L. The blood pressure is not a parameter used in diagnosing SIRS. 'Sepsis' is the term used to represent SIRS in the presence of infection. 'Severe sepsis' represents sepsis with evidence of organ hypoperfusion (e.g. hypoxaemia, oliguria, lactic acidosis, or altered cerebral function); while 'septic shock' refers to severe sepsis with hypotension (systolic blood pressure <90mmHg) despite adequate fluid resuscitation, or the requirement for vasopressors/inotropes to maintain blood pressure. The term 'septicaemia' was previously used to denote the presence of multiplying bacteria in the circulation, but has been replaced with the definitions provided here.

3. Answer: B

Macrophages ingest lipids to become foam cells in the process of atherosclerotic plaque formation. Mature atherosclerotic plaques develop over many years and progress through three main forms: fatty streaks, intermediate plaques, and mature fibrolipid plaques.

Fatty streaks are formed by focal deposition of lipoproteins in the arterial intima with the subsequent migration of monocytes and T cells to the subendothelial space. Monocytes differentiate to macrophages which ingest lipid to form foam cells. Smooth muscle cells then migrate from the media into the affected intima and secrete connective tissue components to form a fibrous cap on the luminal side, resulting in an intermediate plaque. This plaque then breaks down at the base to form a core of extracellular lipid and necrotic debris, which becomes calcified. This is covered by a collagen-rich fibrous cap forming a mature fibrolipid plaque.

4. Answer: E

A Jefferson fracture is a 'bursting type' fracture of the atlas (C1 vertebra). It involves fractures of the anterior and posterior arches, and causes the lateral masses to be displaced laterally. However, a Jefferson fracture does not produce neurological injury, as there is no encroachment on the neural canal. In contrast, atlanto-axial fracture-dislocations result in a posterior dislocation of the axis, causing the odontoid process to compress the spinal cord, thus leading to sudden death. Acute fractures of the axis (C2 vertebra) represent about 18–20% of all cervical spine injuries and approximately 60% of axis fractures involve the odontoid process. Fractures of the axis can be classified as type I (i.e. fractures involving the tip of the odontoid process), type II (i.e. the commonest type; fractures through the base of the dens, involving the junction of the odontoid peg with the body), and type III (i.e. fractures at the base of the dens, extending obliquely into the body of the axis). In type II fractures, the posterior elements of the axis (i.e. the pars interarticularis) may be fractured by a hyperextension injury (a hangman's fracture). Patients with this type of fracture should be maintained in external immobilization until specialized care is available. Odontoid fractures can be seen on plain radiography using a lateral cervical-spine view or open-mouth odontoid views. However, a CT scan may be required to further delineate the type and extent of the fracture.

5. Answer: E

Pierre Robin syndrome is an autosomal recessive disease, affecting approximately 1 in 8500 live births with a male-to-female ratio of 1:1 (except in the X-linked form). The widely accepted aetiological factor for this condition is that during the initial event, mandibular hypoplasia occurs between the 7–11th week of gestation. This keeps the tongue high in the oral cavity, causing a cleft in the palate by preventing the closure of the palatal shelves; this may explain the inverted U-shaped cleft and the absence of an associated cleft lip. Oligohydramnios may also play a role in the aetiology of this condition, since the lack of amniotic fluid could cause deformation of the chin and subsequent impaction of the tongue between the palatal shelves. The prevalence of cleft palate (soft and hard palatal clefts) may be as high as 91%. The cleft is usually U-shaped (80%) or V-shaped. Occasionally, it may present as a bifid or double uvula, or as an occult submucous cleft. Micrognathia is seen in the majority of cases; its features include retraction of the inferior dental arch behind the superior dental arch; and abnormal features of the mandible including a small body, obtuse genial angle and a posteriorly located condyle. The growth of the mandible catches up during the first year. The mandibular hypoplasia resolves and the child attains a normal profile by approximately 5–6 years of age. The combination of micrognathia and glossoptosis may cause severe respiratory and feeding difficulties as well as obstructive sleep apnoea in the newborn. The most common otic abnormality is otitis media (about 80%), followed by auricular anomalies (75%), conductive hearing loss (nearly 50%), and external auditory canal atresia (5%). Delayed eruption of the teeth is not a recognized feature of Pierre Robin syndrome.

6. Answer: C

The normal 24-hour fluid requirements for a 70-kg adult male include 40 mL/kg of water, 2 mmol/kg of sodium and 0.5–1 mmol/kg of potassium.

Normal saline (0.9% sodium chloride) has 150 mmol of sodium and 10 mmol of chloride. It is an isotonic solution but can cause hyperchloraemic metabolic acidosis if overused.

Hartmann's solution is an isotonic balanced salt solution and it does not cause acidosis. Sodium and chloride concentrations are less than in normal saline.

5% dextrose contains 50g/L of glucose and no electrolytes. The glucose gets metabolized to leave free water, which equilibrates across all body fluid compartments. It is ineffective at resuscitating the intravascular space but can be used to replace whole body water loss.

Dextrose saline (4% dextrose, 0.18% saline) reduces the risk of sodium overload but can cause water overload.

7. Answer: D

Traumatic dislocation of the hip is one of the few true orthopaedic emergencies, with 80% being posterior dislocations. It often occurs in road traffic accidents, in which the patient may have been seated in a car and have been thrown forward, hitting their knee against the dashboard and forcing the femoral head upwards and backwards, dislocating the hip joint posteriorly. This mechanism of injury may cause a concomitant fracture of the acetabulum (i.e. being a fracture-dislocation of the hip joint). On examination, the leg at the side of the dislocation is adducted, internally rotated, slightly flexed, and is shorter than the unaffected leg. This injury may be missed if there is a fracture of one of the long bones of the lower limb (e.g. the femur). In order not to miss this injury, pelvic radiography should be performed in all cases of major lower limb trauma. Signs of sciatic nerve injury may also be present. In such instances, the risk of avascular necrosis of the hip increases over time. Due to the force involved in the injury, reduction will be very unlikely in the Emergency Department. The patient must therefore be sent to theatre immediately for closed reduction of the hip.

8. Answer: C

The posterior cricoarytenoid muscles are small, paired laryngeal muscles that extend from the posterior cricoid cartilage to the arytenoid cartilages. By rotating the arytenoid cartilages laterally, these muscles abduct the vocal cords and thereby open the rima glottidis. Their action opposes the lateral cricoarytenoid muscles, which are primarily responsible for vocal cord adduction. Both the posterior and lateral cricoarytenoid muscles are innervated by the recurrent laryngeal nerve. Paralysis of the posterior cricoarytenoid muscles may lead to asphyxiation as they are the only laryngeal muscles to open the true vocal folds, allowing inspiration and expiration.

The cricothyroid muscle originates from the anterolateral cricoid cartilage and inserts into the inferior cornu and lamina of the thyroid cartilage. It is the only laryngeal muscle to be supplied by the external branch of the superior laryngeal nerve (i.e. instead of the recurrent laryngeal nerve). Its contraction produces tension and elongation of the vocal folds, resulting in higher pitched phonation.

The thyroarytenoid is a broad, thin muscle lying parallel and lateral to the vocal fold. It functions to allow fine tonal control of the vocal cords. The transverse arytenoid muscle is an unpaired muscle that crosses transversely between the two arytenoids cartilages, serving to adduct them. Both of these muscles are supplied by the recurrent laryngeal nerve.

9. Answer: A

Continence in maintained by several mechanisms:

- The anorectal angle occurs partly due to the embryological formation of the anorectum and is partly maintained by the pull of the puborectalis, but is not of major functional importance.
- The internal anal sphincter has a constant low resting tone under autonomic control. Reflex increases in tone occur in response to coughing and straining to prevent leakage of gas, fluid and small amounts of solid.
- The endoanal cushions are formed from the submucosal vascular and connective tissue; they function to physically plug the anal canal, ensuring its continence towards gas and fluid.
- The external anal sphincter is under voluntary control. Its tone can usually be increased to defer defaecation until appropriate.

10. Answer: E

The history of smoking, working in the petrochemical industry, and other pertinent signs and symptoms in this patient are highly suggestive of carcinoma of the bladder. Carcinoma of the bladder epithelium is the most common tumour of the genitourinary tract, with transitional cell carcinoma accounting for 90% of all bladder malignancies (about 5% are squamous carcinomas and 2% are adenocarcinomas). The peak incidence is in the seventh decade, and there is a male to female preponderance of 3:1. Some of the recognized risk factors for the development of carcinoma of the bladder include cigarette smoking (more than 20 cigarettes/day increases the risk of developing bladder cancer by 2–6 times), working in the aniline dye industry, rubber industry, petrochemical industry, printing industry, schistosomiasis of the bladder, local radiation therapy, some chemotherapeutic drugs and long-term catheterization. Some recognized bladder carcinogens include benzidine, aromatic amines and nitrosamines, as well as various dyes and solvents. Patients with carcinoma of the bladder most commonly present with painless haematuria but may also present with dysuria, frequency and urgency of micturition. The patient may have symptoms of anaemia such as palpitations, dryness and pallor of the tongue and generalized tiredness. Investigations include urine microscopy and culture (to exclude infection) and cystoscopy. Endoscopic resection of the lesion followed by a 4–6-week course of radiotherapy to the bladder and the pelvic side walls are useful in treating the majority of the tumours. A combination chemotherapy regimen comprising cisplatin, methotrexate, and vinblastine (and adriamycin in some cases) is useful in the treatment of metastatic disease.

11. Answer: C

Supracondylar fractures of the humerus most commonly occur in children as a consequence of falling on the hand with the elbow bent. The distal fragment of bone is displaced backwards and angulated, although anterior displacement may rarely occur. The main complication of such fractures is injury to the brachial artery, which runs in close proximity to the fracture site, and may become kinked over the anterior prominence of the proximal fragment or become lacerated. This may result in oedema of the forearm and subsequent compartment syndrome. The distal circulation must therefore be carefully assessed and documented in the patient's notes. Other complications include transient median nerve injury, tardy ulnar palsy (i.e. a late complication caused by stretching of the ulnar nerve) and malunion, which may lead to the appearance of a 'gunstock deformity'. Initial management includes analgesia and an emergency reduction of the fracture into a good anatomical position; this usually results in unkinking of the brachial artery and restoration of the distal perfusion. If this is unsuccessful, surgical exploration of the brachial artery is warranted, and should be performed by a vascular surgeon. Lacerations of the artery are repaired either primarily (i.e. with sutures) or with vein grafts.

12. Answer: B

Exomphalos (or 'omphalocoele') is a congenital malformation involving of part of the intestine herniating through a defect in the abdominal wall at the umbilicus, with an incidence of 1 in 5000 births. It is due to failure of the intestine to return to the abdomen during early gestation. The herniated bowel is contained within a sac, the wall of which is a thin, semitranslucent membrane, which may remain unruptured. However, a large sac may occasionally rupture during birth, causing peritonitis and death. The sac comprises three layers: amniotic membrane on the outside, Wharton's jelly in the middle and the inner peritoneum. Exomphalos is frequently associated with other conditions—50% of infants have other serious defects involving the gastrointestinal, cardiovascular, genitourinary, musculoskeletal, and central nervous systems. Emergency management includes the insertion of an orogastric tube for gastric decompression and to prevent bowel distension caused by aerophagia. If patient transfer is necessary, the omphalocoele must be covered with a sterile saline-soaked dressing or cling film to prevent fluid loss. The patient's overall condition and associated anomalies must be thoroughly assessed before surgical intervention is undertaken.

The main differential diagnosis is gastroschisis, which also involves evisceration of the bowel through the anterior abdominal wall. However, in gastroschisis, the protruding bowel is not contained with a sac; and there are usually no associated congenital abnormalities. Management involves early prevention of hypothermia, hypovolaemia, and sepsis (i.e. resulting from the exposed bowel) upon delivery. The lower half of the infant should be placed into a sterile bag and fluids administered at two-and-a-half times of that of a normal newborn. An orogastric tube must be used to avoid aerophagia and to aspirate intestinal contents because of the associated paralytic ileus. Parenteral antibiotics should also be given and following reduction of the viscera and closure of the defect, total parenteral nutrition should be continued for 3–4 weeks.

Duodenal atresia is associated with Down's syndrome and presents differently (i.e. profuse bile stained vomiting and gastric distension from birth). It may involve the complete absence of the duodenum, a fibrous band, a diaphragm, or a partial diaphragm; and most commonly occurs at the transition point between foregut and midgut.

Hirschsprung's disease manifests in the immediate neonatal period by the failure to pass meconium, followed by obstructive constipation. It is due to a developmental failure of the parasympathetic plexuses of Auerbach and Meissner in the gut. If only a small segment of the rectum is affected, the accumulation of pressure may permit the occasional passage of stools, resulting in intermittent bouts of diarrhoea.

Imperforate anus is another cause of neonatal intestinal obstruction, and often manifests as failure to pass meconium. It describes a spectrum of abnormalities affecting the anorectal area and is a cause of bladder and sexual dysfunction. It is usually discovered during routine neonatal checking.

13. Answer: D

Diarrhoea associated with enteral feeding may be due to a low temperature of the feed, high osmolarity of the feed, lactose intolerance, fat malabsorption, hypoalbuminaemia, drugs (e.g. antibiotics or sorbitol-containing preparations), contaminated feed (i.e. resulting in gastroenteritis), low fibre intake, and bolus tube feeding regimes (or rapid continuous feeding). Constipation with overflow diarrhoea should also be excluded. It is known that gastric feeding more commonly results in diarrhoea than jejunal feeding. Of these options, only reduced fluid replacement would result in more formed stool. Reduced intestinal absorptive capacity, of any cause, is likely to cause diarrhoea due to the osmotic effect of the enteral feed.

14. Answer: A

This is a typical presentation of bleeding oesophageal varices. Beta-blockers and nitrates have been shown to be useful in the prophylaxis of variceal bleeding. For acutely bleeding varices, current evidence supports endoscopic therapy (sclerotherapy or band ligation) as the most effective means of control. Vasoactive drugs (e.g. vasopressin, terlipressin, octreotide, somatostatin) may also be used, and recent evidence supports their effectiveness when used in combination with endoscopic therapy to control the initial variceal bleed. If endoscopic and drug treatments fail, balloon tamponade (e.g. with a Sengstaken–Blakemore tube) can provide temporary haemostasis. Subsequent definitive management would include radiological (e.g. transjugular intrahepatic porto-systemic shunt or TIPS) or surgical (e.g. oesophageal transection, portosystemic shunting) procedures.

15. Answer: D

The pudendal nerve is a somatosensory nerve in the pelvic region and is a large branch of the sacral plexus (L4–L5, S1–S4). It originates in Onuf's nucleus in the sacral region of the spinal cord and arises from the anterior rami of the 2nd–4th sacral roots. The nerve passes between piriformis and coccygeus, leaving the pelvis through the lower part of the greater sciatic foramen. It crosses the ischial spine and re-enters the pelvis through the lesser sciatic foramen. It then accompanies the internal pudendal vessels upward and forward along the lateral wall of the ischiorectal fossa, being contained in a sheath of the obturator fascia (i.e. the pudendal canal).

The pudendal nerve gives off the inferior rectal nerves before dividing into two terminal branches: the perineal nerve, and the dorsal nerve of the penis (in males) or the dorsal nerve of the clitoris (in females). The inferior rectal nerve innervates the external anal sphincter and the perianal skin. The perineal nerve innervates the sphincter urethrae and other muscles of the anterior compartment via a deep branch, and the skin of the perineum posterior to the clitoris via its superficial branch. The dorsal nerves of the penis and clitoris innervate the skin of the penis and that surrounding the clitoris respectively.

The levator ani muscles are mostly innervated by the pudendal nerve, perineal nerve and inferior rectal nerve in concert. The testes are innervated by the spermatic (or 'testicular') plexus, which is derived from the renal plexus (which itself receives branches from the aortic plexus).

As demonstrated by this case, it is important to remember the structures passing through the greater and lesser sciatic foramina:

- Greater sciatic foramen:
  - Above piriformis: superior gluteal vessels; superior gluteal nerve
  - Below piriformis: inferior gluteal and internal pudendal vessels; inferior gluteal nerve; pudendal nerve; sciatic nerve; posterior femoral cutaneous nerve; nerve to obturator internus; nerve to quadratus femoris
- Lesser sciatic foramen:
  - Tendon of obturator internus; internal pudendal vessels; pudendal nerve; nerve to the obturator internus.

16. Answer: A

When looking at a near object, the lens must accommodate (i.e. round up) in order to create sufficient refraction of light. Activation of the parasympathetic nervous system causes contraction of the ciliary muscles, resulting in a reduced pull on the lens by the suspensory ligaments, thus allowing the lens to remain more spherical. Alterations in the diameter of the pupil in response to changes in the ambient light are mediated solely via the parasympathetic neurons of the oculomotor nerve (CN III). However, in response to a change in emotions such as happiness or increased libido, activation of the sympathetic nervous system can cause pupillary dilatation. Micturition or voiding of the bladder is a parasympathetic reflex; the parasympathetic nerves arising in the sacral regions of the spinal cord (S2, S3, and S4) innervate the detrusor muscle and it compresses the sphincter at the neck of the bladder. Thus, a lesion at the level of T10 would affect the micturition reflex. Increased sympathetic activity, such as that observed during a fight or flight response, results in increased sweating. However, sweat production is unusual as the post-ganglionic sympathetic innervation of the sweat glands is cholinergic rather than adrenergic. Bronchial diameter is very sensitive to changes in the levels of circulating adrenaline. Respiratory frequency, however, is controlled by the medullary brainstem respiratory control centre, which in turn regulates the contraction of skeletal muscles such as the diaphragm and intercostal muscles.

17. Answer: C

Chronic exposure to sunlight increases the risk of occurrence of squamous cell carcinoma, basal cell carcinoma and malignant melanoma. UVB is a small but very dangerous part of sunlight, as it causes direct DNA damage. It is mostly absorbed by the ozone layer but prolonged exposure can increase the incidence of skin cancers.

Other risk factors for skin cancer include dysplastic naevi, fair skin types, immunosuppressed states, strong family history and ionizing radiation. Ultraviolet light exposure is the most important risk factor for developing malignant melanoma.

18. Answer: C

The prothrombin time (PT) and platelet aggregation are usually normal in type I von Willebrand's disease. It is the bleeding time, partial thromboplastin time (APTT) and factor VIII-coagulant (VIIIc) that are likely to be abnormal. Although the bleeding time would serve as a good screening test, the patient's coagulopathy is already known and so this test will not give a quantitative measurement of her bleeding tendency. In the same way, APTT will not be very useful. The most useful test in practice is therefore the von Willebrand's antigen and activity (RICOF) but the factor VIIIc level should also be checked, as as it is also low in von Willebrand's disease.

19. Answer: D

FNAC involves a needle being advanced into a lesion, with suction applied as the needle is moved in different directions within the mass (i.e. stereotactically). In experienced hands, the technique is very accurate with a 1% false positive and a 5% false negative rate. However, FNAC cannot distinguish between follicular adenoma and carcinoma because the principal difference between them is that follicular carcinoma involves capsular invasion (i.e. something that FNAC cannot determine; evaluation by frozen section is required for follicular carcinoma). Core needle (e.g. Trucut) biopsy can provide information about the histology and the hormone receptor status of tumours, which FNAC cannot do. All patients presenting with a breast lump should undergo triple assessment, which includes clinical examination, radiological examination (ultrasound if under 35 years or mammography if over 35 years) and either FNAC or core biopsy. Finally, branchial cysts usually produce an opalescent fluid containing cholesterol crystals or frank pus, whilst thyroglossal cysts commonly contain serous fluid.

20. Answer: C

The right coronary artery arises form the anterior aortic sinus. It proceeds along the right atrioventricular groove and gives rise to the marginal branch, which supplies the right ventricle.

The left coronary artery, which is usually larger than the right coronary artery, arises from the left posterior aortic sinus and divides into the anterior interventricular branch and a circumflex branch in the atrioventricular groove.

Dominance is based on the origin of the posterior interventricular artery. In right dominance (90%) the posterior interventricular artery is a large branch of the right coronary artery. Approximately 3% of hearts are co-dominant.

The sinoatrial node is usually supplied by the right coronary artery but sometimes by the left coronary artery. The AV node is consistently supplied by the right coronary artery.

21. Answer: C

The cardiac action potential of non-nodal cells has the following phases (Figure 5.1):

  Phase 0: rapid depolarization due to rapid influx of sodium ions into the cells.

  Phase 1: fast sodium channels close. The small downward deflection is due to continuing outflow of potassium and chloride.

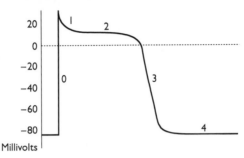

Figure 5.1 Cardiac action potential (for non-nodal cells) demonstrating the five phases of the action potential.

Reproduced from Matthew D. Gardiner and Neil R. Borley, Training in Surgery, 2009, Figure 2.1, p. 13, with permission from Oxford University Press.

Phase 2: plateau phase balancing the slow inflow of calcium and outflow of potassium.

Phase 3: slow calcium channels close while potassium channels remain open. The net current leads to a negative change in membrane potential and the opening of rapid delayed potassium channels. This repolarization returns cells their resting state.

Phase 4: resting membrane potential is restored.

22. Answer: D

The muscles involved in the Achilles tendon reflex are supplied by the tibial nerve (a branch of the sciatic nerve), which is derived from the S1 and S2 nerve roots. The tibial nerve forms in the popliteal fossa, and leaves it running inferiorly on the tibialis posterior muscle. It supplies the posterior muscles of the leg and knee joint, and terminates by dividing into the medial and lateral plantar nerves.

23. Answer: C

This severely malnourished patient has developed refeeding syndrome, as a result of the abrupt reinstitution of nutrition via her nasogastric tube. Individuals with negligible nutrient intake for 5 consecutive days are at risk of this syndrome, which usually occurs within 4 days of recommencing feeding. Refeeding malnourished patients increases basal metabolic rate with glucose being the predominant energy source. This anabolic response causes intracellular shift of minerals, causing serum levels to fall significantly. These rapid metabolic changes and electrolyte movements may lead to severe cardiorespiratory and neurological problems resulting in cardiorespiratory failure, lethargy, confusion, coma, convulsions, and death. The symptoms of refeeding syndrome are thought to be due predominantly to hypophosphataemia but metabolic changes in potassium, magnesium, glucose, and thiamine can also contribute to this. Although calcium depletion is possible, the absence of tetany in this patient makes serum calcium a less urgent test than serum phosphate. Although vitamin B stores may also be depleted in such individuals, this patient's presentation also lacks the neuro-ophthalmological features of vitamin B deficiency, to warrant urgent testing of serum vitamin B levels.

24. Answer: A

Perforation of the oesophagus most commonly occurs during upper GI endoscopy, especially if oesophageal dilatation or stenting is being performed, or if the patient has an unrecognized pharyngeal pouch. The location of the perforation is variable. Iatrogenic perforation may also occur during trans-oesophageal echocardiography and antireflux or thoracic surgery. However, as in this case, perforation may occur as a result of vomiting against a closed glottis, leading to a sudden increase in oesophageal intraluminal pressure (Boerhaave's syndrome). The rupture usually occurs in the lower third of the oesophagus, leading to spillage of highly irritant oesophagogastric contents into the mediastinum and widespread chemical and bacterial mediastinitis. The site of perforation can occasionally be intraperitoneal. Other causes of oesophageal perforation, such as ulcerating oesophageal carcinomas or gunshot/knife injuries, are far less common. Patients present with epigastric pain or shock out of proportion to the apparent injury. Note that Mackler's triad describes the classical features of Boerhaave's syndrome (i.e. vomiting, followed by severe chest pain and subcutaneous emphysema). Delayed presentations may result in collapse, with features of severe sepsis. Initial investigations include basic blood tests and an ECG (i.e. to rule out cardiogenic chest pain), followed by an erect CXR (on which a pathognomonic pneumomediastinum, pleural effusion or pneumothorax may be identified). Perforation of the intra-abdominal oesophagus results in free gas under the diaphragm.

Initial treatment comprises airway management, fluid resuscitation, catheterization, thromboprophylaxis, parenteral analgesia (i.e. ensuring that the patient remains nil-by-mouth), IV broad-spectrum antibiotics, and IV proton pump inhibitor administration. Further investigations may include CT thorax, upper GI endoscopy, and contrast (i.e. water-soluble) swallow. Further management may be non-operative (i.e. especially for iatrogenic perforations with minimal mediastinal contamination) with enteral feeding via a NJT or jejunostomy site, oesophageal stenting, and HDU or ITU support. Operative management may be indicated especially for Boerhaave's syndrome, extensive contamination, or in unstable patients. This may entail primary repair of the ruptured oesophagus with washout of the mediastinal, pleural or peritoneal cavities; establishing a controlled fistula (i.e. with a T-tube, especially if there is uncertainty surrounding the need for primary repair or the degree of contamination); or even oesophagectomy.

25. Answer: D

After performing the wide local incision, a second transverse incision is made in the axilla. Dissection progresses through the subcutaneous fat and the clavipectoral fascia down to the lateral border of the pectoralis major. The axillary vein and thoracodorsal pedicle are identified and preserved. The intercostobrachial nerve (T2) is also protected if possible, but if it gets in the way of the complete excision of lymph nodes then it can be divided. The long thoracic nerve is also preserved. The intercostobrachial nerve is the lateral cutaneous branch of the second intercostal nerve. The medial cutaneous nerve of the arm (C8, T1) arises from the medial cord and is the smallest branch of the brachial plexus. The long thoracic nerve of Bell arises from the C5–C7 nerve roots and supplies the serratus anterior. The thoracodorsal nerve arises from the posterior cord of the brachial plexus and supplies the latissimus dorsi.

26. Answer: B

Gastrin is secreted by the G cells in the antrum of the stomach and the duodenum in response to food entry and vagal stimulation. Gastrin stimulates gastric acid secretion by Parietal cells, pepsinogen secretion by Chief cells, and histamine release by enterochromaffin-like cells. Gastrin acts to increase the lower oesophageal sphincter pressures, relax the pyloric sphincter, and promote gastric and intestinal motility and secretion. Secretin is produced by the S cells of the villi and crypts of the small intestine in response to acidification of duodenal contents. Secretin stimulates pancreatic enzyme and bicarbonate release while inhibiting gastric acid and pepsin secretion. It also potentiates the action of cholecystokinin, which is produced by the I cells of the duodenum and jejunum. This occurs in response to the presence of intraluminal fat, amino acids and peptides, to stimulate gallbladder contraction and the release of pancreatic enzymes and bicarbonate. Vasoactive intestinal peptide is a neurotransmitter which is secreted by the small intestine in response to vagal stimulation. It promotes gallbladder and gastric relaxation and inhibits the secretion of gastric acid and pepsin. It also acts to increase pancreatic and intestinal secretions.

27. Answer: D

Mirizzi syndrome is due to impaction of gallstones either in the cystic duct or Hartmann's pouch of the gallbladder, which leads to external compression of the common hepatic duct and results in symptoms of obstructive jaundice. Impaction of gallstone(s) in Hartmann's pouch or the cystic duct results in Mirizzi syndrome either by: (1) chronic and/or acute inflammatory changes leading to contraction of the gallbladder and stenosis of the common hepatic duct, or (2) cholecysto-choledochal fistula formation due to direct pressure necrosis of adjacent duct walls from large impacted stones. Patients may present with pain over the right upper quadrant of the abdomen, vomiting, fever, recurrent cholangitis, cholecystitis, or pancreatitis. Pale stools and dark urine result from obstruction of the flow of bile into the intestine. Exploration of the common bile duct by either open or laparoscopic cholecystectomy and placement of a T-tube is a recognized method of managing this condition.

28. Answer: D

Three main longitudinal arteries supply blood to the spinal cord it. These comprise an anterior spinal artery and two posterior spinal arteries that are unlikely to be damaged during the proce-dure. The spinal cord also receives arterial supply from branches of the vertebral (directly off the aorta), ascending cervical, deep cervical, intercostal, lumbar and lateral sacral arteries. The circu-lation to much of the inferior portion of the spinal cord is supplied by the anterior and posterior segmental medullary arteries which are located chiefly at the cervical and lumbosacral enlarge-ments. They enter the canal through the intervertebral foramina. The great anterior medullary artery (i.e. artery of Adamkiewicz) supplies blood to the inferior two-thirds of the spinal cord and is found on the left side in 65% of people. The accidental ligation of this artery may result in a loss of function of the lower limbs, bladder and intestines, although patients commonly remain asymptomatic due to adequate collateral blood supply to these areas.

29. Answer: C

The three phases of gastric secretion are:

- Cephalic phase: the excitatory stage (via odours and thoughts, processed in the cerebral cortex, hypothalamus, and medulla) is responsible for saliva production, some pancreatic juice production and 10% of gastric acid secretion.
- Gastric phase: this is mediated via the short gastric reflex (via local neurohormonal pathways in the stomach wall) and the long vagus reflex. It is responsible for 80% of gastric secretion.
- Intestinal phase: this is responsible for 10% of gastric secretion.

Gastric secretion is stimulated by:

- Gastrin
- Histamine, which is produced by mast cells
- Acetylcholine: from parasympathetic vagal neurones, which directly innervate parietal cells

Gastric secretion is inhibited by secretin, cholecystokinin, and somatostatin.

30. Answer: D

Meconium ileus occurs in up to 1 in 5000 live births. Although it occurs in only 15% of neonates with cystic fibrosis, 90% of patients with meconium ileus have cystic fibrosis. Failure of pancreatic secretion causes inspissated meconium, which obstructs the bowel lumen. The colon is small and unused (microcolon) and meconium is not passed. The proximal bowel dilates with subsequent abdominal distension and vomiting in the first day of life. Complications include volvulus, atresia, perforation and/or meconium peritonitis.

Meconium plug syndrome is the commonest cause of bowel obstruction and is seen in 1 in 500 live births. In this condition, inspissated meconium obstructs the distal colon. It has an infrequent association with Hirschsprung's disease and cystic fibrosis.

31. Answer: E

The popliteal fossa is a diamond-shaped region on the posterior aspect of the knee. It is bounded superomedially by the semimembranosus and semitendinosus muscles; superolaterally by the biceps femoris muscle; and inferolaterally and inferomedially by the lateral and medial heads of the gastrocnemius muscle respectively. The fossa is overlain by the popliteal fascia, which is perforated by the short saphenous vein and the sural nerve. The sural nerve is the most superficial structure and is thus most likely to be encountered when the popliteal fossa is explored during surgery. The important contents of the fossa include the popliteal artery and vein, tibial and common peroneal nerves, short saphenous vein, sural nerve, posterior femoral cutaneous nerve, and obturator nerve.

32. Answer: A

Hyperparathyroidism is classified as primary, secondary or tertiary disease.

Primary hyperparathyroidism is usually due to a parathyroid adenoma and is characterized by high circulating levels of PTH resulting in excessive resorption of calcium and phosphate from bone. Most patients are asymptomatic but symptoms may be related to elevated PTH or hypercalcaemia, which can be remembered as 'stones, bones, abdominal groans, and psychic moans'.

Symptoms of raised PTH include: urinary tract stones due to excessive calcium excretion, bone pains, and pathological fractures due to osteopenia.

Symptoms of hypercalcaemia include fatigue, abdominal pain, vomiting, constipation, polyuria, polydipsia, and psychiatric disturbances (depression, confusion).

33. Answer: C

Malignant parotid tumours would metastasize to the deep cervical nodes. These nodes form a chain along the course of the internal jugular vein from the skull to the root of the neck. Table 5.1 demonstrates the patterns of lymphatic drainage from the head and neck.

Table 5.1 Head and neck lymphatic drainage patterns

Lymph node group	Anatomical sites drained
Submandibular	Oral cavity
Preauricular	Scalp and skin
Posterior cervical	Scalp, neck, upper thoracic skin
Deep cervical	(to jugular trunk)
Superficial cervical	Larynx, tongue, oropharynx, anterior neck
Supraclavicular	Gastrointestinal tract, genitourinary tract and pulmonary regions

34. Answer: A

The scenario describes the features of a malignant melanoma. Further to the features described, characteristics which are suggestive of malignant melanoma include: increase in size, spread of pigmentation, red halo around the lesion, satellite lesions and pain.

The feature which most accurately describes the risk of regional or distant metastasis is the depth of the primary lesion. This is called Breslow's thickness, first described by Alexander Breslow, who found a correlation between the thickness of the tumour on histological examination and 10-year survival without nodal or distant metastasis (Table 5.2).

Table 5.2 Tumour thickness and risk of metastasis

Tumour thickness	Risk of regional metastasis	Risk of distant metastasis	10-year survival without nodal or distant metastasis
<1 mm	3–5%	3–5%	95%
1–4 mm	25–60%	10–20%	60–75%
>4 mm	>60%	70%	45%

Options B, C, and D are poor prognostic indicators of malignant melanoma. Scalp lesions tend to recur locally. Lesions on the head, neck and trunk carry a worse prognosis than those of the extremities. Other prognostic factors include: pathological stage, number and size of lymph node metastasis, and gender—females with thick lesions fare better than males.

35. Answer: E

There are numerous lymphatic vessels that drain lymph from the thyroid gland. Due to this, there is a high propensity for metastasis of thyroid malignancies. The lymph from the thyroid gland is drained by: (1) the pre-laryngeal nodes (that lie above thyroid isthmus) via the tracheal plexus; (2) the pre-tracheal nodes (that lie along the recurrent laryngeal nerve); (3) the paratracheal nodes (that also lie along the recurrent laryngeal nerve); (4) the brachiocephalic nodes (that lie in the superior mediastinum); (5) the deep cervical nodes via the superior thyroid vessels; and (6) the thoracic duct (directly). The pectoral nodes, which lie along the inferior border of the pectoralis minor, drain most of the breast (and not the thyroid).

36. Answer: B

This patient has the classical clinical history, signs and symptoms of Boerhaave's syndrome. This is the spontaneous, complete (i.e. transmural) rupture of a non-diseased oesophagus, usually induced by episodes of vigorous vomiting, and frequently seen in alcoholics. The dramatically raised intra-oesophageal pressure caused by vigorous vomiting and associated failure of the cricopharyngeal sphincter to relax may lead to sudden spontaneous rupture of the oesophagus. The most common anatomical location of the tear is at the left posterolateral wall of the lower third of the oesophagus, 2–3 cm proximal to the gastro-oesophageal junction, along the longitudinal wall of the oesophagus. The signs and symptoms include sudden pain in the thorax and epigastrium following forceful protracted vomiting, pain radiating to the neck, progressive dyspnoea, tachypnoea, cyanosis, hypotension and shock. Subcutaneous emphysema may be present, palpable in the neck or chest, but this sign may take time to develop. The triad of vomiting, chest pain, and subcutaneous emphysema is also known as 'Mackler triad'; however, this should not always be relied upon since only one or two of the listed symptoms are present in the majority of patients in the early stages. Examination of the chest may reveal decreased breath sounds on the side of the perforation (usually the left side). Chest radiography may reveal an abnormal left cardiac border with free fluid within the left hemithorax, as well as air in the mediastinum and under the diaphragm. A definitive diagnosis may be made with gastrografin swallow to show the site of the perforation; CT scanning may be considered. Treatment is ideally surgical, and should be instituted within 6 hours of diagnosis and stabilization of the patient. After this time, the metabolic effects and damage to the oesophagus make survival less likely. Surgery entails draining the pleural cavity, searching for concomitant pathology at thoracotomy, e.g. tumours, oversewing the lesion, and closing the chest with an underwater seal drain. Oesophagectomy may be required for extensive stenosing lesions. Parenteral feeding or a feeding gastrostomy may be required.

37. Answer: C

The recurrent laryngeal nerve (RLN) is a branch of the vagus nerve. It is described as recurrent due to its roundabout route: it descends down into the thorax before ascending to supply the larynx. It provides motor innervation to all the laryngeal muscles (except for the cricothyroid) and sensation to the larynx. In the neck, it is found behind the thyroid towards the inferior pole, in close association with the inferior thyroid artery. The nerve can pass above, below, or through the branches of this artery. The RLN can be easily damaged during thyroid and parathyroid surgery. Unilateral damage to the RLN will result in unilateral paralysis of the vocal cords and hoarseness of voice. Bilateral damage will present as marked dysphonia and difficulty in breathing. The right RLN lies more medially than the left and is therefore more likely to be damaged.

The external laryngeal nerve is a small branch of the superior laryngeal nerve, which descends on the larynx to supply the cricothyroid muscle. Damage to this nerve will present with difficulty in producing high pitched sounds and alteration in the fundamental speaking frequency, especially in women or professional singers.

Many surgeons recommend that patients undergoing parathyroid and thyroid surgery routinely undergo preoperative laryngoscopy to assess the vocal cords.

38. Answer: C

Fournier's gangrene is necrotizing fasciitis of the scrotum and perineum. Its aetiology and risk factors as follows:

- Anorectal causes: perianal abscess, bowel injury, inflammatory bowel disease.
- Urogenital causes: urethral injury (may be iatrogenic following urethral stricture manipulation), bulbourethral gland infection, lower urinary tract infections.
- Dermatological causes: hidradenitis suppurativa, trauma, surgical wounds (and subsequent infection).
- Other: HIV, systemic lupus erythematosus.

The patient is usually septic and will need resuscitation with intravenous fluid. The sepsis is usually caused by a combination of micro-organisms and should therefore be treated with broad-spectrum antibiotics. Such patients should inevitably be taken to theatre for debridement of devitalized skin and subcutaneous tissue. Most will need a re-look operation and secondary input from the plastic surgical team. It is associated with a 50% mortality rate.

39. Answer: E

This patient has the classical features of injury to the spinal accessory nerve. The superficial course of the spinal accessory nerve in the posterior cervical triangle makes it susceptible to both trauma and surgical injuries. Iatrogenic injury to the nerve can result from surgery to this region such as during radical neck dissection (for removal of pathological lymph nodes), cervical lymph node biopsy, cannulation of the internal jugular vein, and carotid endarterectomy. The spinal accessory nerve provides motor innervation to the sternocleidomastoid and the upper part of the trapezius muscles. The sternocleidomastoid muscle helps in the side-to-side movement of the neck, and tilts and rotates the head, whilst the trapezius muscle elevates, laterally rotates and retracts the scapula. Patients with injury to the spinal accessory nerve (and subsequent dysfunction of the trapezius) present with an asymmetric neckline, drooping shoulder and winging of the scapula (also seen in serratus anterior muscle palsy due to weakness or paralysis of the long thoracic nerve). However, long thoracic nerve injury does not cause drooping of the shoulder.

40. Answer: E

Courvoisier's law states that, in the presence of jaundice, an enlarged gallbladder is unlikely to be due to gallstones. In such cases, carcinoma of the pancreas or of the lower biliary tree are more likely. Gallstones form over a longer period of time, causing chronic irritation, fibrotic thickening and a shrunken gallbladder. In this scenario, given the history of weight loss, carcinoma of the pancreatic head is the most likely cause. All other causes result in pain or tenderness within the right upper quadrant. If the gallbladder outflow tract is obstructed with a stone, the gallbladder becomes distended with mucous and is referred to as a mucocoele, and is often palpable and tender. When its contents become infected, an abscess develops and is known as an empyema.

41. Answer: D

Ludwig's angina describes infection within the submandibular space. It is most common caused by odontogenic infections (>90%). Once developed, it can spread to the retropharyngeal space. The most life-threatening complication of Ludwig's angina is airway obstruction and therefore airway management is the foundation of its treatment. In the era prior to the development of antibiotics, mortality from this condition exceeded 50%.

The submandibular space lies between the floor of the mouth and the investing layer of fascia, bounded by the mandible superiorly till the mastoid process and the two bellies of the digastric muscle. The submandibular space is divided by the mylohyoid muscle into the sublingual space superiorly and submaxillary space inferiorly.

The retropharyngeal space lies between the prevertebral fascia and the fascia covering the pharynx. Abscesses in the retropharyngeal space can cause oedema and dysphagia. The prevertebral space lies between the prevertebral fascia and the vertebral bodies. An abscess in this space can extend as far down as the thoracic vertebrae.

42. Answer: B

The female lifetime risk for developing breast cancer in the UK is 1 in 9. Many risk factors are thought to act by increasing lifetime exposure to oestrogen:

- High risk: increasing age, family history of breast cancer
- Medium risk: high socioeconomic status, late first pregnancy (>30 years), past history of breast cancer, breast irradiation <20 years
- Low risk: early menarche (<11 years), nulliparity, late menopause (>55 years), oral contraceptive therapy, and postmenopausal use of hormone replacement therapy, obesity, alcohol.

43. Answer: C

The inguinal canal contains the spermatic cord and the ilioinguinal nerve. The spermatic cord is ensheathed in the following three layers:

- External spermatic fascia (extension of the innominate fascia overlying the aponeurosis of the external oblique)
- Cremasteric muscle (extension of the internal oblique and transversus abdominis)
- Internal spermatic fascia (continuation of the transversalis fascia)

The spermatic cord contains the following structures:

- Arteries: testicular artery, artery to the vas deferens, cremasteric artery

- Nerves: genital branch of the genitofemoral nerve and sympathetics (note that the ilioinguinal nerve runs within the inguinal canal but lies outside of the spermatic cord)
- Other structures: vas deferens, pampiniform plexus, and lymphatics

44. Answer: A

The main complications of subarachnoid haemorrhage are:

- Mortality: 50% in the first month; many patients die before reaching hospital.
- Rebleeding: without intervention, 10% of patients rebleed within hours, 30% within 4 weeks, and 50% within 6 months. Apnoea occurs in 30% of all cases, and assisted ventilation can be used to restore spontaneous respiration in most cases. Emergency clipping is the mainstay of treatment for such rebleeding.
- Cerebral ischaemia: usually insidious and diffuse. A declining level of consciousness is observed in most cases, with half of patients exhibiting focal neurological signs. Cerebral perfusion must be increased by expanding plasma volume and/or inducing hypertension with dopamine or dobutamine. Transluminal angioplasty is rarely performed because of the associated risks.
- Hydrocephalus: this occurs acutely within the first few days in 15–20% of cases. Gradual obtundation is suggestive, and spontaneous improvement is seen in about half of patients within 24 hours, as long as massive intraventricular haemorrhage is absent. An external ventricular catheter may be beneficial but carries an increased risk of rebleeding. Lumbar puncture may obviate the need for a shunt if the obstruction lies in the subarachnoid space rather than the ventricular system.

45. Answer: E

Zygomatic fractures are the commonest fractures of the upper cheek. Diplopia suggests misalignment of the visual axis and injury to the eyeball and orbit. The most serious form of zygomatic fractures are tripod fractures that involve fractures through the infra-orbital canal into the infra-orbital groove, fractures through the zygomaticoparietal suture and through the zygomatic arch. The zygomatic arch usually fractures at its narrowest point or at the suture between the zygomatic process of the temporal bone and the temporal process of the zygomatic bone.

46. Answer: E

The renin-angiotensin-aldosterone system is a hormonal axis which regulates fluid and electrolyte balance, and blood pressure. When there is decreased renal perfusion, the juxtaglomerular cells in the kidney release renin. Renin cleaves the zymogen angiotensinogen, converting it into angiotensin I. Angiotensin I acts on receptors within the heart (increasing contractility and ventricular hypertrophy), vasculature (vasoconstriction, angiogenesis), kidneys (reduced GFR due to vasoconstriction of efferent glomerular vessels, inhibition of renin release, and increased proximal tubular sodium transport) and in the adrenal glands, where it stimulates aldosterone biosynthesis and catecholamine secretion. Angiotensin I is then converted to angiotensin II by angiotensin converting enzyme (ACE) found in lung and renal endothelium. Angiotensin II stimulates the secretion of aldosterone from the adrenal cortex. Aldosterone acts by increasing the reabsorption of sodium and water, thereby increasing the blood pressure. Angiotensin II also stimulates the release of antidiuretic hormone from the posterior pituitary gland, to act on the central nervous system to stimulate thirst.

Renal artery stenosis has been implicated in 1% of all hypertensive patients. In such individuals (i.e. especially those with bilateral renal artery stenoses), ACE inhibitors would inhibit the production of angiotensin II, and thereby eliminate its ability to constrict the glomerular efferent arterioles to maintain the glomerular filtration rate. This often results in acute renal failure and can be detected as a progressively rising serum creatinine level in such patients.

47. Answer: C

The symptoms and signs in this patient are clearly suggestive of non-Hodgkin's lymphoma, a malignancy of the lymphatic system. Approximately 85% of non-Hodgkin's lymphomas are derived from a clone of B cells, and the remainder have a T-cell origin. Non-Hodgkin lymphoma may develop in any organ associated with the lymphatic system such as the spleen, lymph nodes and tonsils. The disease spreads from one lymph node group to another, and the patients develop systemic symptoms with advanced disease. The common clinical presentations of non-Hodgkin lymphoma include pyrexia of unknown origin, night sweats, anorexia, weight loss, fatigue, and the development of painless, generalized lymphadenopathy. Abdominal involvement of the disease may lead to abdominal pain, hepatomegaly or splenomegaly, nausea and vomiting. Lactate dehydrogenase levels are usually elevated in patients with non-Hodgkin lymphoma. Ann Arbor staging criteria (Stage I: involvement of a single lymph node area; Stage II: involvement of two or more lymph node regions on same side of the diaphragm; Stage III: involvement of lymph node regions on both sides of the diaphragm ± spleen; Stage IV: disseminated extralymphatic spread) is used to stage the disease.

48. Answer: A

Undescended testes or 'cryptorchidism' may imply incomplete testicular descent (i.e. the testis fails to descend fully and may truly be incompletely descended or retractile); or it may imply abnormal descent (i.e. the testis does not lie along its normal path of descent, but in an ectopic position). The condition affects 3% of full-term boys, with the majority of such testes lying in the inguinal canal. Approximately 75% of undescended testes descend into the scrotum during the first year of life; surgery should therefore be considered during the second year of life. The condition is associated with an increased risk of testicular malignancy, which develops in 5% of intra-abdominal testes. Amongst males with initially undescended testes, 80% with bilateral descended testes are fertile but only 30% with bilateral undescended testes have normal fertility. Boys with a palpable testis should undergo a routine orchidopexy, whilst impalpable testes should undergo exploratory laparoscopy. Clinicians should be alerted to the possibility of female virilization if hypospadias and cryptorchidism are found to coexist in a patient.

49. Answer: C

Tissue typing is usually limited to looking for six HLA antigens, i.e. one inherited from each parent at the HLA-A, HLA-B, and HLA-DR loci. Each locus has a high number of possible alleles. A mismatch is used to describe the difference in HLA phenotype between individuals and is recorded in the form A–B–DR. A perfectly matched donor-recipient pair will have a 0–0–0 mismatch. A donor–recipient pair with no common phenotype will have a 2–2–2 mismatch. HLA-DR is the most important match as a mismatch here is associated with the highest incidence of transplant rejection.

50. Answer: A

Despite recent advances in minimally invasive techniques, oesophageal cancer still harbours one of the poorest prognoses of gastrointestinal malignancies. Patients with oesophageal malignancy tend to present late with progressive dysphagia, weight loss and anaemia. Definitive treatment (i.e. oesophagectomy) is reserved for early cancers that do not exhibit local invasion. Malignant dysphagia in advanced cancer and in patients unfit for surgery was traditionally managed with serial endoscopic dilatations. However, endoscopically inserted self-expanding metal stents have recently become the mainstay of treatment in such malignant dysphagia. Despite evidence of good symptom relief, stent insertion may be complicated in the early stages by stent malposition, migration, bleeding and oesophageal perforation. Late complications commonly involve tumour overgrowth or obstruction by food bolus. The initial management of the latter involves the ingestion of a carbonated drink, which assists in dissolving the obstructing bolus. If this fails, endoscopy is required to ascertain the cause of obstruction, and to dislodge the food bolus, if necessary.

Basic sciences: Applied anatomy

1. **Which of the following nerves does not arise from the medial cord of the brachial plexus?**
   A. Medial cutaneous nerve of the forearm
   B. Medial pectoral nerve
   C. Musculocutaneous nerve
   D. Ulnar nerve
   E. Median cutaneous nerve of the arm

Basic sciences: Physiology

2. **Which of the following statements concerning lung volumes in a healthy male subject is incorrect?**
   A. A typical value for tidal volume is approximately 500–600 mL
   B. The volume of alveolar dead space is approximately 150 mL
   C. The helium dilution method is an appropriate way of measuring functional residual capacity
   D. A typical alveolar ventilation rate may be in the region of 5000–6000 mL/min
   E. Inspiratory reserve volume is often nearly double the size of the expiratory reserve volume

Basic sciences: Pathology

3. **A 60-year-old man present with dysphagia and heartburn. He undergoes a gastroscopy, which shows evidence of Barrett's oesophagus. Which of the following options best describes the pathological process in the development of Barrett's oesophagus?**
   A. Squamous metaplasia
   B. Dysplasia
   C. Hyperplasia
   D. Columnar metaplasia
   E. Hypertrophy

Common surgical conditions and the subspecialties:
Trauma and orthopaedics

4. A 23-year-old soldier is referred by his **GP** to the vascular surgeon for
    a 6-week history of progressively worsening symptoms of unilateral
    calf claudication. He has no significant risk factors for cardiovascular
    disease. Neurovascular examination of the affected leg at rest reveals
    no significant findings. The **ABPI** of the affected limb is normal at
    rest (1.04) but decreases after 5 minutes of treadmill testing, to 0.69.
    Doppler ultrasonography of the posterior tibial pulse reveals arterial
    obstruction with resisted plantarflexion, but no obstruction when
    active plantarflexion is discontinued. A CT arteriogram of the limb
    demonstrates complete blockage of the popliteal artery with passive
    dorsiflexion of the ankle. What is the most likely diagnosis?

    A. Popliteal arteriovenous malformation
    B. Deep venous thrombosis
    C. Rupture of a popliteal artery aneurysm
    D. Thrombosis of a popliteal artery aneurysm
    E. Popliteal artery entrapment syndrome

Common surgical conditions and the subspecialties:
Trauma and orthopaedics

5. A 24-year-old male involved in a high speed road traffic collision is
    brought to the Emergency Department. He is noted to be bleeding
    from his nose, and he describes a salty taste in his mouth. Closer
    inspection reveals bruising over the left mastoid process and bilateral
    periorbital haematomas. Otoscopic examination reveals visible
    bleeding behind the left tympanic membrane. Which of the following
    options is the most likely diagnosis in this case?

    A. Open skull fracture
    B. Basal skull fracture
    C. Extradural haematoma
    D. Subarachnoid haemorrhage
    E. Subdural haematoma

Perioperative care: Metabolic and endocrine disorders

6. A 60-year-old man who underwent a distal gastrectomy 2 months
    previously, presents to his GP with symptoms of dizziness, nausea,
    sweating, and palpitations a few hours after eating. What is the cause
    of his symptoms?

    A. Hyperglycaemia
    B. Increased secretion of secretin
    C. Hypertension
    D. Hypoglycaemia
    E. Increased secretion of gastrin

The assessment and management of the surgical patient:
Clinical decision-making

7. **A 31-year-old teacher presents to her GP 7 weeks postpartum with a painful and swollen left breast. Examination reveals erythema, tenderness and fluctuance just above the left nipple–areolar complex. What is the most appropriate management of this patient?**
    A. Incision and drainage of abscess
    B. Intravenous antibiotics and rehydration
    C. Radiography-guided needle aspiration
    D. Trucut biopsy of breast lump
    E. Ultrasound-guided needle aspiration

Basic sciences: Applied anatomy

8. **An adolescent boy is seen in the Emergency Department after experiencing a sharp pain in his throat after eating bony fish. The ENT surgical registrar on call manages to retrieve the fish bone non-surgically but is unsure if there may have been damage to the mucosa of the piriform fossa. Which nerve constitutes the afferent (sensory) supply to the piriform fossa?**
    A. External laryngeal nerve
    B. Glossopharyngeal nerve
    C. Hypoglossal nerve
    D. Internal laryngeal nerve
    E. Recurrent laryngeal nerve

Basic sciences: Physiology

9. **Which of the following is not true about calcium homeostasis?**
    A. PTH causes increased tubular reabsorption of calcium but decreased reabsorption of phosphate
    B. 1,25-dihydroxycholecalciferol increases gut and renal absorption of calcium and phosphate
    C. PTH causes renal conversion of 25-hydroxycholecalciferol to 1,25-dihydroxycholecalciferol
    D. PTH inhibits osteoblastic and osteoclastic activity
    E. Calcitonin is not essential for calcium homeostasis

Basic sciences: Pathology

10. **Which of the following factors does not contribute to the formation of thrombus?**
    A. Atheroma
    B. Thrombocytosis
    C. Hypergammaglobulinaemia
    D. Megaloblastic anaemia
    E. Inherited protein S deficiency

Common surgical conditions and the subspecialties:
Trauma and orthopaedics

11. A 25-year-old acrobat presents to the Emergency Department with an 'unusual feeling' in his left arm, one week after falling from height during his trapeze routine. He describes being fully conscious throughout the incident, having hit his left arm on a number of sharp structures during the fall, and landing on his outstretched left hand. Examination reveals multiple healed lacerations over the left forearm but good vascular perfusion of the limb. However, there is visible extension at the metacarpophalangeal joints, and marked flexion at the interphalangeal joints of the ring and little fingers. Furthermore, abduction and adduction of the fingers is markedly weaker in the affected hand. No radial or ulnar deviation is noted, and the patient remains systemically well. Which of the following mechanisms of injury is most likely to have caused this presentation?

   A. Laceration near the elbow
   B. Laceration near the wrist
   C. Blunt trauma to the forearm
   D. Supracondylar fracture of the humerus
   E. Delayed compartment syndrome

Common surgical conditions and the subspecialties: Endocrine disease

12. A 40-year-old man presents with a 2-week history of progressively worsening central abdominal pain and constipation. Examination reveals a haemodynamically stable patient with a soft, diffusely tender abdomen and decreased bowel sounds. Initial blood tests are unremarkable except for a raised serum adjusted calcium level. Which of the following pathologies may have caused such hypercalcaemia?

   A. Secondary hyperparathyroidism
   B. Pseudohypoparathyroidism
   C. Thyrotoxicosis
   D. Hyperventilation
   E. Osteomalacia

Perioperative care: Postoperative care

13. A 67-year-old male undergoes an emergency hip hemiarthroplasty. The procedure is complicated by a fracture of the femoral shaft following the insertion of the prosthesis. Postoperatively, he is found to be unsteady on his feet and depressed. He remains bedbound for 3 weeks and is slow to progress despite adequate physiotherapy. Which of the following physiological changes is not seen following prolonged immobilization?

   A. Eventual loss of potassium
   B. Reduction in autonomic nervous system activity
   C. Bradycardia
   D. Demineralization of bone
   E. Increased risk of deep venous thrombosis

The assessment and management of the surgical patient:
Planning investigations

14. A 63-year-old retired teacher with no significant past medical history presents to his GP with a 3-month history of progressively worsening lethargy and malaise. Physical examination reveals a blood pressure of 150/95 mmHg but no other significant signs. Initial blood tests reveal: Hb 8.5 g/dL, MCV 80 fL, urea 8.3 mmol/L, creatinine 220 µmol/L, ESR 45 mm/hour, and CRP 35 mg/L. Subsequent abdominal ultrasound scanning reveals bilateral hydronephrosis. Which of the following investigations is likely to be most beneficial in diagnosing the underlying pathology?

A. Computed tomography scan of the abdomen
B. Intravenous urogram
C. Renal biopsy
D. Renal perfusion scan
E. Retrograde urogram

Basic sciences: Applied anatomy

15. A patient presents with left-sided facial weakness, loss of sensation to the anterior two-thirds of the tongue, and hyperacusis. Tear production is normal in both eyes and there is no vestibular dysfunction. At which of the following regions would a lesion to the facial nerve result in the symptoms described?

A. Left stylomastoid foramen
B. Left parotid gland
C. Left facial canal
D. Left geniculate ganglion
E. Left cerebellopontine angle

Basic sciences: Physiology

16. Which of the following statements is incorrect regarding magnesium homeostasis?

A. The majority of the body's magnesium is contained within bone
B. In healthy individuals, serum magnesium concentration is contained within a narrow range of 0.7–1.05 mmol/L
C. Aldosterone reduces renal excretion of magnesium
D. Parathyroid hormone increases magnesium absorption from the small intestine
E. Severe forms of hypomagnesaemia result in respiratory insufficiency and cardiac arrest

Common surgical conditions and the subspecialties:
Gastrointestinal disease

17. **Which of the following is not true about gastrinomas?**
    A. The majority of gastrinomas are located in the gastrinoma triangle
    B. 25% of all gastrinomas are associated with MEN 2
    C. Calcium stimulation tests are used to differentiate gastrinomas from other causes of hypergastrinaemia
    D. Gastrinomas associated with MEN are usually located in the duodenum
    E. Sporadic gastrinomas are most commonly located in the pancreas

Perioperative care: Postoperative care

18. **A 25-year-old man with a longstanding history of well-controlled Crohn's disease presents to the Emergency Department with acutely peritonitic abdomen. An emergency laparotomy reveals a perforated caecum with free fluid in the abdominal cavity. A bowel resection with primary anastomosis and a thorough washout are performed. The patient is transferred to ITU postoperatively. In addition to the standard antimicrobial and supportive therapy, which of the following therapeutic measures is most likely to improve this patient's outcome in ITU?**
    A. Intravenous corticosteroids (high dose)
    B. Intravenous corticosteroids (low dose)
    C. Recombinant antiendotoxin antibody
    D. Recombinant human antithrombin III
    E. Recombinant human tissue-factor pathway inhibitor

The assessment and management of the surgical patient:
Clinical decision-making

19. **An active 75-year-old gentleman presents with a 4-hour history of acute-onset pain and paraesthesia of his right upper limb. He denies any similar symptoms previously but describes a 10-year history of atrial fibrillation, for which he takes digoxin and aspirin. He has no other significant medical history. Examination reveals a cold right hand, absent right radial, ulnar, and brachial pulses, and reduced power and sensation to the right hand and forearm. What is the most appropriate definitive management for this patient?**
    A. Embolectomy
    B. Intravenous heparin infusion
    C. Reassurance and discharge home with analgesia and urgent follow-up arranged in the vascular clinic
    D. Thrombolysis
    E. Urgent duplex scanning of the affected limb

Basic sciences: Applied anatomy

20. **A 52-year-old lady presents with a 'band like' across her upper abdomen, at the level of L1. While examining her abdomen, the surgical trainee attempts to remember all the organs found at this level. Which one of the following structures is not found in this plane?**

A. Neck of the pancreas

B. Pylorus of the stomach

C. Origin of the coeliac trunk

D. Fundus of the gallbladder

E. Origin of the superior mesenteric artery

Basic sciences: Physiology

21. **Which of the following causes a left shift of the oxygen–haemoglobin dissociation curve?**

A. Blood in storage

B. Exercise

C. Reduced pH

D. Raised temperature

E. High altitude

Common surgical conditions and the subspecialties: Cardiovascular and pulmonary disease

22. **A 35-year-old female with cystic fibrosis and a complex history of opportunistic chest infections develops adult respiratory distress syndrome, and is subsequently ventilated on intensive care. Her inspired oxygen fraction is 100%, positive end-expiratory pressure is 15 cmH$_2$O and peak airway pressure is 40 cmH$_2$O. Her current arterial blood gas results demonstrate a PaO$_2$ of 6 kPa, PaCO$_2$ of 6.9 kPa, and SpO$_2$ 88%. Which further adjunct to ventilation is likely to be of greatest benefit to this patient?**

A. High-frequency oscillatory ventilation

B. Increasing the tidal volume and respiratory rate on the ventilator

C. Inhaled nitric oxide therapy

D. Intravenous oxygenation

E. Adopted a prone position

Perioperative care: Postoperative care

23. **A previously healthy 80-year-old gentleman is diagnosed with gastric adenocarcinoma. The surgeon believes that the tumour is amenable to a subtotal gastrectomy with Roux-en-Y reconstruction and invites the patient for preoperative counselling. Which of the following is an important complication of subtotal gastrectomy if Roux-en-Y reconstruction is not concurrently performed?**
    A. Abdominal compartment syndrome
    B. Bilious vomiting
    C. Constipation
    D. Gut sepsis from bacterial overgrowth
    E. Haemolytic anaemia

Assessment and management of patients with trauma (including the multiply injured patient): Shock

24. **A 55-year-old man is brought into the Emergency Department having suffered a road traffic accident. On arrival, he is tachycardic with a pulse rate of 130/min, blood pressure of 80/40 mmHg, and a respiratory rate of 34/min. His urine output is 5–10 mL per hour. There is an obvious deformity of his left femur visible through blood-soaked clothing. What is the most likely amount of blood loss?**
    A. 500 mL
    B. 750 mL
    C. 1000 mL
    D. 1750 mL
    E. 2500 mL

Basic sciences: Applied anatomy

25. **A 50-year-old man undergoes open carpal tunnel decompression for carpal tunnel syndrome. After his operation, he complains of difficulty in moving his thumb. Which nerve is likely to have been injured to cause this?**
    A. Anterior interosseous branch of the median nerve
    B. Recurrent branch of the median nerve
    C. Palmar cutaneous branch of the median nerve
    D. Superficial branch of ulnar nerve
    E. Deep branch of ulnar nerve

Basic sciences: Physiology

26. The clinical history of a 75-year-old patient reveals a vagotomy performed in 1985 for peptic ulcer disease. Which of the following statements is incorrect regarding the physiological effects of vagotomy?

    A. Vagotomy reduces gastric acid secretion by decreased stimulation of oxyntic cells
    B. Vagotomy reduces gastric acid secretion by reducing mucosal histamine and gastrin release
    C. After vagotomy, reduced coordination of the myenteric plexus may lead to delayed emptying and gastric stasis
    D. After vagotomy, the pylorus fails to relax prior to the peristaltic emptying wave
    E. Vagotomy increases pancreatic exocrine function

Common surgical conditions and the subspecialties: Endocrine disease

27. A 56-year-old male presents to his GP with a 3-week history of sweating, headaches, constipation, and itchy lesions over his back. On examination, his blood pressure is 166/94 mmHg and his pulse rate is 104/min. Twenty-four-hour urinary catecholamines, metanephrines and vanillylmandelic acid are found to be elevated. A CT scan and a 131I-meta-iodo-benzyl-guanidine scan confirm the presence of a phaeochromocytoma. The patient is subsequently also found to have a medullary carcinoma of the thyroid. Which of the following is the most likely diagnosis?

    A. Multiple endocrine neoplasia type 1
    B. Carcinoid tumour
    C. Multiple endocrine neoplasia type 2A
    D. Secondary hyperparathyroidism
    E. Multiple endocrine neoplasia type 2B

Basic sciences: Applied anatomy

28. A 55-year-old female presents with pain in her right inner thigh and a swelling in her right groin. Examination reveals this swelling to be inferior to the medial third of the inguinal ligament, and lateral to the pubic tubercle (i.e. over the femoral ring). Which of the following statements regarding the femoral canal is incorrect?

    A. It is a short and blind-ending potential space in the medial compartment of the femoral sheath
    B. The femoral sheath is an extension of the transversalis fascia and fascia iliaca
    C. It contains lymphatic vessels and the node of Cloquet
    D. It is bounded by the femoral nerve laterally
    E. It is bounded by the lacunar ligament medially

Basic sciences: Physiology

29. When the pH falls, the oxygen–haemoglobin dissociation curve shifts to the right. Which of the following phenomena best describes this shift?

    A. Haldane effect
    B. Bohr effect
    C. Pasteur effect
    D. Rebound effect
    E. Breuer effect

Common surgical conditions and the subspecialties: Endocrine disease

30. A 58-year-old woman presents to her GP seven weeks after her renal transplant procedure, with polyuria, polydipsia and abdominal pain. Her blood tests show the following: corrected calcium 2.90 mmol/L (2.2–2.6 mmol/L), phosphate 0.69 mmol/L (0.8–1.4 mmol/L). Which of the following is the most likely diagnosis?

    A. Primary hyperparathyroidism
    B. Paget's disease
    C. Multiple myeloma
    D. Secondary hyperparathyroidism
    E. Tertiary hyperparathyroidism

Basic sciences: Applied anatomy

31. When interpreting a CT scan of the abdomen, which of the following structures is usually seen as a posterior relation of the first part of the duodenum?

    A. Cystic artery
    B. Hilum of the right kidney
    C. Hepatic portal vein
    D. Superior mesenteric vessels
    E. Transverse colon

Common surgical conditions and the subspecialties: Cardiovascular and pulmonary disease

32. **A 60-year-old woman with no significant past medical history undergoes a right hemicolectomy for colorectal cancer. Three days postoperatively, she develops shortness of breath and chest tightness. Which of the following features would be consistent with the presence of a systemic inflammatory response syndrome in this patient?**

A. Temperature of 37.5°C and heart rate of 100/min

B. Respiratory rate of 22/min and systolic blood pressure of 90 mmHg

C. $PaCO_2$ of 4.2 kPa and neutrophil count of 12.5×10^9/L

D. Temperature of 38.5°C and respiratory rate of 19/min

D. Heart rate of 100/min and temperature of 36.1°C

Basic sciences: Applied anatomy

33. **Which of the following statements is true regarding the anatomy of the parotid gland?**

A. The parotid duct emerges from the anterior border of the gland and pierces the buccinator to enter the buccal cavity at the level of the second lower molar tooth

B. The external carotid artery gives off its branches prior to passing through the gland

C. The facial nerve lies within the superficial lobe of the parotid gland

D. The retromandibular vein passes through the gland

E. Facial nerve palsy from lesions within the parotid gland results in sensory loss to the affected side of the face

Common surgical conditions and the subspecialties: Skin, head, and neck

34. **A 30-year-old male presents with a right-sided frontal headache and right-sided periorbital oedema, erythema and sensory loss. Examination reveals a furuncle over his right cheek, a dilated right pupil that reacts sluggishly to light, and lateral gaze palsy of the right eye. What is the most likely diagnosis?**

A. Brain abscess

B. Cavernous sinus thrombosis

C. Orbital sepsis

D. Periorbital sepsis

E. Frontal sinusitis

Basic sciences: Applied anatomy

35. A 6-year-old boy is brought to the Emergency Department with a painful and swollen right elbow after falling awkwardly from a bouncy castle. Examination reveals an obviously deformed and tender elbow, and a weak radial pulse. The boy is unable to flex his right index finger and has loss of sensation over the thenar eminence and thumb. Plain radiography of the limb reveals a supracondylar fracture of the right humerus with the proximal fragment penetrating the skin. Which nerve is most likely to be injured in this child?

A. Radial nerve

B. Median nerve

C. Posterior interosseous nerve

D. Ulnar nerve

E. Musculocutaneous nerve

Common surgical conditions and the subspecialties: Endocrine disease

36. A 28-year-old lady is referred from the fertility centre to the medical outpatient clinic with a history of secondary amenorrhoea for 8 months and galactorrhoea for 6 months. She takes paracetamol tablets occasionally for headaches and does not have any significant past medical history. She had her menarche at 14 years of age. She has been living with her partner for 5 years and is now keen to start a family. Her baseline blood investigations are unremarkable. Her serum levels of LH, FSH, and thyroid hormones are within normal limits but her serum prolactin level is 1500 mU/L (normal range: <450 mU/L). A MRI scan of the pituitary gland reveals a hypodense lesion suggestive of a microadenoma. What will be the most appropriate treatment at this stage to restore her gonadal function and fertility?

A. Somatostatin

B. *In vitro* fertility therapy

C. Octreotide

D. Bromocriptine

E. Pituitary surgery

Basic sciences: Applied anatomy

37. **A previously fit and healthy 37-year-old lady undergoes a prolonged laparoscopic cholecystectomy due to multiple equipment-related complications. In the immediate postoperative period, she develops biphasic stridor and cyanosis upon extubation, and is therefore immediately re-intubated. The surgical registrar present at the time diagnoses this as possible bilateral vocal cord paralysis and prepares to perform an open tracheostomy. Which of the following structures are not encountered during this procedure?**

    A. Deep investing fascia
    B. Platysma
    C. Strap muscles (sternothyroid and sternohyoid)
    D. Superior thyroid artery
    E. Thyroid isthmus

Common surgical conditions and the subspecialties: General presenting symptoms or syndromes

38. **A 60-year-old man attends the urology clinic as part of his routine follow-up for metastatic prostate cancer. Examination reveals a grossly distended, ascitic abdomen. A hard, non-tender, ulcerated nodule is noted to arise from the umbilicus. The nodule demonstrates no overlying erythema, warmth, or palpable cough impulse, and is not reducible. Which of the following options is this nodule most likely to represent?**

    A. Umbilical hernia
    B. Fluid-filled urachal sinus
    C. Para-umbilical hernia
    D. Sister Mary Joseph nodule
    E. Caput medusae

Basic sciences: Applied anatomy

39. A 43-year-old man is referred by his **GP** to the ophthalmology outpatient clinic with a 2-month history of intermittently blurred vision. This symptom occurred immediately after a head injury, for which the patient did not seek medical attention. Examination reveals head-tilt towards the left shoulder and normal bilateral visual acuity with the Snellen chart. Although no nystagmus is observed when testing eye movements, the patient reports double vision when looking downwards and outwards. Further examination reveals vertical and torsional diplopia. Which of the following extraocular muscles is most likely affected?

A. Superior oblique muscle
B. Inferior oblique muscle
C. Superior rectus muscle
D. Inferior rectus muscle
E. Lateral rectus muscle

Common surgical conditions and the subspecialties: Breast disease

40. A 54-year-old male presents to the breast clinic with a 6-month history of bilaterally enlarging breast tissue. He denies any pain or family history of breast cancer. Which of the following factors is not known to be a risk factor for the development of gynaecomastia?

A. Alcohol excess
B. Digoxin
C. Obesity
D. Renal failure
E. Klinefelter's syndrome

Basic sciences: Applied anatomy

41. A 48-year-old lady with central invasive breast cancer underwent a mastectomy and axillary clearance of level I and level II nodes. On the postoperative ward round, she complained of numbness in the medial aspect of the upper arm. Which nerve is most likely to have been damaged to cause the described symptoms?

A. Intercostobrachial nerve
B. Long thoracic nerve
C. Thoracodorsal nerve
D. Axillary nerve
E. Musculocutaneous nerve

Common surgical conditions and the subspecialties:
Gastrointestinal disease

42. **A 65-year-old male presents to the colorectal surgical clinic after his right hemicolectomy. He is informed of the histology results of the resected specimen, which confirm the presence of adenocarcinoma of the right colon. The surgeon explains that although the resection margins were clear, the tumour was found to have spread through the bowel wall into the extrarectal and extracolic tissues, without lymph node involvement. The patient now enquires about his prognosis. What is the patient's chance of 5-year survival?**

A. 95%

B. 80%

C. 60%

D. 30%

E. 5%

Basic sciences: Applied anatomy

43. **A 35-year-old woman undergoes a laparoscopic cholecystectomy for recurrent biliary colic. During the operation, the surgeon seeks to identify Calot's triangle. Which structure is not bound by, or does not lie within, Calot's triangle?**

A. Common hepatic duct

B. Common bile duct

C. Cystic duct

D. Cystic artery

E. Inferior edge of the liver

Common surgical conditions and the subspecialties: General presenting symptoms or syndromes

44. **A 58-year-old bartender presents to the Emergency Department with a 4-hour history of acute abdominal pain. He has a temperature of 39.2°C, a heart rate of 133/min and a blood pressure of 83/60 mmHg. Abdominal examination reveals right upper quadrant tenderness and features of localized peritonism. Initial blood tests reveal a Hb of 13.5 g/dL, WCC of 22.3 × 10⁹/L, platelet count of 190 × 10⁹/L, and CRP of 316 mg/dL. A plain abdominal radiograph suggests pneumatobilia. What is the most likely diagnosis?**

A. Acute pancreatitis

B. Ascending cholangitis

C. Acute cholecystitis

D. Gallstone ileus

E. Sclerosing cholangitis

Common surgical conditions and the subspecialties:
Gastrointestinal disease

45. **A 24-year-old male is referred to the colorectal clinic following the incidental finding of bilateral retinal pigmentations. Further questioning reveals that he has been passing a small amount of blood with his stool, which he has attributed to recent constipation. A subsequent colonoscopy reveals hundreds of colonic polyps, and the patient is diagnosed with familial adenomatous polyposis (FAP). Which of the following statements regarding this condition is false?**
    A. It is an autosomal dominant condition
    B. It is caused by a deletion mutation of the long arm of chromosome 5
    C. Congenital hypertrophy of the retinal pigment epithelium occurs in 10% of these patients
    D. In the presence of osteomas, fibromas and sebaceous cysts, the condition is termed Gardner's syndrome
    E. The multiple colonic polyps resulting from this condition are inherently benign

Common surgical conditions and the subspecialties:
Gastrointestinal disease

46. **A 49-year-old gentleman presents to the Emergency Department with an 8-hour history of severe epigastric and central abdominal pain radiating through to his back. He has also had three episodes of bilious vomiting. He has experienced previous episodes of colicky abdominal pain but never as severe as on this occasion. On examination, his temperature is 37.6°C, pulse rate is 92/min and respiratory rate is 18/min. Abdominal examination reveals epigastric tenderness and guarding but no rigidity. Plain radiographs of the chest (erect) and abdomen (supine) are unremarkable. What is the most likely diagnosis?**
    A. Mechanical intestinal obstruction
    B. Mesenteric ischaemia
    C. Acute pancreatitis
    D. Perforated peptic ulcer
    E. Ruptured abdominal aortic aneurysm

Common surgical conditions and the subspecialties: Endocrine disease

47. **A 52-year-old estate agent presents to his GP with a 4-week history of upper abdominal pain and diarrhoea. He also describes a few episodes of 'dark-coloured' vomitus during this period. General examination is unremarkable. Oesophagogastroduodenoscopy reveals multiple ulcers in the stomach and duodenum. What is the most likely diagnosis?**

   A. Vasoactive intestinal peptide secreting tumour
   B. Adrenocorticotropin secreting tumour
   C. Somatostatinoma
   D. Carcinoid tumour
   E. Gastrinoma

Common surgical conditions and the subspecialties:
Gastrointestinal disease

48. **The mother of a 2-day-old neonate is worried as her infant has failed to pass meconium in the first 24 hours after birth, and has now developed abdominal distension and vomiting. The paediatrician suspects Hirschsprung's disease and obtains consent for a digital rectal examination. Which of the following options is most suggestive of Hirschsprung's disease?**

   A. Absolute constipation and large-bowel obstruction at 1 month of age
   B. Gross dilatation of the affected bowel segment as visualized on contrast imaging
   C. Large bowel obstruction in a neonate
   D. Occasional passage of redcurrant jelly stools
   E. Persistent vomiting in a neonate

Professional behaviour and leadership: Evidence and guidelines

49. **A pharmaceutical company testing a drug against postoperative pain wishes to compare the mean scores for pain between standard analgesia and the new drug. Which one of the following is the most appropriate statistical test?**

   A. Chi-squared test
   B. Life table analysis
   C. Paired t-test
   D. Pearson's correlation
   E. Unpaired t-test

Basic sciences: Microbiology

50. A 7-year-old girl presents to the Emergency Department with acute pain over her right proximal tibia. She has no past medical history of note, and has not suffered any recent trauma to the affected limb. Examination reveals the child to be febrile and refusing to move her leg. After a series of radiographs, a provisional diagnosis of osteomyelitis is made. Which of the following organisms is the most likely cause of the infection?

A. *Haemophilus influenzae*
B. *Pseudomonas aeruginosa*
C. *Salmonella typhii*
D. *Staphylococcus aureus*
E. *Streptococcus pneumoniae*

1. Answer: C

The following nerves arise from the medial cord of brachial plexus: the medial cutaneous nerve of the forearm (C8 and T1); the median cutaneous nerve of the arm (C8 and T1); the medial root of the median nerve (C8 and T1); the medial pectoral nerve (C8 and T1); and the ulnar nerve (C8 and T1). The musculocutaneous nerve (C5, C6, and C7) arises from the lateral cord of the brachial plexus. The other nerves which arise from the lateral cord of the brachial plexus are the lateral pectoral nerve (C5, C6, C7) and the lateral root of the median nerve (C5, C6, C7).

2. Answer: B

An appropriate value for the tidal volume (as quoted by many physiology textbooks) in a healthy adult male is about 500–600 mL. However, it should be recognized that what is 'normal' for a healthy subject varies widely depending on the gender and age, as well as the individual's anatomical make-up. The alveolar dead space is typically zero in a healthy subject. The anatomical dead space is approximately 150 mL. (Thus the physiological dead space is also about 150 mL since physiological dead space = alveolar dead space + anatomical dead space.) In order to measure the functional residual capacity, the subject is connected to a spirometer of known volume, containing a known concentration of helium. As helium does not cross the alveolar/capillary interface, inspiration of helium will result in distribution of helium throughout the spirometer and lungs. Measurement of helium concentration throughout this closed system at the end of a normal expiration will allow calculation of the functional residual capacity/volume. Assuming a tidal volume of 500–600 mL and an anatomical dead space of 150 mL, for a respiratory frequency (respiratory rate) of between 12 and 16/min, the resulting alveolar ventilation values will be in the range of about 4500–7000 mL. The lungs are always left partially inflated with the functional residual capacity from which the expiratory reserve volume (ERV) is drawn. The ERV is typically about 2000 mL. Assuming our subject has a typical value for vital capacity of 6000 mL, the inspiratory reserve capacity would be of the order of 3500 mL, which is well in excess of the ERV.

3. Answer: D

Metaplasia is the replacement of one differentiated cell type by another. Barrett's oesophagus is defined as the presence of columnar epithelium lining the distal oesophagus, replacing normal squamous epithelium.

Barrett's oesophagus is a premalignant disease and surveillance must be considered in patients with the condition.

Squamous metaplasia is said to occur when the epithelial lining is replaced by squamous epithelium, as is seen in the bladder or cervix. Dysplasia, which is usually a premalignant state, refers to the abnormal development of cells. Hyperplasia refers to an increase in cell number, while hypertrophy refers to an increase in cell size.

4. Answer: E

Popliteal artery entrapment syndrome is a rare cause of exercise-induced leg pain due to an abnormal relationship between the popliteal artery and the surrounding myofascial structures in the popliteal fossa. Compression of the artery within the fossa, especially in those with muscular calves (e.g. male athletes and soldiers), causes arterial insufficiency manifesting as exertional leg claudication. Repeated popliteal artery compression causes trauma to the arterial wall, leading to premature localized atherosclerosis. The natural progression of the syndrome includes arterial thrombosis occurring in some individuals, leading to acute limb ischaemia, although the majority of patients simply experience exercise-induced leg pain (or acute-on-chronic ischaemia). Up to 85% of all patients who are clinically diagnosed are males, aged between 25–30 years. Bilateral popliteal artery entrapment is noted in 25% of cases, resulting in a significant functional loss for active individuals. The diagnosis involves examination of the dorsalis pedis and posterior tibial pulses, Doppler ultrasonography, and arteriography. The treatment of functional popliteal artery entrapment usually includes surgical exploration, release of the popliteal artery and a myomectomy of the medial gastrocnemius head.

5. Answer: B

This patient presents with the classical signs and symptoms of a basal skull fracture. Trauma is the commonest cause of such fractures, which usually involve the roof of the orbits, the sphenoid bone, or portions of the temporal bone. Frequent signs and symptoms of basal skull fractures include 'Raccoon eyes' (periorbital haematoma), subconjunctival haemorrhage (i.e. where the posterior margins cannot be seen), Battle's sign (post auricular bruising, and blood behind the eardrum; this sign may develop after 24–48 hours of injury) and rhinorrhoea/otorrhoea (i.e. a haemoserous mixture of blood and CSF that does not clot; this is caused by damage to the cribriform plate). The management of such patients depends on the finding of other associated injuries and the results of relevant investigations such as CT or MRI scanning. Indications for a CT scan include a falling GCS score or a GCS score of lower than 13, depressed skull fracture, lateralizing neurological signs and convulsions. Patients with a GCS score under 8 warrant intubation to protect their airway. With any skull fracture, especially basal skull fractures, prophylactic antibiotics are indicated to prevent meningitis. Some recognized complications of basal skull fractures include an increased risk of infection (especially following CSF rhinorrhoea), facial palsy (which usually responds well to steroids), and isolated VI nerve palsy.

6. Answer: D

The clinical presentation of this patient is consistent with late dumping syndrome.

Dumping syndrome results from rapid gastric emptying after pyloroplasty or gastrectomy. It can be classified as 'early dumping' or 'late dumping'.

Early dumping is characterized by nausea, vomiting, dizziness, diarrhoea and abdominal cramps; and manifests within 5–45 minutes of eating. It occurs due to a hypertonic load in the small intestine, causing large-volume fluid shifts.

Late dumping is characterized by an autonomic response (faintness, tachycardia, sweating, palpitations) owing to a late reactive hypoglycaemia secondary to postprandial insulin release.

7. Answer: E

The postpartum pathology of breast abscess is not uncommon in breastfeeding women. This usually results from *Staphylococcus aureus* introduced through cracks in the nipple–areolar complex; the foci of infection are usually situated peripherally. Infection may also result at the time of weaning, due to engorgement of the breast, or due to development of dentition in the infant.

Early breast infections (i.e. before pus formation) may be treated successfully with antibiotics. However, delayed presentations involving collections of pus usually necessitate ultrasound-guided needle aspiration; radiography-guided aspiration would require compression of the painful breast between radiographic plates, and is therefore contraindicated. In addition, incision and drainage of the abscess may result in cutaneous fistulae; this is therefore only indicated if the abscess is highly loculated, if it fails to respond to repeated guided aspirations, or if the overlying skin is necrotic.

8. Answer: D

The piriform fossae are recesses on either side of the laryngeal orifices, which are involved in speech. They are bounded medially by the aryepiglottic fold, and laterally by the thyroid cartilage and thyrohyoid membrane. The internal laryngeal nerve (a branch of the superior laryngeal nerve) supplies sensory innervation to the area (and also the mucous membrane to the rest of the larynx), and may become damaged if the mucous membrane is inadvertently punctured. The nerve ends by anastomosing with branches of the recurrent laryngeal nerve behind (or within) the posterior cricoarytenoid muscle; and the connection may pierce the inferior constrictor of the pharynx.

In contrast, the external laryngeal nerve is the smaller, external branch of the superior laryngeal nerve. It descends on the larynx beneath the sternothyroid muscle, to supply the cricothyroid muscle. It also gives branches to the pharyngeal plexus and the superior portion of the inferior pharyngeal constrictor, and communicates with the superior cardiac nerve behind the common carotid artery. The commonest modes of damage to the external laryngeal nerve include thyroidectomy and cricothyroidotomy, as the nerve lies immediately deep to the superior thyroid artery.

The glossopharyngeal nerve generally provides sensory innervation to the skin of the external ear, the internal surface of the tympanic membrane, the walls of the upper pharynx, and the posterior third of the tongue. The recurrent laryngeal nerve provides sensory innervation to the larynx, while the hypoglossal nerve does not carry a sensory component.

9. Answer: D

Calcium is absorbed by the intestine and excreted by the kidney. Parathyroid hormone is released by the chief cells of the parathyroid gland in response to hypocalcaemia. It causes increased tubular reabsorption of calcium, decreased reabsorption of phosphate and increased activation of vitamin D. It inhibits osteoblasts, thereby activating osteoclasts. It causes increased intestinal absorption of calcium due to increasing conversion of 25-hydroxycholecalciferol to 1,25-dihydroxycholecalciferol (activated vitamin D). Activated vitamin D increases absorption of calcium and phosphate in the kidney, stimulates osteoblasts to form new bone, and increases calcium and phosphate absorption in the intestine.

Calcitonin is not essential for calcium homeostasis. It is secreted by the parafollicular cells of the thyroid gland in response to hypercalcaemia. It acts by inhibiting the reabsorption of calcium and phosphate by the kidney and osteoclast activity in bone.

10. Answer: D

Thrombus is a solid material formed from various haematological constituents of blood. Thrombus formation is primarily a function of platelets, although the clotting cascade is also involved. Some important factors that contribute to thrombus formation can be grouped into three main areas. They are: (I) changes in the vessel wall, such as atheroma, causing a change in the speed and flow through the arteries; (II) changes in the constituents of blood, such as thrombocytosis; increases in coagulation factors (e.g. fibrinogen and procoagulant factors released from malignancies); hyperviscosity from conditions such as hypergammaglobulinaemia and polycythaemia (*not* anaemia); and inherited deficiencies of protein C, protein S, and anti-thrombin; (III) changes in the blood flow—reduction in blood flow in patients who have compromised venous drainage, such as in the deep veins of the leg; local stasis in aneurysms; and turbulence from artificial valves, stents and implanted devices. These three factors contribute to thrombus formation, and are known collectively as 'Virchow's triad'.

11. Answer: B

This patient has presented with an 'ulnar claw', following denervation of the medial two lumbricals of the hand. The lumbricals normally induce flexion at the metacarpophalangeal (MCP) joints and so their denervation causes extension at the MCP joints due to the unopposed action of the digital extensor muscles (i.e. extensor digitorum and extensor digiti minimi). If the ulnar nerve lesion occurs distally (e.g. at the level of the wrist), the innervation of the medial half of flexor digitorum profundus (FDP), which is responsible for flexing the medial two interphalangeal (IP) joints, is unaffected. It is thus the extension of the MCP joints coupled with the slight flexion of the IP joints that gives the hand the claw-like appearance. However, if the ulnar nerve lesion occurs more proximally (e.g. near the elbow), the medial half of FDP may also be denervated, causing decreased flexion at the medial two IP joints and reducing the claw-like appearance of the hand. This is known as the 'ulnar paradox', as a more debilitating injury from a proximal lesion would normally be associated with a more abnormal appearance, unlike in this case. In addition, a more proximal lesion may cause denervation of flexor carpi ulnaris, resulting in radial deviation, which this patient does not feature. The weakness of finger adduction and abduction is a result of denervation of the palmar and dorsal interossei respectively, which are also supplied by the ulnar nerve. If this patient had sustained a supracondylar fracture of the humerus instead, other neurovascular signs of injury would probably have been apparent. Delayed compartment syndrome is very unlikely, primarily because of the patient's relative lack of pain.

12. Answer: C

Hypercalcaemia is seen in up to 5% of hospital inpatients. The causes of hypercalcaemia are as follows:

- Malignancy: bone metastases, primary tumours secreting PTH-related peptide, multiple myeloma, lymphoma
- Hyperparathyroidism: primary hyperparathyroidism, familial hypocalciuric hypercalcaemia, multiple endocrine neoplasia type I, lithium
- Increased bone turnover: prolonged immobilization, hyperthyroidism, thiazide diuretics
- Excess vitamin D: vitamin D intoxication, sarcoidosis
- Renal failure

In secondary hyperparathyroidism, the serum PTH is high with low or normal calcium levels.

Hyperventilation leads to respiratory alkalosis. As the pH of blood increases, the protein in the blood becomes increasingly ionized into anions. This causes the free calcium present in blood to bind strongly with protein (mainly albumin), resulting in an apparent hypocalcaemia.

13. Answer: C

Following the fifth day of immobilization, there is a reduction in lean body mass, which is seen in the excretion of nitrogen by protein catabolism. Potassium is the major intracellular cation in muscles and after the initial hyperkalaemia from tissue breakdown, potassium is seen to fall as it is excreted with the loss of total body lean tissue mass. The muscle mass is then replaced by adipose tissue.

With prolonged immobilization, the heart rate gradually increases while the stroke volume falls due to cardiac atrophy. The cardiac output and blood pressure, however, are maintained due to the compensatory changes mentioned earlier.

With a reduction in the overall activity of the autonomic nervous system coupled with a fall in inotropic and cardiac output response, the patient's adaptation to postural changes becomes impaired, making him unsteady on his feet. The bones eventually demineralize and calcium, phosphate, and hydroxyproline will be excreted in the urine.

In addition to the increased risk of DVT, these patients are also at increased risk of developing decubitus ulcers.

14. Answer: A

The clinical picture presented in this scenario is most suggestive of retroperitoneal fibrosis (or 'peri-aortitis'): a rare condition characterized by intense, progressive fibrosis of the connective tissue behind the peritoneal cavity. The majority of cases are idiopathic, although the condition has been known to occur with certain drugs (e.g. methysergide, bromocriptine, methyldopa, beta-blockers), carcinoid tumours, and certain fibrotic diseases (e.g. mediastinal fibrosis). In addition, it bears an association with inflammatory aortic aneurysms (e.g. chronic aortitis) and occasionally with radiotherapy. The progressive pathology usually leads to hypertension, renal impairment (i.e. as fibrosis compresses the ureters, resulting in bilateral hydronephrosis and eventual kidney failure), and, occasionally, inferior vena caval obstruction. As in this patient, initial investigations tend to reveal anaemia and uraemia in the context of raised inflammatory markers; intravenous urography will demonstrate bilateral hydronephrosis with drawing together of the ureters towards the midline. Subsequently, computed tomography (or magnetic resonance) scanning of the abdomen is useful in excluding other intra-abdominal pathology, whilst revealing a peri-aortic mass. Diagnosis is by biopsy of the retroperitoneal tissue (i.e. and not of renal tissue) at the time of operation. Treatment commonly involves the placement of double J stents to maintain ureteric patency; and dissection of ureters from the retroperitoneal fibrosis and resiting them within the peritoneal cavity, to discourage recurrence of fibrosis. They may be wrapped in omentum as a protective measure. Steroid therapy may assist in suppressing oedema in cases of recurrence.

15. Answer: C

The facial nerve (VII) serves primarily as a motor nerve to the muscles of facial expression, although it also transmits sensory fibres from the external acoustic meatus, fibres controlling salivation (i.e. to the submandibular and sublingual glands), and taste fibres from the anterior two-thirds of the tongue (via the chorda tympani) (Figure 6.1). As it also supplies stapedius, complete nerve lesions may alter auditory acuity on the affected side. From the facial nerve nucleus in the brainstem, fibres loop around the nucleus of the abducens nerve before leaving the pons medial to the vestibulocochlear nerve, and passing through the internal acoustic meatus. The facial nerve then passes through the facial canal (of the petrous temporal bone), widens to form the geniculate ganglion (which mediates taste and salivation) on the medial side of the middle ear. At this point, it deviates sharply (giving off the chorda tympani) to emerge through the stylomastoid foramen, to supply all of the muscles of facial expression (including the platysma).

It is important to remember that in partial facial nerve paralysis, the lower face is generally affected to a greater degree; in severe paralysis, there is often demonstrable loss of taste over the front of the tongue and intolerance to high-pitched or loud noises. This may cause mild dysarthria and difficulty with eating.

Lower motor neuron lesions of the facial nerve may be differentiated from upper motor neuron lesions as follows:

- In a lower motor neuron lesion, the patient generally cannot wrinkle his/her forehead, as the final common pathway to the muscles is defunct. Such lesions must be either in the pons or outside the brainstem (e.g. posterior fossa, bony canal, middle ear or outside skull).
- In an upper motor neuron lesion, the patient should be able to wrinkle his/her forehead (unless there is a bilateral lesion), since the upper facial muscles are partially spared due to alternative pathways in the brainstem.

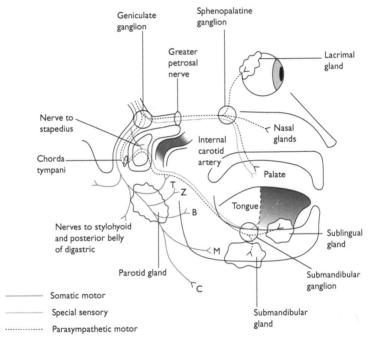

Figure 6.1 Diagram showing the anatomy of the facial nerve (CNVN). The greater petrosal nerve, nerve to stapedius and chorda tympani branch inside the facial canal. The somatic motor branch emerges from the stylomastoid foramen and then branches to supply the muscles of facial expression (T – temporal, Z – zygomatic, B – buccal, M – mandibular, C – cervical).

Reproduced from Matthew D. Gardiner and Neil R. Borley, *Training in Surgery*, 2009, Figure 11.24, p. 307, with permission from Oxford University Press.

16. Answer: C

Magnesium is the second most abundant intracellular cation and only 0.5% of the total body magnesium is found in the plasma. The measurement of serum magnesium is therefore a poor indicator of total body magnesium levels. Magnesium is found within common elements of the diet including chlorophyll in green vegetables. The vast majority of magnesium is reabsorbed in the ascending limb of the loop of Henle. Renal excretion of magnesium is increased by aldosterone and decreased by PTH. PTH also increases the absorption of magnesium from the small intestine. Magnesium is important in over 300 enzyme systems, most aspects of cellular physiology, neural function and hormone excretion. Hypomagnesaemia may present as nausea, vomiting, muscle wasting, and, in severe cases, respiratory insufficiency and cardiac arrest.

17. Answer: B

Gastrinomas are rare gastrin-secreting tumours of non-beta pancreatic islet cells. Most tumours are sporadic and are commonly found in the pancreas. About 25% are associated with MEN type 1 and tend to be found in the duodenum. Sporadic tumours have greater malignant potential.

Overall, the majority of the tumours are located in the gastrinoma triangle, which is bounded superiorly by the cystic duct, inferiorly by the second and third parts of the duodenum, and medially by the head of the pancreas.

The biochemical diagnosis of gastrinoma is based on three tests:

- High fasting serum gastrin level of >150 pg/mL
- High basal acid output >10 mEq/hour
- Secretin and calcium stimulation tests are used to differentiate gastrinomas from other conditions associated with hypergastrinaemia

18. Answer: B

Although the use of corticosteroids in sepsis remains largely controversial, meta-analyses have confirmed no benefit, or even occasional adverse effects of high-dose steroid use in septic patients. However, recent randomized controlled trials have suggested a benefit of lower doses of steroids in such instances of sepsis. The precise mechanism behind this is not fully understood but it is known that septic patients have innately low levels of endogenous steroids, and do better if supplemented in this respect. The production of recombinant human anticoagulants has evolved in recent years and there have been several randomized trials of recombinant human antithrombin III (KyberSept trial) and tissue-factor pathway inhibitor (OPTIMIST trial). However, of these, only recombinant activated protein C has shown significant survival benefit at 28 days.

19. Answer: A

This gentleman has suffered an acute ischaemic event to his right upper limb. Upper limb ischaemia is most commonly due to emboli following trauma or from known embolic sources (e.g. the heart, in atrial fibrillation); atherosclerotic occlusions are rarely a cause of such acute ischaemia. Although this gentleman's hand is currently viable, urgent intervention is necessary to prevent deterioration to beyond a non-salvageable state. In such cases, it is common for the embolus to have lodged at the level of the brachial artery. The 'fresh' embolus from this recent event should be definitively dealt with by surgical exploration and embolectomy using a Fogarty catheter. If distal material cannot be removed by the catheter, intraoperative thrombolysis may be attempted.

If available, an urgent arterial duplex scan may prove useful in identifying the site of vascular occlusion prior to endovascular intervention; however, duplex scanning is merely an imaging modality and is not a form of definitive management. This patient will also need a clotting screen and echocardiogram as basic initial tests for his thromboembolic event.

20. Answer: C

The transpyloric plane lies at the level of the L1 vertebra and bisects the line joining the suprasternal notch and the pubic symphysis. Numerous important abdominal structures lie along this plane, making it a vital anatomical landmark. These structures include the L1 vertebral body, gastric pylorus, hila of the kidneys, duodenojejunal flexure, fundus of the gallbladder, neck of the pancreas, origin of the hepatic portal vein, transverse mesocolon, second part of the duodenum, origin of the superior mesenteric artery, hilum of the spleen, 9th costal cartilage, and the end of the spinal cord (i.e. at the level of L1/L2). Note that coeliac trunk originates at the level of T12, and the inferior mesenteric artery originates at the level of L3.

21. Answer: A

The oxygen–haemoglobin dissociation curve has a sigmoid shape. The main factors that can shift the oxygen dissociation curve are as follows:

- Left shift: fall in $PaCO_2$, rise in pH, fall in temperature, fall in 2,3-DPG.
- Right shift: rise in $PaCO_2$, fall in pH, rise in temperature, rise in 2,3-DPG.
- Stored blood has low 2,3-DPG and hence a reduced ability to release oxygen to the tissues. This effect is reduced if the blood is stored in a citrate-phosphate-dextrose (CPD) solution rather than an acid-citrate-dextrose (ACD) solution.
- Exercise causes a rise in 2,3-DPG in addition to a rise in $PaCO_2$, rise in temperature and fall in pH, thereby causing a right shift of the curve.
- A significant rise in 2,3-DPG is seen with ascent to high altitude, thereby reducing the affinity of haemoglobin for oxygen.

22. Answer: E

This patient remains hypoxic despite maximal ventilation therapy. Her high CO_2 level is a reflection of permissive hypercapnoea to prevent overdistension of the lungs with high tidal volumes. None of the therapeutic options listed have been proven to improve mortality. However, laying the patient in a prone position in such a situation will aid ventilation/perfusion mismatch and temporarily improve oxygenation. Some clinicians would move immediately to high-frequency oscillatory ventilation without setting the patient in a prone posture, due to the challenging orientation of the latter. Intravenous oxygenation is complicated, requires specialist equipment and has not yet proven its benefit. Nitric oxide therapy is used infrequently to improve hypoxic pulmonary vasoconstriction.

23. Answer: B

The subtotal gastrectomy procedure (e.g. Polya gastrectomy for gastric malignancy) usually involves the formation of a simple retrocolic loop gastro-jejunostomy to the remaining stomach. The absence of a functioning pylorus allows bile to reflux into the stomach, which is now of reduced capacity, thereby increasing the chance of bilious vomiting. Severe bile reflux may require revision of the gastro-jejunostomy to a Roux-en-Y formation. In the latter case, the proximal jejunum is disconnected from the loop gastro-jejunostomy and reattached at least 30 cm distally. Peristalsis should then direct the bile distally rather than back into the stomach.

Although constipation is not specifically recognized as a complication of gastrectomy, diarrhoea can occur as a result of large volumes of highly osmotic chyme entering the duodenum, due to impaired motility secondary to vagus nerve division. A macrocytic anaemia may be consequent to vitamin B12 deficiency (i.e. due to lack of intrinsic factor production); and a microcytic anaemia may be the result of iron deficiency, as the post-gastrectomy stomach does not convert iron from Fe^{3+} to Fe^{2+}, thereby impairing its absorption from the terminal ileum.

'Dumping syndrome' is another important and relatively common complication, and is characterized by postprandial faintness, sweating, abdominal pain and tachycardia. It is caused by transient hypovolaemia following the passage of large volumes of highly osmotic food into the duodenum, and by impaired glucose control as a result of large carbohydrate loads entering the small bowel.

24. Answer: D

Haemorrhage is associated with a physiological response mediated by the autonomic nervous system that aims to maintain the perfusion of vital organs. Haemorrhagic shock can be classified according to the estimated volume of blood loss:

- Class 1: loss of 0–15% of circulating blood volume. The patient may seem uncomfortable and restless.
- Class 2: loss of 15–30% of circulating blood volume. It is associated with a pulse rate of >100/min, respiratory rate of 20–30 breaths/min, and urine output of 20–30 mL per hour. The blood pressure remains normal; however, the pulse pressure is reduced.
- Class 3: loss of 30–40% of circulating blood volume. It is associated with a pulse rate of >120/min, reduction of pulse pressure and blood pressure. The urine output can fall to 10–20 mL/hour.
- Class 4: loss of >40% of circulating blood volume. The patient may seem irritable and confused, with a pulse rate of >130/min and respiratory rate of >40/min. The blood pressure and pulse pressure will remain low and the patient may be anuric.

25. Answer: B

Weakness of thumb movements after carpal tunnel decompression is related to paralysis of the thenar muscles. The thenar muscles of the hand are supplied by the recurrent branch of the median nerve, which usually lies just distal to the transverse carpal ligament. It is therefore at risk of damage during carpal tunnel decompression. The palmar cutaneous nerve is also at risk of injury during this operation as it can be damaged while placing the distal part of the skin incision. It is the commonest nerve to be injured during carpal tunnel decompression. Injury can lead to neuroma formation, which in turn leads to pain. Care is therefore taken to avoid injury to this nerve during surgery. The superficial branch of the ulnar nerve passes superficially to the carpal tunnel. The deep branch of the ulnar nerve enters the hand through Guyon's canal (or the 'ulnar canal'). The ulnar nerve supplies all the intrinsic muscles of the hand except for the thenar muscles and the first two lumbricals.

26. Answer: E

All of the statements regarding vagotomy are correct except for E. The reduced coordination of myenteric activity may also lead to early hyperactive emptying, particularly if a gastric drainage procedure (e.g. pyloroplasty) has been performed. Another potential side effect of vagotomy is vitamin B12 deficiency, as it impairs gastric secretions and the production of intrinsic factor. Since the discovery of *Helicobacter pylori* to be the causative agent of peptic ulcer disease, vagotomy procedures have been made redundant and less invasive treatment strategies have been adopted.

27. Answer: C

Multiple endocrine neoplasia type 2 (MEN 2) is an autosomal dominant disorder caused by mutations in the *RET* proto-oncogene. MEN 2 has 3 distinct subtypes—MEN 2A, MEN 2B and familial medullary thyroid carcinoma. MEN 2A describes the association of medullary thyroid carcinoma, phaeochromocytomas and parathyroid tumours. MEN 2B is characterized by MEN 2A plus Marfanoid features and mucosal neuromas. In MEN 2B, the medullary cancer is very aggressive with most patients dying before developing either a phaeochromocytoma or hyperparathyroidism. A patient with medullary carcinoma of the thyroid may present with diarrhoea due to elevated prostaglandin or calcitonin levels. Patients with hypercalcaemia may present with constipation, polyuria, polydipsia, depression, nephrolithiasis, glucose intolerance, gastro-oesophageal reflux, loss of bone density and fatigue. Patients with phaeochromocytoma may present with hypertension, tachycardia, sweating and headaches. Cutaneous lichen amyloidosis in patients with MEN 2A manifests as multiple pruritic scaly skin lesions in the scapular area of the back.

28. Answer: D

The femoral sheath contains three main compartments. The lateral compartment contains the femoral artery, the intermediate compartment contains the femoral vein, and the medial compartment contains the femoral canal. The femoral canal is a short, 0.5 cm wide blind-ending potential space containing loose areolar tissue, lymphatics and the node of Cloquet. It allows for the expansion of the femoral vein when there is increased venous return from the lower limbs or increased intra-abdominal pressure. The femoral canal has the following boundaries:

- Anteriorly: inguinal ligament
- Posteriorly: pectineal ligament
- Medially: lacunar ligament
- Laterally: femoral vein

The femoral nerve lies lateral to the femoral artery, and is considered to be external to the femoral sheath.

29. Answer: B

The Bohr effect describes the reduction in affinity of haemoglobin for oxygen in active tissues in response to a drop in pH caused by increased CO_2 production. As a result, oxygen is readily offloaded to these active tissues.

The Haldane effect describes the increased CO_2 carrying capacity of deoxygenated blood. This means that for any given $PaCO_2$, the CO_2 content of deoxygenated blood is greater than that of oxygenated blood.

The Pasteur effect describes the inhibitory effect of oxygen on fermentation.

The rebound effect is the tendency of a medication to cause a more severe return of symptoms when discontinued.

30. Answer: E

Tertiary hyperparathyroidism is the autonomous hypersecretion of parathyroid hormone (PTH) without an abnormal stimulus. It occurs in patients with longstanding secondary hyperparathyroidism caused by chronic renal failure. Following renal transplantation, there is resolution of renal stimuli and normalization of serum calcium, but continued hypersecretion of PTH. Most cases resolve spontaneously. Parathyroidectomy is indicated if there is no resolution by 1 year. Secondary hyperparathyroidism is caused by excessive PTH secretion in response to an abnormal stimulus, such as chronic renal failure and vitamin D deficiency. It is associated with high serum PTH and phosphate levels, with low or normal serum calcium levels.

31. Answer: C

Traditional anatomy describes the duodenum as being divided into four sections. The posterior relations of the first part of the duodenum include the portal vein, common bile duct and gastroduodenal artery (behind which lies the inferior vena cava). The abdominal aorta crosses behind the third part of the duodenum, whilst the superior mesenteric vessels are related anteriorly to the third part of the duodenum. The main pancreatic duct opens into the second part of the duodenum at the ampulla of Vater. The second part of the duodenum is crossed by the transverse colon.

32. Answer: C

Systemic inflammatory response syndrome (SIRS) is characterized by the presence of two or more of the following:

- Core temperature > 38°C or <36°C
- Heart rate >90/min

- Respiratory rate >20/min or $PaCO_2$ <4.3 kPa
- WCC >12 ×10^9/L or < 4 × 10^9/L

'Sepsis' implies the presence of SIRS with a proven source of infection.

'Severe sepsis' implies sepsis with evidence of organ failure due to inadequate perfusion.

'Septic shock' implies severe sepsis with hypotension (systolic blood pressure <90 mmHg) despite adequate fluid resuscitation, or the requirement for vasopressors/inotropes to maintain blood pressure

The term 'multiple organ dysfunction syndrome' (MODS) implies the requirement of organ support for two or more organ systems in the presence of SIRS.

33. Answer: D

The parotid gland is the largest salivary gland in humans. The gland extends from the zygomatic arch to the angle of the mandible. Superior to it lie the external auditory meatus and the temporomandibular joint; inferiorly, the posterior belly of the digastric muscle; medially, the styloid process; and posteriorly, the masseter and sternocleidomastoid muscles.

The facial nerve runs through the parotid gland, dividing it into superficial and deep lobes. The superficial lobe is larger and is the site of a greater proportion of tumours. The facial nerve supplies the muscles of facial expression, rather than facial sensation, which is supplied by the trigeminal nerve. The retromandibular vein and the internal carotid artery pass through the parotid gland, where the latter divides into its terminal branches (maxillary and superficial temporal arteries). The parotid duct (or Stensen's duct) opens within the buccal cavity opposite to the second upper molar.

34. Answer: B

A furuncle (or boil) is a *Staphylococcus* abscess which develops within a hair follicle. A furuncle in the infra-orbital region or the lateral aspect of the nose drains into the cavernous sinus via the facial vein and inferior ophthalmic vein. The cavernous sinus is an irregularly shaped cavity, which is located lateral and superior to the sphenoidal sinus and posterior to the optic chiasm. The cavernous sinus receives venous blood from the facial vein (via the superior and inferior ophthalmic veins) as well as the sphenoidal and middle cerebral vein. It empties into the superior and inferior petrosal sinusus (and subsequently into the internal jugular vein). This complex of veins does not contain valves, thereby permitting blood to flow in any direction, potentially distributing infections from the face, nose, orbits and tonsils to the cavernous sinus. Within the sinus also lie the internal carotid artery and its associated sympathetic nervous plexus. The 3rd, 4th and 6th cranial nerves, and ophthalmic and maxillary divisions of the 5th cranial nerve are embedded within the lateral wall of the sinus. Infection within this sinus may therefore result in associated cranial nerve palsies as described in this scenario.

35. Answer: B

The nerve that is most likely to be injured in this child is the median nerve. The median nerve is derived from the C5–C7 roots from the lateral cord of the brachial plexus and from the C8 and T1 roots from the medial cord. In the arm, it runs in close proximity to the brachial artery and may be injured following supracondylar fractures of the humerus. Thus the radial pulse may be feeble or absent with such injuries. In the cubital fossa, the median nerve passes between the two heads of the pronator teres. It then travels between the muscle bellies of flexor digitorum superficialis and flexor digitorum profundus before emerging between flexor digitorum superficialis and flexor pollicis longus. The median nerve then passes through the carpel tunnel, where it may be compressed to cause carpal tunnel syndrome.

36. Answer: D

Dopamine agonist therapy with bromocriptine will be useful to reduce this patient's elevated prolactin levels and induce normal ovulatory function, restoring her fertility. It has been shown that treatment with bromocriptine can shrink pituitary microadenomas by up to 90% within 1 year of commencing therapy. Somatostatin and octreotide are used in the treatment of growth hormone-secreting tumours. Although smaller tumours are best treated by conservative correction of the underlying hormonal disturbances, large tumours usually require surgical debulking via a trans-sphenoidal, trans-ethmoidal or trans-frontal (i.e. for tumours with large frontal or lateral extensions, a craniotomy flap is required) approach. Surgery is then followed by radiotherapy and correction of the underlying endocrine abnormalities, with steroid cover prior to surgery.

37. Answer: D

The commonest reason for an open tracheostomy is the need for long-term mechanical ventilation. To perform an open tracheotomy, the patient should be positioned supine with their neck extended. The neck is prepared and draped, and a 2–3 cm transverse incision is made 2 cm above the sternal notch in the midline (i.e. at the level of the 3rd tracheal ring). The skin, deep fascia and the platysma are divided and the strap muscles retracted to expose the thyroid isthmus. The thyroid isthmus is then either pushed down or divided and ligated to achieve haemostasis. The trachea is incised either between the 2nd and 3rd or the 3rd and 4th tracheal rings. The anaesthetist is then asked to withdraw the endotracheal tube until above this level. The incision is widened and a tracheostomy tube is inserted and secured.

38. Answer: D

Sister Mary Joseph nodule refers to a palpable umbilical nodule that is indicative of metastatic spread of abdominopelvic malignancy. It is suggestive of a poor prognosis. The underlying malignancy tends to be gastrointestinal, gynaecological or urological in origin. It is thought to result from transperitoneal spread of malignant cells via the lymphatics travelling around the obliterated umbilical vein to the umbilicus.

39. Answer: A

This patient experiences diplopia on downward and outward gaze (vertical and torsional diplopia—torsional rotation of the eye refers to keeping the eye oriented straight up and down when the head tilts from side to side), and thus the superior oblique muscle is most likely to be affected. The muscle is probably affected due to paralysis of the trochlear nerve (from the head injury). The long course of the nerve makes it especially susceptible to injury in association with severe head injury. The superior oblique muscle abducts the eye and moves the eye downwards (it intorts, depresses and abducts the globe). It originates from the posterior orbit and travels along the superomedial wall of the orbit to the trochlea. Its tendon passes through a pulley-like structure at the superior orbital rim and then courses back toward the globe, inserting upon the posterosuperior quadrant of the eye.

40. Answer: C

Gynaecomastia is the benign hypertrophy of glandular tissue in the male breast resulting from the physiological/pathological alteration in the body's oestrogen/androgen balance. Causes of gynaecomastia include:

- Physiological causes: seen in neonates, adolescents, and elderly men.
- Pathological causes: congenital anorchia, Klinefelter's syndrome, testicular feminization, hermaphroditism, pituitary tumours, adrenal tumours, liver disorders, and malnutrition.

- Pharmacological causes:
  - ◆ Drugs that function like oestrogen: diethylstilbestrol, oral contraceptive pills, digoxin, oestrogen-containing cosmetics.
  - ◆ Drugs that enhance endogenous oestrogen formation: gonadotropins, progesterone, clomiphene.
  - ◆ Drugs which inhibit testosterone synthesis and function: ketoconazole, metronidazole, cimetidine.
  - ◆ Unknown mechanism: isoniazid, methyldopa, captopril, tricyclic antidepressants, diazepam, cannabis, heroin.

41. Answer: A

Patients should be specifically warned of neurovascular damage prior to surgery. In particular they should be consented for possible numbness on the medial aspect of the upper arm.

The long thoracic nerve supplies the serratus anterior muscle and damage to this will result in winging of the scapula.

Thoracodorsal nerve innervates the latissimus dorsi muscle and should be preserved particularly in those who are undergoing latissimus dorsi flap reconstructions.

Axillary nerve supplies the deltoid and teres minor muscles and the small patch of skin on the lateral aspect of the upper arm, called the 'regimental badge patch'.

Musculocutaneous nerve supplies sensation to the skin on the lateral aspect of the forearm.

42. Answer: C

A good understanding of the modified Dukes classification is required to answer this question. The Dukes classification describes the staging and survival rates of patients with treated colorectal carcinoma:

- Dukes A describes a tumour which is confined to the bowel wall with no extension into the extrarectal or extracolic tissue, and without any lymphatic metastasis. The 5-year survival of these patients is between 95–97%.
- Dukes B describes a tumour which has spread through the muscularis propria into the extrarectal and extracolic tissues by direct continuity but without lymphatic spread. These patients have a 5-year survival of 80%.
- Dukes C implies the presence of lymph node metastasis. If only a few lymph nodes are involved near the primary, the 5-year survival is 60%. If there is a continuous string of involved lymph nodes up to the proximal limit of resection, then the 5-year survival falls to 30%.
- Dukes D implies the presence of distant metastasis, which suggests that the lesion is surgically incurable. The 5-year survival in such cases is less than 5%.

43. Answer: B

Calot's triangle is formed by the inferior border of the liver, the cystic duct, and the common hepatic duct. Within it lies the cystic artery, which is usually a branch of the right hepatic artery. By identifying this triangle, the surgeon is able to safely dissect and ligate the cystic duct and cystic artery without damaging the common bile duct. The famous lymph node that lies within Calot's triangle is named Mascagni's lymph node (or node of Lund), and is the sentinel lymph node of the gallbladder.

44. Answer: B

Ascending cholangitis is an acute inflammation of the biliary tree due to infection of an obstructed common bile duct. This is in contrast to sclerosing cholangitis, which presents less acutely and is of non-infective aetiology. The biliary obstruction from ascending cholangitis is usually due to gallstones (80%), although it may also result from strictures, tumours or damage following ERCP. The causative organisms are usually gut-derived coliform bacteria. Management involves intravenous fluid resuscitation and broad-spectrum antibiotics while awaiting microbial sensitivities from blood culture. Emergency ERCP and decompression of the common bile duct is usually necessary to relieve the obstruction and to encourage the evacuation of pus from the biliary tree. Nearly all patients who do not receive treatment for ascending cholangitis will die, thereby emphasizing the need for a high index of clinical suspicion and prompt intervention in such patients.

45. Answer: C

Familial adenomatous polyposis (FAP) is a rare autosomal dominant condition which results from the deletion of the long arm of chromosome 5. This gives rise to hundreds of colorectal adenomatous polyps that are inherently benign. The adenomatous polyposis coli (APC) gene is a tumour suppressor gene that is usually located in the long arm of the chromosome 5. Congenital hypertrophy of the retinal pigment epithelium occurs in as many as 95% of individuals with FAP. Its presence is therefore used as a screening tool, alongside colonoscopy and gene testing, in relatives of patients with FAP.

46. Answer: C

The signs and symptoms of this patient are suggestive of acute pancreatitis. Gallstone disease accounts for about 40–60% of all cases of acute pancreatitis. In this case, the patient seems to have experienced past episodes of biliary colic leading up to this. The other important cause of acute pancreatitis (though usually acute-on-chronic) is alcohol abuse (30–40%). Approximately 25% of patients presenting with acute pancreatitis may have associated cardiovascular (tachycardia) or respiratory (tachypnoea) symptoms. Pancreatitis is thought to result from early activation of pancreatic enzymes, producing autodigestion of the pancreas and surrounding tissues. The severity of acute pancreatitis is validated using various prognostic scoring systems. Currently in the UK, the Glasgow-Imrie scoring system is widely used for assessing the severity and predicating the prognosis in acute pancreatitis (age >55 years, WCC >15 × 10^9/L, glucose >10 mmol/L, urea >16 mmol/L, PaO$_2$ <60 mmHg or 7.9 kPa, calcium <2 mmol/L, albumin <32 g/L, lactate dehydrogenase >600 IU/L, aspartate aminotransferase >200 IU/L. Serum CRP, although not part of the Glasgow criteria, has an independent prognostic value if the peak level is >210 mg/L in the first 4 days of the attack). Serum amylase is another useful indicator of acute pancreatitis; a diagnosis of acute pancreatitis is likely if the level is three times the upper limit of normal, although this may vary between laboratories, and depending on individual hospital policy/guidelines (i.e. a serum amylase level of over 1000 IU/L is widely regarded as indicating pancreatitis). To this effect, serum lipase is more sensitive and specific, and has a longer half-life than serum amylase; it is therefore used in preference to amylase, where available. An ultrasound of the abdomen is indicated in all patients with acute pancreatitis to determine the presence/absence of biliary calculi, which urgent ERCP may be required to relieve. A CT scan of the abdomen should be performed on all patients with severe acute pancreatitis, preferably between days 3–10 following the onset of symptoms, to rule out pancreatic necrosis and subsequent abscess formation.

In addition, it is worth noting that perforated duodenal ulcers can present in a similar fashion to acute pancreatitis, demonstrating a normal CXR (i.e. without evidence of pneumoperitoneum) in up to a third of cases.

47. Answer: E

Gastrinomas primarily occur in the pancreas and duodenum, and are malignant in nearly two-thirds of cases. The patients may present with upper abdominal pain and vomiting; the vomitus may be 'coffee-ground' due to the digestion of blood (from the ulcers) within the stomach. Ninety per cent of patients with gastrinomas develop peptic ulceration. Gastrinomas may either arise sporadically or as part of Zollinger–Ellison syndrome (i.e. peptic ulceration, gastric acid hypersecretion, and islet cell tumours of the pancreas). Sporadic Zollinger–Ellison syndrome occurs most frequently in the fifth decade of life. Approximately 20% of patients with Zollinger–Ellison syndrome have multiple endocrine neoplasia type 1. An elevated basal gastric acid output >15 mEq/h and a serum gastrin level of >1000 pg/mL are suggestive of a gastrinoma. If it is difficult to make a diagnosis, a secretin stimulation test may be indicated. Lesions are localized by somatostatin-receptor scintigraphy. CT scanning may be indicated to exclude metastases. The treatment of this condition is either medical (e.g. with high-dose proton pump inhibitors) or surgical. Surgical resection may be aided by intraoperative ultrasound and/or intraoperative endoscopy.

48. Answer: C

Hirschsprung's disease is a well-described cause of neonatal large bowel obstruction, resulting from the failure of migration of ganglion cells to the affected bowel segment. This invariably involves the distal colon and may occasionally involve proximal segments; rarely, the entire large bowel may be affected. The affected segment is histologically devoid of ganglion cells in the Meissner's (submucosal) and Auerbach's (myenteric) plexus but demonstrates immunohistochemical evidence of increased acetylcholinesterase activity. Contrast imaging tends to reveal tonic contraction of the affected segments. Rectal irrigation or emergency colostomy formation may be required before a definitive 'pull-through' procedure is performed. Eighty per cent of cases present in the neonatal period, typically with constipation, and subsequently with vomiting and other features of obstruction.

49. Answer: E

It is vital that clinicians have a basic grasp of the various statistical tests used in evidence-based medicine to be able to appraise the literature and also to facilitate the conduct of their own research. The two-sample unpaired t-test is used to test the null hypothesis that the two populations corresponding to the two random samples are equal. For a paired t-test, the data are dependent (i.e. there is a one-to-one correspondence between the values in the two samples; e.g. the same subject measured before and after a process change, or the same subject measured at different times).

50. Answer: D

The commonest infective cause of acute osteomyelitis in children over the age of 4 years is *Staphylococcus aureus*, a Gram-positive anaerobic coccus that is frequently part of the skin flora (note that 20% of the human population are long-term carriers of *S. aureus*). *S. aureus* is incidentally also the organism most commonly isolated from all forms of osteomyelitis. After diagnosis (which is usually based on radiological findings of lytic bone with a ring of sclerosis) and culture from a bone biopsy, prolonged antibiotic therapy (i.e. usually for at least 4–6 weeks, via central venous access) is warranted. The primary treatment of such cases is with a combination of penicillinase-resistant synthetic penicillin and a third-generation cephalosporin (e.g. ceftriaxone). Alternative therapy is with vancomycin or clindamycin and a third-generation cephalosporin, particularly if methicillin-resistant *S. aureus* (MRSA) is likely.

Salmonella species are the characteristic cause of osteomyelitis in patients with sickle cell disease (together with *S. aureus*); treatment for such cases is primarily with a fluoroquinolone antibiotic (but not in children) or a third-generation cephalosporin. *Pseudomonas* infection is most commonly seen in haemodialysis patients, intravenous drug abusers, and, for example, when a nail puncture occurs through an athletic shoe. In such cases, treatment should include ceftazidime or ciprofloxacin. Trauma-induced osteomyelitis may commonly be attributed to *S. aureus*, *P. aeruginosa*, and coliform bacilli, and may be treated as described above. Cases of haematogenous osteomyelitis due to *H. influenza* have almost completely been eradicated with immunization.

Basic sciences: Applied anatomy

1. **Which of the following tendons form the ulnar border of the anatomical snuff box?**
   A. Tendon of extensor digitorum longus
   B. Tendon of extensor indicis proprius
   C. Tendon of extensor pollicis longus
   D. Tendon of abductor pollicis longus
   E. Tendon of extensor pollicis brevis

Basic sciences: Physiology

2. **Which of the following statements regarding oxygen delivery to the tissues is correct?**
   A. Typical arteriovenous difference of oxygen partial pressure for a healthy 21-year-old male at rest would be approximately 75%
   B. Arterial oxygen partial pressure is reduced in women with iron deficiency anaemia
   C. In subjects living at high altitude, the oxygen dissociation curve is shifted to the left
   D. Use of erythropoietin stimulates greater dissociation of oxygen from haemoglobin
   E. An increase in the acidity of the blood would promote greater oxygen delivery to the tissues

Basic sciences: Pathology

3. **A 45-year-old diabetic man presents to his GP with a 2-week history of progressively worsening sweating from the left side of his face during meals. Six months prior to this, he underwent excision of a pleomorphic adenoma from his left parotid gland. The GP diagnoses Frey's syndrome and advises the patient about the various management options. Which of the following statements is correct regarding Frey's syndrome?**
   A. A positive starch-iodine test is diagnostic
   B. It can lead to sialolithiasis if left untreated
   C. It is caused by growth of the divided sympathetic nerve fibres into the skin
   D. It occurs in about 65% of patients who have undergone surgery to the parotid gland
   E. Treatment using 1% glycopyrrolate lotion is based on a sympatholytic effect

Common surgical conditions and the subspecialties:
Trauma and orthopaedics

4. A 33-year-old motorcyclist is brought to the Emergency Department
    following a high-speed road traffic accident. On examination, his
    pulse rate is 110/min, blood pressure is 100/74 mmHg and his Glasgow
    Coma Scale score is 15. Examination reveals swelling and tenderness
    over the left lower leg, and subsequent plain radiography confirms a
    closed but comminuted fracture of the left tibia. Whilst the patient
    is being transferred to the orthopaedic ward, he complains of severe,
    unremitting pain in his left lower leg and numbness in his left foot. The
    dorsalis pedis and posterior tibial pulses are palpable. The pain in his
    foot is made worse by passive dorsiflexion of the ankle. What is the
    most likely cause of this patient's signs and symptoms?

    A. Torn gastrocnemius and soleus
    B. Common peroneal nerve palsy
    C. Deep venous thrombosis
    D. Ruptured Achilles tendon
    E. Compartment syndrome

Common surgical conditions and the subspecialties: Endocrine disease

5. A 31-year-old man is referred to the urology clinic following numerous
    episodes of renal colic. His blood test results reveal a serum adjusted
    calcium level of 2.9 mmol/L, a phosphate level of 0.7 mmol/L, and
    on subsequent tests, a PTH level of 45 pmol/L. The patient later
    describes headaches and loss of peripheral vision, and on further
    questioning, reveals that his sister had undergone parathyroid surgery
    at 33 years of age. What is the most likely diagnosis of this patient?

    A. Primary hyperparathyroidism
    B. Secondary hyperparathyroidism
    C. Tertiary hyperparathyroidism
    D. Multiple endocrine neoplasia type 1
    E. Multiple endocrine neoplasia type 2

Perioperative care: Preoperative assessment and management

6. Which of the following statements is true of bariatric surgery?

    A. It is contraindicated in patients aged under 20 years
    B. It is associated with a postoperative mortality of between 5–10%
    C. It is associated with nutritional deficiencies
    D. It is indicated in selected patients with a body mass index (BMI) greater than 30 kg/m^2
    E. It reduces cardiovascular morbidity and mortality

The assessment and management of the surgical patient:
Clinical decision-making

7. **A 47-year-old female with a new diagnosis of early breast cancer undergoes wide local excision and axillary node clearance of the right breast. Eight hours postoperatively, she complains of increasing pain from the operated breast. Examination reveals a swollen and tender right breast, with the single axillary drain having drained 40 mL of haemoserous fluid. Which of the following options describes the most appropriate management for this patient?**
    A. Continue titrated analgesia and observe
    B. Discontinue thromboprophylactic medication
    C. Operative haemostasis and washout
    D. Percutaneous insertion of drain into swollen area
    E. Ultrasound-guided needle aspiration

Basic sciences: Applied anatomy

8. **A vascular surgeon attempts to palpate the femoral pulse prior to femoral artery cutdown for an endovascular aneurysm repair. What is the posterior relation of the femoral artery against which the surgeon compresses the artery to feel its pulsation?**
    A. Adductor longus
    B. Iliac bone
    C. Inguinal ligament
    D. Psoas tendon
    E. Superior pubic ramus

Basic sciences: Physiology

9. **Which of the following is responsible for controlling testicular descent in the inguinoscrotal phase?**
    A. Mullerian inhibiting substance
    B. Calcitonin gene-related peptide (CGRP)
    C. Testosterone and CGRP
    D. Mullerian inhibiting substance and CGRP
    E. Testosterone and Mullerian inhibiting substance

Common surgical conditions and the subspecialties: Trauma and orthopaedics

10. **A 60-year-old-woman slips on an icy pavement and falls onto her outstretched hand. Radiography of her wrist reveals a Smith's fracture. Which one of the following best describes a Smith's fracture?**

    A. Intra-articular distal radius fracture with dorsal angulation of distal fragment

    B. Extra-articular distal radius fracture with dorsal angulation of distal fragment

    C. Intra-articular distal radial fracture with volar angulation of distal fragment

    D. Extra-articular distal radial fracture with volar angulation of distal fragment

    E. Complete displacement of an intra-articular fracture involving the volar lip of the distal radius

Common surgical conditions and the subspecialties: Genitourinary disease

11. **A 90-year-old retired GP incidentally discovers a swelling in his right scrotum. Self-examination reveals a semi-firm lump that cannot be palpated separately from the vas deferens, does not demonstrate a cough impulse, and does not transilluminate. What is the most likely diagnosis of this lump?**

    A. Epididymal cyst

    B. Inguinal hernia (direct)

    C. Inguinal hernia (indirect)

    D. Neoplasm of the vas deferens

    E. Testicular seminoma

Perioperative care

12. **A 30-year-old male suffering from hypersplenism due to idiopathic thrombocytopenic purpura is scheduled for an elective splenectomy. Which of the following is the best time to administer his vaccination?**

    A. 1 week before surgery

    B. 2 weeks before surgery

    C. 48 hours before surgery

    D. Immediately after surgery

    E. 6 weeks before surgery

The assessment and management of the surgical patient:
Clinical decision-making

13. **A 53-year-old man undergoes internal fixation (intramedullary nailing)
of his right tibia after sustaining a comminuted fracture of the tibia in
a road traffic accident. Twenty-hours after surgery, he complains of
severe pain in his right leg. Examination reveals a blood pressure of
122/82 mmHg and a heart rate of 84/min. His right calf is swollen and
mildly tender, and his foot pulses are present. There is some altered
sensation over the dorsum of his foot, and pain is worsened when the
foot is actively dorsiflexed. Which of the following options will most
likely improve this patient's outcome?**

A. Amputation
B. Analgesia and prophylactic antibiotics
C. Embolectomy
D. Fasciotomy
E. Thrombolysis

Basic sciences: Applied anatomy

14. **An upper gastrointestinal surgeon dissects around the oesophageal
hiatus of the diaphragm during a minimally invasive oesophagectomy
for an early oesophagogastric tumour. Which of the following
statements is correct regarding the thoracic diaphragm?**

A. It has an oesophageal hiatus at vertebral level T8
B. It has a central tendon that transmits the right phrenic nerve
C. It is partly derived from the pleuroperitoneal membranes
D. It originates partly from the body of the sternum
E. The intercostal nerves supply it with accessory motor innervation

Basic sciences: Physiology

15. **Which of the following statements is correct regarding the physiology
of fluid balance?**

A. An average 70 kg man will have 11 L of plasma in his intravascular circulation
B. On average, the stomach produces about 750–1000 mL of fluid daily
C. When a 1 L bag of normal saline is infused into a patient, only 500 mL will stay within the
intravascular compartment
D. When 1 L of 5% dextrose is administered to a patient, the plasma volume effectively
increases by no more than 80 mL
E. Colloids have approximately the same composition and osmolality as plasma

Common surgical conditions and the subspecialties:
Trauma and orthopaedics

16. A 4-year-old girl presents to the Emergency Department with her parents after falling from the top of the slide at the playground a few hours previously. She has since refused to walk. On examination, the child is unable to weight bear on her right leg, is tender over the right mid-tibia, but has no obvious limb deformity. Of the following options, what is plain radiography of the affected limb most likely to reveal?

A. Butterfly fracture
B. Comminuted fracture
C. No evidence of fracture
D. Salter–Harris fracture
E. Spiral fracture

Common surgical conditions and the subspecialties: Breast disease

17. A 55-year-old lady presents to the breast clinic with a 1-week history of a left breast lump. She was involved in a car accident 1 month previously, when the car she was driving was hit in the rear by another car. She only suffered minor symptoms of whiplash injury after the accident. Her past medical history includes diabetes and hypertension. Her sister was recently diagnosed with breast cancer. Examination reveals a small, mildly tender nodule in the upper outer quadrant of the left breast. Biopsy reveals numerous large foamy cells with small multiple nucleoli. What is the most likely diagnosis?

A. Periductal mastitis
B. Ductal carcinoma
C. Fat necrosis
D. Fibrocystic disease
E. Lobular carcinoma

Perioperative care

18. A 28-year-old man with hereditary spherocytosis is preoperatively assessed for elective splenectomy. When should the pneumococcal vaccine (e.g. Pneumovax) be administered?

A. A month before surgery
B. A week before surgery
C. A week after surgery
D. A month after surgery
E. In the immediate postoperative period

The assessment and management of the surgical patient: Case work-up and evaluation

19. A 25-year-old builder lands on his head after falling 20 feet from a ladder, losing consciousness for an unknown duration. He is brought to the Emergency Department by ambulance, where primary and secondary surveys are largely unremarkable. CT imaging confirms a non-displaced skull fracture and excludes intracranial haemorrhage. The patient is resuscitated and stabilized before being transferred to the high-dependency unit for monitoring. Twelve hours later, his blood tests reveal the following results: sodium 163 mmol/L (137–144), potassium 3.5 mmol/L (3.5–4.9), chloride 125 mmol/L (95–107), urea 3.4 mmol/L (2.5–7.5) and creatinine 82 μmol/L (60–110). Which one of the following statements is most accurate in this case?

A. Urgent crystalloid rehydration is indicated
B. Syndrome of inappropriate antidiuretic hormone secretion (SIADH) is likely
C. Salt restriction is a priority
D. A hyperchloraemic acidosis is likely to be present
E. The patient's urine osmolality is likely to be low

Basic sciences: Applied anatomy

20. A 47-year-old male presents to hospital with perianal pain and swelling. Physical examination reveals a tender, erythematous swelling in his right ischioanal fossa. The junior surgical trainee attempts to perform an incision and drainage of abscess. Which of the following structures is most vulnerable to injury during this surgery?

A. Superficial perineal nerve
B. Pudendal nerve
C. Nerve to obturator internus
D. Perineal branch of S4
E. Deep perineal nerve

Basic sciences: Physiology

21. A 7-week-old boy presents with projectile, non-bilious vomiting after feeding. Examination during feeding reveals an olive-shaped mass in the right upper quadrant. Which of the following biochemical abnormalities is most likely to manifest in this patient?

A. Hyperchloraemic, hypokalaemic metabolic acidosis with a low urinary pH
B. Hypochloraemic, hyperkalaemic metabolic alkalosis with a high urinary pH
C. Hypochloraemic, hypokalaemic metabolic alkalosis with high urinary pH
D. Hypochloraemic, hypokalaemic metabolic alkalosis with a low urinary pH
E. Hyperchloraemic, hyperkalaemic metabolic acidosis with low urinary pH

Common surgical conditions and the subspecialties: Endocrine disease

22. **A 30-year-old woman presents with a 6-week history of weight loss and anxiety. She takes no regular medication and has smoked 10 cigarettes daily for 6 years. Examination reveals a resting heart rate of 108/min, a fine resting tremor of the hands, lid lag, and periorbital oedema. A diffusely enlarged diffuse goitre is noted, with a non-tender 2 cm nodule on the right thyroid lobe. No obvious lymphadenopathy is noted but a thyroid bruit is found on auscultation. Initial blood tests reveal a free T4 level of 31.5 pmol/L (10–22), TSH level of 0.10 mU/L (0.4–5), and the presence of thyroid peroxidase antibodies. Radioisotope scanning of the thyroid reveals a diffuse uptake with no uptake in right nodule. What is the most likely diagnosis in this patient?**
    A. De Quervain's thyroiditis
    B. Follicular carcinoma of the thyroid
    C. Graves' disease
    D. Papillary carcinoma of the thyroid
    E. Toxic multinodular goitre

Perioperative care: Preoperative assessment and management

23. **A 60-year-old gentleman is seen in the preoperative assessment clinic prior to a laparoscopic cholecystectomy. He has a significant past medical history of ischaemic heart disease but is also found to have clinical signs of aortic regurgitation. Which of the following is not a feature of aortic regurgitation?**
    A. Early diastolic murmur
    B. Austin Flint murmur
    C. Quincke's sign
    D. De Musset's sign
    E. Slow rising pulse

Assessment and management of patients with trauma (including the multiply injured patient): Shock

24. **A 30-year-old man is involved in a road traffic accident. He presents to the Emergency Department appearing mildly anxious, after losing a significant amount of blood, with tachycardia (113/min), tachypnoea (25/min) and oliguria (20 mL/hour). Which of the following statements is true about his degree of hypovolaemic shock?**
    A. Class I hypovolaemic shock
    B. Class II hypovolaemic shock
    C. Class III hypovolaemic shock
    D. Class IV hypovolaemic shock
    E. None of the above

Basic sciences: Applied anatomy

25. A 30-year-old lady with symptomatic varicose veins undergoes a right leg sapheno-popliteal ligation and stripping of the short saphenous vein. Which nerve is at risk of injury in this procedure?

A. Saphenous nerve
B. Sural nerve
C. Common peroneal nerve
D. Superficial peroneal nerve
E. Deep peroneal nerve

Basic sciences: Physiology

26. A 24-year-old female presents to her GP with symptoms of recurrent renal colic. Basic blood tests reveal the presence of hypercalcaemia. Which of the following statements is incorrect regarding calcium homeostasis?

A. Parathyroid hormone increases serum calcium by increasing renal tubular reabsorption and lowering serum phosphate
B. Vitamin D3 increases serum calcium by promoting absorption through the terminal ileum, and by renal tubular reabsorption
C. Calcitonin lowers serum calcium and serum phosphate
D. Acidosis increases protein binding and decreases ionized calcium levels
E. The commonest cause of hypercalcaemia is malignancy

Common surgical conditions and the subspecialties: Gastrointestinal disease

27. Which among the following statements regarding Dukes' staging for cancer of the colon is incorrect?

A. Dukes' stage A implies carcinoma limited to the bowel wall
B. The 5-year survival rate following surgical resection for Dukes A tumours can be over 90%
C. Dukes' stage C implies malignant spread to the regional lymph nodes
D. The 5-year survival rate of patients with Dukes' stage D tumours is approximately 30%
E. Dukes' stage B implies tumour extension through the muscularis mucosae

Basic sciences: Applied anatomy

28. A 14-year-old gymnast sustains a deep laceration to her distal forearm during a training-related accident. Examination of the injured hand and wrist reveal intermittent spurts of blood from the lateral aspect of her wound, which are easily controlled with pressure. Closer examination reveals two transected tendons. She is able to adduct her thumb but is unable to oppose it. She is unable to produce fine movements of her 2nd and 3rd digits, and she describes diminished sensation over the lateral aspect of her palm and digits. Further examination reveals weakened wrist flexion, with associated ulnar deviation. Which one of the following structures is unlikely to have been damaged in the scenario described?

    A. Palmaris longus tendon
    B. Tendon of the flexor carpi radialis
    C. Radial artery
    D. Superficial palmar branch of the radial artery
    E. Median nerve
    F. Ulna nerve

Basic sciences: Physiology

29. What is the main mode of transport of carbon dioxide within the blood?

    A. As bicarbonate ions
    B. Bound to plasma proteins
    C. Bound to haemoglobin
    D. Dissolved in solution
    E. Bound to hydrogen ions

Common surgical conditions and the subspecialties: Gastrointestinal disease

30. A 60-year-old man who was recently diagnosed with non-metastatic colorectal cancer undergoes a left hemicolectomy. The histopathology report for the resected specimen reveals a tumour extending into the muscularis propria but not breaching the subserosa. Six out of 16 lymph nodes are found to be positive for tumour spread. What is the TNM staging for this tumour?

    A. T2N1M0
    B. T2N2M0
    C. T3N1M0
    D. T3N2M0
    E. T4N2M0

Basic sciences: Applied anatomy

31. **A 5-year-old girl presents to the Emergency Department after falling off her bed and landing on her left upper limb. Plain radiographs of her left elbow demonstrate a displaced supracondylar fracture of the humerus. Which of the following nerves is most likely to be injured with this mechanism of fracture?**

    A. Anterior interosseous
    B. Musculocutaneous
    C. Medial cutaneous
    D. Posterior interosseous
    E. Ulnar nerve

Common surgical conditions and the subspecialties: Endocrine disease

32. **A 50-year-old man presents to his GP with a 4-week history of a neck lump, abdominal pain, back pain, sweating, headaches, palpitations, and constipation. Examination reveals a blood pressure of 170/80 mmHg and a pulse rate of 104/min. Examination of the abdomen is unremarkable. Laboratory tests showed a raised serum calcium and raise urine metanephrines and vanillylmandelic acid. Serum calcitonin levels are also elevated. Which of the following is the most likely diagnosis?**

    A. Multiple endocrine neoplasia type 1
    B. Multiple endocrine neoplasia type 2A
    C. Multiple endocrine neoplasia type 2B
    D. Phaeochromocytoma
    E. Primary hyperparathyroidism

Basic sciences: Applied anatomy

33. **A 65-year-old female presents to the endocrine clinic with an 8-week history of anorexia, nausea, constipation, polydipsia, polyuria and symptoms of intermittent renal colic. Investigations reveal the presence of a parathyroid adenoma, which the patient wishes to be removed. During surgical exploration of the patient's neck, the surgeon promptly locates the two superior parathyroid glands and one inferior parathyroid gland, which appear to be normal. He systematically searches the anterior part of the neck for the 4th parathyroid gland. Which of the following statements is false regarding the parathyroid glands?**

    A. The superior parathyroid glands are derived from the 3rd pair of the pharyngeal pouches while the inferior ones are derived from the 4th pair
    B. The inferior glands are more likely to be ectopic
    C. Ectopic parathyroid glands are commonly found in association with the thymus   .
    D. 5% of patients have more than four parathyroid glands
    E. If the gland cannot be found in the neck, the surgeon should explore the superior mediastinum following dyed or imaged localization

Common surgical conditions and the subspecialties:
Gastrointestinal disease

34. **A 35-year-old man is admitted with severe epigastric pain after an episode of heavy drinking. On arrival at the Emergency Department his observations include a temperature of 37.0°C, a pulse of 108/min, a blood pressure of 89/69 mmHg, and a respiratory rate of 27/min. Initial blood tests reveal a haemoglobin level of 13.1 g/dL (13.0–18.0), platelet count of 185 × 10⁹/L (150–400) and WCC of 3.9 × 10⁹/L (4–11). Which of the following can most accurately be diagnosed, given the above clinical findings?**

A. Acute gastritis
B. Multiorgan dysfunction syndrome
C. Pancreatitis
D. Septic shock
E. Systemic inflammatory response syndrome

Basic sciences: Applied anatomy

35. **A 63-year-old gentleman undergoes a repair of his right popliteal artery aneurysm by the vascular surgeons. The popliteal fossa is opened during the procedure to gain access to the popliteal artery. He has an uneventful postoperative recovery but shortly before discharge, he complains of diminished sensation over the lateral aspect of his right ankle, foot, and the lateral aspect of his little toe. His knee jerk and ankle jerk reflexes are normal. He has full range of movement of his leg. Which nerve is most likely to have been injured causing the described symptoms?**

A. Tibial nerve
B. Posterior femoral cutaneous nerve
C. Saphenous nerve
D. Common peroneal nerve
E. Sural nerve

Common surgical conditions and the subspecialties:
Gastrointestinal disease

36. **A 69-year-old South-Asian man presents to his GP with a 3-month history of tiredness, evening pyrexia, night sweats, and abdominal discomfort. He also experiences nausea and vomiting, and states that he might have lost about 10 kg in weight during this period. On examination, his temperature is 37.8°C. Abdominal examination reveals tenderness over the right iliac fossa and a non-tender mass in this region. His haemoglobin is 9.4 g/dL, WCC 15 × 10⁹/L, and the ESR 112 mm/hour. An ultrasound scan of the abdomen reveals thickening of the mesentery and mesenteric lymphadenopathy. Plain chest radiography demonstrates evidence of right apical fibrosis. What is the most likely diagnosis?**

A. Crohn's disease

B. South American blastomycosis

C. Intestinal tuberculosis

D. Non-Hodgkin lymphoma

E. Yersiniosis

Basic sciences: Applied anatomy

37. **A 58-year-old man, who is on chemotherapy for metastatic gastric cancer, is brought into the Emergency Department with acute general deterioration. On examination, he is found to be confused, with a blood pressure of 80/45 mmHg and pulse rate of 110/min. Chest examination reveals an elevated jugular venous pressure, normal breath sounds and muffled heart sounds with no cardiac murmurs. Which of the following procedures is likely to be most beneficial to the patient?**

A. Insertion of a large-bore needle in the 2nd intercostal space, along the mid-clavicular line

B. Large-bore needle insertion between the xiphoid process and the left 7th costal cartilage, aiming towards the left shoulder tip

C. Inserting a needle through the cricothyroid membrane, attached to a bag valve device

D. Inserting a chest drain in the left 5th intercostal space, along the mid-axillary line

E. Large-bore needle insertion in the 4th intercostal space, aiming towards the right shoulder tip

Common surgical conditions and the subspecialties: Skin, head, and neck

38. A 57-year-old man is found by his GP to have a non-healing ulcer on his left lower leg. He recalls having suffered a burn to this area over 20 years ago. Despite debridement and skin grafting, the slowly progressive chronic leg ulcer has not resolved. On examination, bilateral pedal pulses are palpable and there is no evidence of venous insufficiency. The ulcer is painless with an irregular, everted edge. The surrounding skin appears chronically inflamed and exhibits non-pitting oedema. What is the most likely diagnosis?

   A. Arterial ulcer

   B. Basal cell carcinoma

   C. Marjolin's ulcer

   D. Neuropathic ulcer

   E. Venous ulcer

Basic sciences: Applied anatomy

39. A 17-year-old male is brought to the Emergency Department after having sustained blunt trauma to his chest. On examination, he is tachypnoeic with a respiratory rate of 36/min, heart rate of 120/min and systolic blood pressure of 70 mmHg. Chest examination reveals bruising over his right lower ribs, tracheal deviation to the left, with right-sided hyper-resonance to percussion and decreased breath sounds. The surgical registrar diagnoses a tension pneumothorax and prepares to perform needle decompression. Whilst attempting to locate the second intercostal space, he palpates for the manubriosternal junction. Which of the following anatomical structures does not lie at this level?

   A. The hemiazygos vein passing from left to right to join the azygos vein

   B. Between the T4 and T5 vertebral bodies

   C. Bifurcation of the trachea

   D. Entry of the azygos vein into the superior vena cava

   E. Beginning and end of the aortic arch

Common surgical conditions and the subspecialties:
Gastrointestinal disease

40. **A 35-year-old lawyer is referred to the surgical assessment unit with a 2-day history of constant, worsening right upper quadrant pain, occasional rigors and vomiting. She is a heavy smoker and consumes an average of 3 units of alcohol daily. On examination, she appears dehydrated and jaundiced, with a temperature of 38°C. Her abdomen is soft but exquisitely tender in the right hypochondrium. Her blood tests reveal: bilirubin 45 µmol/L, ALT 60 µmol/L, ALP 655 µmol/L, amylase 250 U/L, WCC 15×10⁹/L, and CRP 35 mg/L. What is the most likely diagnosis?**
   A. Cholelithiasis
   B. Choledocholithiasis
   C. Cholecystitis
   D. Cholangitis
   E. Pancreatitis

Basic sciences: Applied anatomy

41. **A 45-year-old lady is awaiting a mastectomy and axillary node clearance for a central, invasive breast tumour. After careful consideration, the surgeon decides to excise the level I and level II nodes during the procedure. Which of the following structures best defines the level of axillary clearance?**
   A. Clavicle
   B. Axillary artery
   C. Axillary vein
   D. Pectoralis minor
   E. Pectoralis major

Common surgical conditions and the subspecialties: Neurology and Neurosurgery

42. A 29-year-old woman collapses in the supermarket after experiencing an acute, severe headache associated with nausea. She has no significant past medical history. Upon arrival to the Emergency Department, her GCS level is 12/15 (Eyes 3, Voice 3, Motor 6). Her blood pressure is 145/85 mmHg, pulse is 90/min and regular, and temperature is 37.1°C. Cardiovascular, respiratory and neurological examinations are grossly normal, although nuchal rigidity is present together with bilateral extensor plantar responses. Initial blood tests are normal, and a CT scan of the brain is equivocal. A lumbar puncture yields straw-coloured fluid at an opening pressure of 17 cmH$_2$0 (normal 6–18 cmH$_2$0), a cerebrospinal fluid (CSF) white cell count of 6/mL (normal <5/mL), CSF red cell count of 1210/mL (normal <5/mL), and CSF protein of 0.50 g/L (normal 0.15–0.45 g/L). What is the next most appropriate step in managing this patient?

A. Arrange a four-vessel cerebral angiogram
B. Arrange a magnetic resonance angiogram
C. Arrange an urgent magnetic resonance brain scan
D. Commence intravenous cefotaxime and acyclovir therapy
E. Refer to neurosurgeons for urgent assessment

Basic sciences: Applied anatomy

43. A 45-year-old hypothyroid lady presents to the orthopaedic clinic with pain and paraesthesia over the lateral three-and-a-half digits of her right hand. Her symptoms are often worse at night. Examination reveals wasting of the thenar eminence and a positive Tinel's sign, suggesting carpal tunnel syndrome. Which of the following structures does not pass through the carpel tunnel?

A. Tendon of flexor digitorum superficialis
B. Tendon of flexor digitorum profundus
C. Tendon of flexor pollicis longus
D. Median nerve
E. Palmar cutaneous branch of the median nerve

Common surgical conditions and the subspecialties: Neurology
and Neurosurgery

44. **A 78-year-old woman with a history of cervical canal stenosis slips
    and falls down a flight of twelve stairs. The paramedics conduct a
    primary survey, immobilize her cervical spine, and ascertain that she
    did not lose consciousness at any point. Upon arrival at the Emergency
    Department, examination reveals loss of motor function of all four
    limbs, with the upper limbs affected to a much greater degree than the
    lower limbs. Which spinal cord syndrome is this patient most likely
    to have?**

    A. Anterior cord syndrome
    B. Brown–Sequard syndrome
    C. Central cord syndrome
    D. Complete cord transection
    E. Posterior cord syndrome

Common surgical conditions and the subspecialties: Endocrine disease

45. **A 27-year-old man with no significant past medical history is found to
    be hypertensive at 180/120 mmHg at a routine health visit. Further
    questioning reveals a 4-month history of weight loss, intermittent
    palpitations, headaches, nausea and shortness of breath. Physical
    examination is unremarkable except for a fine hand tremor.
    Subsequent ultrasound imaging of the abdomen reveals no renal
    abnormalities but a small nodule within the centre of the right adrenal
    gland. What is the most likely diagnosis?**

    A. Adrenocortical adenoma
    B. Adrenocortical carcinoma
    C. Carcinoid tumour
    D. Neuroblastoma
    E. Phaeochromocytoma

Common surgical conditions and the subspecialties: Breast disease

46. **Which among the following statements concerning pathologies of the
    breast is correct?**

    A. A breast cyst is considered to be an aberration of normal development and involution
    B. Fibroadenomas have a high preponderance for lymphatic spread
    C. Early menopause is a risk factor for the development of breast cancer
    D. Invasive ductal carcinoma accounts for 20% of breast cancers
    E. The nipple–areolar complex is spared when undertaking a simple mastectomy
       procedure

Common surgical conditions and the subspecialties: General presenting symptoms or syndromes

47. **A 42-year-old barmaid presents to the Emergency Department with an 8-hour history of severe right upper quadrant pain and vomiting. She describes the pain as radiating to her right scapula and exacerbated by breathing. She appears pale but exhibits no evidence of jaundice. Examination reveals a pulse rate of 96/min, blood pressure of 126/82 mmHg, and temperature of 37.7°C. Abdominal examination reveals tenderness over the right hypochondrium and no palpable masses. Plain radiographs of the abdomen (supine) and chest (erect) are unremarkable. What is the most likely diagnosis?**

A. Acute cholecystitis

B. Acute hepatitis

C. Biliary colic

D. Perforated duodenal ulcer

E. Right lower lobe pneumonia

Common surgical conditions and the subspecialties: Gastrointestinal disease

48. **A 20-year-old man is referred by his GP to the gastroenterologist for a 3-month history of abdominal pain, weight loss and intermittent bloody diarrhoea. Barium enema and colonoscopy reveal multiple ulcers extending from the rectum to the mid-transverse colon. Biopsy specimens show mucosa-centric disease with goblet cell depletion and with no evidence of granuloma formation. What is the most likely diagnosis?**

A. Crohn's disease

B. Ulcerative colitis

C. *Clostridium difficile* colitis

D. *Salmonella* gastroenteritis

E. Ischaemic colitis

Professional behaviour and leadership: Evidence and guidelines

49. In a study of patients receiving medical treatment for thyrotoxicosis, the patient cohort receiving carbimazole (n=7000) suffered a 7% symptom recurrence rate, whereas the patient cohort receiving propylthiouracil (n=9000) suffered a 11% symptom recurrence rate, over a 5-year study period (p=0.025). The risk of symptom recurrence in an untreated population with thyrotoxicosis over this time was 25%. Which of the following percentages is the annual incidence of symptom recurrence in the treated population in this study?

   A. 1.85%
   B. 2.10%
   C. 2.35%
   D. 2.50%
   E. 2.75%

Common surgical conditions and the subspecialties: Endocrine disease

50. Which of the following statements is true in a patient with primary hyperaldosteronism?

   A. Plasma noradrenaline level is high
   B. Plasma renin level is high
   C. Conn's syndrome is the commonest cause
   D. It is associated with hyperkalaemia
   E. Plasma angiotensin levels are high

1. Answer: C

The anatomical snuffbox lies distal to the styloid process of the radius. The floor of the snuffbox is formed by the scaphoid and the trapezium. Three tendons form the ulnar (medial) and radial (lateral) boundaries of the anatomical snuff box. The tendon of extensor pollicis longus forms the ulnar border while the tendons of abductor pollicis longus and extensor pollicis brevis form the radial border. The radial artery lies in the snuff box and runs in the space between the 1st and 2nd metacarpals to contribute to the superficial and deep palmar arches. The cephalic vein arises within the anatomical snuffbox, while the dorsal cutaneous branch of the radial nerve can be palpated by stroking along the extensor pollicis longus tendon.

2. Answer: E

The typical arteriovenous difference for a healthy 21-year-old male at rest would be approximately 25% (i.e. in a healthy subject at rest, only about 25% of the oxygen delivered to the tissues is utilized therein.) In a patient with simple iron-deficiency anaemia, arterial oxygen partial pressure should remain at normal levels but the decreased haemoglobin (Hb) levels result in a decrease in the total oxygen transported per unit time. In order to maintain sufficient delivery of oxygen, the arteriovenous difference will increase due to the production of molecules such as 2,3 diphosphoglycerate (DPG). The arteriovenous difference is increased and the dissociation curve shifts to the *right* in subjects living at high altitude, which is again due to the increased production of molecules such as 2,3 DPG. Erythropoietin (EPO), whether endogenously or exogenously administered, promotes oxygen delivery by promoting increased maturation of red blood cells. However, it has no effect on the dissociation of oxygen from Hb. An increase in the concentration of hydrogen ions (e.g. in acidosis) has the same effect on the oxygen dissociation curve as an increase in temperature or 2,3 DPG levels—all these factors shift the curve to the *right* thereby increasing the oxygen dissociation and increasing the oxygen delivery to the tissues.

3. Answer: A

Gustatory sweating associated with the parotid gland was first described by Duphenix in 1853. In 1923, Lucja Frey, a Polish neurologist, reported a case of parotid gland infection complicated by gustatory sweating and suggested a possible role of the auriculotemporal nerve. Since then, gustatory sweating related to parotid surgery or infection has been known as Frey's syndrome. It presents as localized flushing and sweating of the skin overlying the surgical site. It is caused by sprouting of the divided parasympathetic nerve branches to the parotid into the divided sympathetic nerve fibres to the sweat glands. The reported incidence ranges from 7–50%. Gustatory sweating is also a rare complication of diabetes mellitus, when sweating may occur on both sides of the head, with mild or substantial severity. It is thought to be due to axonal regeneration within the autonomic nervous system.

The diagnosis is usually made from the presenting history but can be confirmed by the starch-iodine test (Minor's test—the affected skin is painted with iodine and dusted with starch. The appearance of a bluish discoloration during eating is diagnostic. A positive test is due to a reaction of the starch and iodine in the presence of moisture/sweat). The symptoms are usually a minor problem. Occasionally, treatment may be required if the symptoms are significant. Medical treatment consists of topical scopolamine (this may have significant central nervous system side effects if systemically absorbed), or 1% glycopyrrolate, a parasympatholytic cream. The other treatment option is the injection of botulinum toxin into the affected area; however, this procedure does not provide a durable solution and will need to be repeated every 4–6 months. Surgical options are less commonly employed. These include: (1) re-elevating the skin flap and placing temporalis fascia or a dermal flap in the intervening space or (2) Jacobsen's neurectomy, i.e. division of the preganglionic parasympathetic nerve in the middle ear.

4. Answer: E

Compartment syndrome is defined as an increase in the interstitial fluid pressure within an osteofascial compartment sufficient to cause a compromise of the microcirculation, potentially leading to necrosis of the affected nerve(s) and muscle(s). It is a devastating early complication of fractures and crush injury, commonly in the lower limb. It can also be caused by deep thermal burns, electrical injuries, restricting tourniquets, venom from snake bites and fluid extravasation (e.g. intravenous regional anaesthesia). Early in its development, the peripheral pulses are normal as are colour of the affected limb, temperature, and capillary refill (since it is the microvasculature which is initially affected.) The loss of peripheral pulses is usually a late and often sinister sign. The patient may complain of unremitting pain that is not relieved even by high doses of opioid analgesia. Severe pain in response to passive stretch of the ischaemic muscles is by far the most dramatic and reliable clinical sign of compartment syndrome. Sensory loss (distal paraesthesia) occurs before motor loss since the thin cutaneous nerve fibres are more susceptible to ischaemia than the motor fibres. With progression of the condition, the limb becomes tense and swollen, and if left treated, the muscle weakness progresses to paralysis. Irreversible myoneural necrosis within 6–8 hours, even with compartment pressures in the range of 30–35 mmHg (taken in conjunction with the patient's diastolic blood pressure; see later). The areas of muscle may also infarct giving rise to rhabdomyolysis, hyperkalaemia, hyperphosphataemia, hyperuricaemia and metabolic acidosis. Classically, the compartment pressures are measured using a slit catheter device. The normal resting pressure within the compartment tissues is estimated to be about 3–4 mmHg. Compartment pressures in excess of 30–35 mmHg in a normally perfused patient previously suggested the need for open compartment fasciotomy. Recent evidence, however, suggests that fasciotomy should be undertaken if the difference between the diastolic pressure and the measured compartment pressure is less than 30 mmHg. Hence, if the patient is in hypovolaemic shock (e.g. as frequently happens in trauma victims), even a modestly increased compartment pressure warrants fasciotomy. Compartment syndrome can also affect the upper limb, commonly the forearm. In compartment syndromes affecting the anterior forearm, the greatest neurological damage is to the median nerve as it is located in the centre of the muscle mass to be infarcted, whereas the ulnar nerve lies along the periphery of the compartment and is thus subject to a lower risk of ischaemic damage.

5. Answer: D

Primary hyperparathyroidism occurs due to the autonomous overactivity of the parathyroid glands. This may be due to an adenoma, hyperplasia or carcinoma of the gland.

Secondary hyperparathyroidism results from reactive compensation of the parathyroid glands for hypocalcaemia caused by non-parathyroid pathology, such as renal failure.

Tertiary hyperparathyroidism occurs when an abnormal hyperplastic parathyroid gland continues to over-secrete PTH in the absence of an abnormal stimulus (e.g. hypocalcaemia). This usually occurs in patients with chronic renal failure who have had secondary hyperparathyroidism for a long while. After they undergo a renal transplant, for example, the hypocalcaemic stimulus is removed but the parathyroid gland continues to over-secrete PTH.

Multiple endocrine neoplasia (MEN) syndromes are rare disorders characterized by the presence of two or more endocrine tumours, and are inherited in an autosomal dominant pattern:

- MEN 1: tumours of parathyroid (95%), pancreas (40%) and anterior pituitary (30%)
- MEN 2A: medullary thyroid carcinoma, phaeochromocytoma and primary hyperparathyroidism
- MEN 2B: medullary thyroid carcinoma, phaeochromocytoma, Marfanoid body habitus and gastrointestinal ganglioneuromatosis

6. Answer: C

Bariatric surgery is a form of gastrointestinal surgery that has become commonplace in many parts of the UK and Europe. Although it raises social, psychological and developmental issues in adolescents, they are not excluded from surgery based on their age; on the contrary, some hospitals have specialized programmes for younger patients. Potential candidates for surgery are those with a BMI exceeding 40 kg/m^2, or BMI greater than 35 kg/m^2 with serious comorbidities (e.g. type 2 diabetes mellitus, sleep apnoea syndrome, etc.) Postoperative mortality ranges between patient cohorts from 0.1–2 %. The common risks associated with this form of surgery include vomiting, dumping syndrome and nutritional deficiencies. To date, there is no evidence that bariatric surgery reduces cardiovascular mortality in patients, although obesity-related morbidity may be reduced significantly.

7. Answer: A

Postoperative haematoma formation is a common complication of breast conservation surgery, such as the procedure that this patient has undergone for malignancy. Surgical drains are often left in the wound to prevent the accumulation of blood from continual haemorrhage after wound closure. For this reason, meticulous haemostasis must be ensured prior to wound closure as such drains may become blocked and therefore ineffective. An organizing haematoma stretches the overlying skin and causes pain. As long as the patient's clotting ability is unaffected, the bleeding will regress spontaneously from tamponade. Needle aspiration is usually unsuccessful as the haematoma is clotted and therefore cannot be aspirated. The most appropriate management of such postoperative haematomas is therefore analgesia and close observation. Necrosis (or imminent necrosis) of the overlying skin and wound dehiscence are indications for re-operation.

8. Answer: D

The femoral artery is palpated at the mid-inguinal point, which is midway between the anterior superior iliac spine and the pubic symphysis. This is not to be confused with the midpoint of the inguinal ligament, which is located midway between the anterior superior iliac spine and the pubic tubercle, and signifies the surface anatomy of the deep inguinal ring.

The femoral artery is located within the femoral triangle, which is bounded superiorly by the inguinal ligament, medially by the medial border of adductor longus, and laterally by the medial border of sartorius. The floor of the femoral triangle is composed laterally of psoas major and iliacus, and medially by pectineus and adductor longus. The fascia lata forms the roof of the triangle.

The contents of the femoral triangle (from lateral to medial) include the femoral nerve and its branches (i.e. the femoral branch of the genitofemoral nerve and lateral cutaneous nerve of the thigh); the femoral artery, femoral vein, and femoral canal (which contains lymphatic vessels and deep inguinal lymph nodes).

The femoral artery, which is palpated in this region against the tendon of psoas major, is simply the continuation of the external iliac artery after it passes under the inguinal ligament. It passes through the femoral triangle, giving off the profunda femoris, and continuing as the superficial femoral artery before entering the adductor canal. It subsequently enters the popliteal fossa as the popliteal artery.

9. Answer: C

The descent of the testes has four phases:

- Indeterminate phase (up to 8 weeks): the urogenital ridge and development of male and female gonads is similar up to 8 weeks.
- Transabdominal phase (weeks 8–15): this phase in controlled by Mullerian inhibiting substance secreted by the Sertoli cells. It causes regression of the cranial suspensory ligament of the testes and enlargement of the gubernaculums.
- Processus vaginalis (weeks 20–25): this is a peritoneal diverticulum attached to the lower pole of the testis, which elongates further along with the gubernaculum towards the base of the scrotum.
- Inguinoscrotal phase (weeks 28–35): under the guidance of the gubernaculum, the testis descends with the processus vaginalis along the inguinal canal and into the scrotum. The descent is controlled by testosterone and CGRP. CGRP is released by the genitofemoral nerve in response to androgen. It causes rhythmic contraction and shortening of the gubernaculums.

10. Answer: D

A Smith's fracture is an extra-articular fracture of the distal radius with volar angulation of the distal fragment. It usually occurs following a fall on an outstretched hand with the wrist flexed. In contrast, a Colles' fracture is an extra-articular fracture of the distal radius, which is usually 1 cm proximal to the wrist joint. There is dorsal angulation (with dorsal displacement) of the distal fragment. This is usually sustained by falling on an outstretched hand with the wrist extended. A Barton's fracture is a fracture-dislocation of the distal radius that may occasionally be mistaken for a Colles' fracture. It is an intra-articular fracture (i.e. the fracture line runs across the volar lip of the radius into the wrist joint), with the hand and distal radial fragment undergoing a proximal and volar displacement.

11. Answer: C

This gentleman is most likely to have an inguinoscrotal hernia. The fact that the vas deferens cannot be palpated separately suggests that the swelling is arising from above the testis and cord. Inguinoscrotal hernias are almost invariably the consequence of indirect inguinal hernias. Direct inguinal hernias are almost always limited to the inguinal canal and do not enter the scrotum. The lack of a cough impulse suggests the possibility of incarceration of the hernia. In contrast to this, an epididymal cyst would partially transilluminate and should be palpable separately from the testis and vas. Similarly, the vas deferens should be distinctly palpable from testicular tumours. Neoplasms of the vas deferens are extremely rare and so are less likely than hernias in this scenario.

12. Answer: B

The British Committee for Standards in Haematology guidelines recommend that prophylactic treatment should be administered 2 weeks before elective splenectomy; and as soon as possible after emergency splenectomy. This therapy includes:

- *Haemophilus influenzae* type B (HIB) vaccine in unimmunized patients and annual influenza vaccination.
- Pneumococcal vaccine.

- Meningococcal serogroup C conjugated vaccine for unimmunized patients.
- Lifelong prophylactic antibiotics (penicillin V) are recommended, although the first 2 years are most important due to the increased risk of infections during this time.

13. Answer: D

This patient has the classical features of compartment syndrome. Compartment syndrome is defined as an increase in the interstitial fluid pressure within an osteofascial compartment that leads to microcirculatory compromise and subsequent myoneural necrosis. It is a serious and limb-threatening complication seen after long-bone fractures (and after surgery for fixation of long-bone fractures), crush injury, deep thermal burns and other forms of trauma. It can also be caused by electrical injuries, restricting tourniquets, fluid extravasation (e.g. intravenous regional anaesthesia), snake venom, and infections such as meningococcal septicaemia. Severe pain in response to passive stretch of the affected group of muscles is a classical and reliable clinical sign. Sensory loss occurs before motor loss, since the thin cutaneous nerve fibres are more susceptible to ischaemia than the motor fibres. The peripheral pulses are frequently normal during the early stages of the condition since it is the microvasculature which is initially affected. The loss of peripheral pulses is usually a late and sinister sign. If left untreated, the limb becomes tense and swollen, soon progressing to weakness and subsequent paralysis of the affected group of muscles. Compartment pressures in excess of 30–35 mmHg (normal value 3–4 mmHg) in a normally perfused patient suggests the need for open compartment fasciotomy, although recent evidence suggests that fasciotomy should be undertaken if the difference between the diastolic pressure and the measured compartment pressure is under 30 mmHg.

14. Answer: C

The diaphragm develops from the dorsal oesophageal mesentery, pleuroperitoneal membranes, lateral body walls and the septum transversum (i.e. which forms the central tendon). The sternal attachments of the diaphragm include two muscular slips from the back of the xiphoid process (i.e. not the sternal body). The costal attachments include the inner surfaces of the lower six ribs and costal cartilages on either side (interdigitating with the transversus abdominis). The lumbar attachments include the medial and lateral arcuate ligaments and the crura, which are attached to the upper three lumbar vertebrae on the right and upper two on the left.

The motor innervation to the diaphragm is from the cervical roots C3, C4 and C5, via the phrenic nerves. The lower intercostal nerves merely provide proprioceptive supply to the periphery of the diaphragm. The right phrenic nerve leaves the thorax by passing through the caval opening of the diaphragm, while the left phrenic nerve pierces the muscular left dome of the diaphragm separately.

The caval opening lies within the central tendon at the level of T8 and transmits the inferior vena cava and branches of the right phrenic nerve. The oesophageal hiatus lies at the level of T10, in the right crus of the diaphragm, and transmits the oesophagus, vagus nerves, and the oesophageal branch of the left gastric artery. At the level of T12, the aorta (with the azygos vein and thoracic duct to the right of the aorta) passes through the diaphragm in the midline.

The abdominal surface of the diaphragm is mainly perfused by the right and left inferior phrenic arteries (from the aorta), while its costal margins are supplied by the lower five costal and intercostal arteries.

15. Answer: D

The physiological fluid load in a healthy adult is distributed within the intracellular compartment (two-thirds) and extracellular compartment (one-third). A 70-kg man would therefore have 28 L as intracellular fluid, 11 L as extracellular fluid and 3 L as plasma volume. A 70 kg man would also produce an average of 1.5 L of saliva and 2 L of gastric secretions daily.

Following the infusion of 1 L of normal saline in a healthy adult, only 25% (250 mL) will stay in the intravascular space. The remaining 75% will be distributed within the interstitial space.

When 1 L of 5% dextrose is infused, only 8% (80 mL) will remain in the intravascular space and 92% will be redistributed in the interstitial and intracellular space.

In contrast, colloids are made of natural or synthetic protein particles of high osmolality. Infusions of colloid increase the intravascular oncotic pressure, thereby shifting fluid from the interstitial space into the intravascular space.

16. Answer: E

The mechanism of injury, together with the tenderness elicited in the mid-tibial region without any obvious deformity, suggests a spiral fracture as the most likely pathology in this child. This pattern of injury is one in which the plane of the fracture varies with distance along the bone. It is caused by a twisting movement about the long axis of the bone, which can be induced by falls. These fractures are unstable and tend to slip and re-displace even if the bone is splinted. The tips of the spike themselves may commonly break to produce a triangular fragment referred to as a butterfly fragment. In contrast, a 'butterfly fracture' in itself refers to a fracture, typically of long bones, in which the centre fragment is triangular. For instance, a butterfly fracture of the pelvis is one in which there is an 'X', the centre of which comprises the symphysis pubis, which is detached by four fractures. Salter–Harris fractures are known to occur in children but they involve the epiphyseal plate of a bone, by definition, and are therefore unlikely to result in mid-shaft tenderness, as in this case. The simple mechanism of injury makes a comminuted fracture far less likely than a spiral fracture; and the fact that the child cannot weight bear is indicative that there is probably underlying trauma to the bone (i.e. the option of 'no fracture' is unlikely to be true).

17. Answer: C

Trauma to the breast can trigger local inflammation of the glandular tissue and subsequent fat necrosis. The mechanism of injury may be minimal (e.g. seat-belt injury) and initial symptoms may go unnoticed. The presentation is often similar to that of a malignant lump and so triple assessment is required.

Periductal mastitis presents with non-cyclical mastalgia, nipple discharge and periareolar inflammation. It may result in a mammary fistula and non-lactating breast abscess.

Duct ectasia can occur with periductal mastitis. It affects the subareolar breast ducts, which dilate and shorten with age. Women with excessive changes present with slit-like nipple retraction or inversion, and cheese-like nipple discharge. Although breast cancer must always be excluded in patients with risk factors (e.g. age, family history), this patient's recent history of trauma makes fat necrosis the most likely diagnosis.

18. Answer: A

The pneumococcal vaccine should be administered at least 2 weeks before elective splenectomy in order to ensure an optimal antibody response. In emergency splenectomy, the patient should be immunized as soon as possible after recovery from the operation, and before discharge from hospital. When discovered, unvaccinated patients with a history of splenectomy should be vaccinated as soon as possible. In cases of elective splenectomy for haematological malignancy, vaccination is delayed for at least 6 months after immunosuppressive chemotherapy or radiotherapy, during which time prophylactic antibiotics should be administered.

19. Answer: E

Shortly after this patient's head injury, his blood tests reveal marked hypernatraemia with elevated levels of chloride and normal levels of potassium, urea and creatinine. The most likely explanation for this, in the context of low urine osmolality, is the acute development of diabetes insipidus. This would result in a low urine osmolality from pure water loss via the kidneys. A hyperchloraemic acidosis cannot be confirmed as the serum bicarbonate level is unavailable. However, a normal anion gap would suggest that the bicarbonate is elevated, thereby suggesting either a metabolic alkalosis or respiratory acidosis with compensation. Although restoration of normovolaemia and osmolality will be required, the rapid administration of crystalloids may exacerbate any existing cerebral oedema and so correction should be gradual.

20. Answer: B

Infection may spread through a small crack or lesion in the anal canal into the ischioanal fossa and form an ischiorectal abscess. The following are the boundaries of the ischioanal fossa:

- Medial: anal canal and levator ani
- Lateral: ischium and the inferior part of the obturator internus
- Posterior: sacrotuberous ligament and gluteus maximus
- Anterior: external urethral sphincter, deep transverse perineal muscle and fascia
- The fossa contains mainly fat, the pudendal nerve and the internal pudendal vessels, which pass in the pudendal canal lying in the lateral wall of the ischioanal fossa. Posteriorly, these nerves and vessels become the inferior rectal nerve and vessels respectively. Damage to the inferior rectal nerve results in impairment of this voluntary anal sphincter.

21. Answer: D

The signs and symptoms in this patient are highly suggestive of infantile hypertrophic pyloric stenosis.

The profuse vomiting leads to the loss of gastric juices and fluid depletion, which leads to a hypochloraemic metabolic alkalosis. The alkalosis is due to the loss of unbuffered hydrogen ions from gastric juice.

In addition, chloride ions are are lost during vomiting. The kidneys try to increase chloride ion resorption, but there is insufficient chloride in the glomerular filtrate to be absorbed along with sodium.

The volume depletion stimulates aldosterone secretion and subsequent renal retention of sodium in exchange for potassium ions, causing further hypokalaemia. This forces sodium ions to preferentially be exchanged for hydrogen ions, causing the paradoxically acidic urine seen in these patients.

Hypokalaemia results from the loss of potassium ions from gastric juice, their exchange for sodium ions in the kidney (i.e. to normalize the extracellular fluid volume) and their exchange for hydrogen ions in an attempt to normalize the pH.

22. Answer: D

The prominent nodule that is 'cold' on radioisotope scanning is highly suggestive of thyroid carcinoma, and in association with the diffuse goitre, periorbital puffiness and thyroid bruit, the mostly likely diagnosis is Graves' disease associated with papillary thyroid carcinoma. Although both options are offered in this question, the most important issue is not to miss the underlying malignancy (that is likely a consequence of her Graves' disease), which could be fatal. Thyroid cancer associated with Graves' disease is not uncommon and is usually due to papillary carcinoma (i.e. which is also more common than follicular carcinoma in this age group). Thyroid peroxidase antibodies are found in more than 70% of cases of Graves' disease, and this is another clue to diagnosis in this question.

23. Answer: E

Aortic regurgitation is characterized by wide pulse pressure with a collapsing 'water hammer' pulse. The circulation is hyperdynamic, which is evident from the following signs:

- Quincke's sign—nail-bed capillary pulsation
- Corrigan's sign—visible neck pulsation
- De Musset's sign—head nodding
- Duroziez's sign—femoral diastolic murmur

The apex beat is found to be displaced laterally, and auscultation reveals an early diastolic murmur loudest at the left sternal edge in the 4th intercostal space. In contrast, the Austin Flint murmur is a mid-diastolic murmur owing to the regurgitant stream hitting the anterior mitral valve cusp.

A slow rising, low volume pulse ('anacrotic pulse') is felt in aortic stenosis.

24. Answer: B

This patient exhibits signs of class II hypovolaemic shock.

Hypovolaemic shock can be classified as shown in Table 7.1.

Table 7.1 Classification of hypovolaemic shock

	Class I	Class II	Class III	Class IV
Blood loss (mL)	<750	750–1500	1500–2000	>2000
Blood loss (% volume)	<15	15–30	30–40	>40
Pulse rate (/min)	<100	>100	>120	>140
Blood pressure	Normal	Normal	Decreased	Decreased
Pulse pressure	Normal or increased	Decreased	Decreased	Decreased
Respiratory rate (/min)	14–20	20–30	30–40	>35
Urine output (mL)	>30	20–30	5–15	Negligible
Mental state	Slightly anxious	Mildly anxious	Anxious/ confused	Confused/lethargic
Fluid replacement	Crystalloid	Crystalloid	Crystalloid and blood	Crystalloid and blood

25. Answer: B

The sural nerve is formed by the union of the medial (branch of the tibial nerve) and lateral (branch of the common peroneal nerve) sural cutaneous nerves. It runs with the short saphenous vein in the posterior aspect of the leg and supplies the lateral aspect of the foot. In symptomatic varicose vein disease involving the short saphenous system, the short saphenous vein is usually ligated at the sapheno-popliteal junction. It is rarely stripped out due to potential damage to the sural nerve. Injury to the saphenous nerve causes loss of sensation in the medial aspect of the leg and can be a complication of long saphenous vein stripping.

26. Answer: D

Parathyroid hormone (PTH) stimulates the action osteoclast cells on bone osteoid, allowing bone resorption and the release of calcium. In the kidney, PTH acts on the distal tubules and the thick ascending limb, to increase calcium reabsorption and decrease phosphate reabsorption. The overall action of 1,25-dihydrocholecalceferol results in a rise in serum calcium and phosphate. It is eventually inactivated in the kidney by 24-hydroxylation. Calcitonin is produced by the C-cells of the thyroid gland and is activated by a rise in the serum calcium levels. Calcitonin decreases the reabsorption of calcium and phosphate by renal tubules and activates osteoblasts to promote bone mineralization, thereby lowering the serum calcium and phosphate levels (calcitonin also decreases intestinal absorption of calcium).

It must also be remembered that in acidosis, the decrease in protein binding (i.e. albumin binding) with calcium leads to an increase in ionized calcium. The converse is also true (i.e. decreased ionized calcium levels with alkalosis) and may result in symptoms of hypocalcaemic tetany in alkalosis.

27. Answer: D

The Dukes' staging system is a widely used staging system for colorectal carcinoma. Dukes' stage A implies carcinoma *in situ* or tumour limited to the mucosa or the submucosa (it has a 90% 5-year survival rate following surgical resection); Dukes' stage B implies cancer that extends through the bowel wall (transmural extension; the 5-year survival rate is about 70–85% following resection, with or without adjuvant therapy); Dukes' stage C implies malignant spread involving the regional lymph nodes (the 5-year survival rate is approximately 30–60% following resection and adjuvant chemotherapy); and Dukes' stage D implies cancer that has metastasized to distant sites such as the liver, lung or bone (the 5-year survival rate is very poor, approximately 5–10%).

28. Answer: C

All structures that are vulnerable to injury from an incision at the distal transverse wrist crease are listed as follows (from radial to ulnar):

- Superficial branch of the radial nerve
- Abductor pollicis longus
- Radial artery
- Superficial palmar branch of the radial artery
- Flexor carpi radialis
- Flexor pollicis longus
- Median nerve with its palmar cutaneous branch
- Palmaris longus
- Flexor digitorum superficialis
- Ulna artery
- Ulna nerve
- Flexor carpi ulnaris
- Dorsal/deep branch of the ulna nerve

In this clinical scenario, small spurts of blood that are easily controlled with pressure suggest a cut to the small superficial palmar branch of the radial artery. A cut to the radial artery would have resulted in more severe bleeding. The median nerve supplies sensation to the radial three-and-a-half digits and motor supply to the first two lumbricals, opponens pollicis, abductor pollicis brevis and flexor pollicis brevis. Therefore, numbness of the lateral aspect of the hand, weakness in fine movements of the 2nd and 3rd digits and inability to oppose the thumb indicate potential injury to the median nerve. As the posterior interosseous nerve, which is a branch of the radial nerve, is preserved, the patient is still able to abduct her thumb using the abductor pollicis longus. As the deep branch of the ulna nerve supplying the adductor pollicis is preserved, the patient remains able to adduct her thumb.

Cutting the palmaris longus and the flexor carpi radialis wound weaken the wrist flexion and produce an ulna deviation upon attempted flexion, due to the contraction of flexor carpi ulnaris, since ulnar nerve function is preserved.

29. Answer: A

Carbon dioxide is transported in the bloodstream by three mechanisms:

1. As bicarbonate ions (85%)
2. Bound to proteins (e.g. haemoglobin) to form carbamino compounds (10%)
3. Dissolved in solution

Carbon dioxide is 24 times more water-soluble than oxygen. Red blood cells contain carbonic anhydrase, which accelerates the hydration of carbon dioxide.

The Haldane effect describes the increased CO_2 carrying capacity of deoxygenated blood. This enhances the removal of CO_2 from respiring deoxygenated tissues and its release from the oxygenated blood within the pulmonary vasculature.

30. Answer: B

The TNM Classification colorectal cancer is as follows:

- Primary tumour:
  - T1: tumour invades submucosa
  - T2: tumour invades muscularis propria
  - T3: tumour invades through muscularis propria into subserosa or into non-peritonealized pericolic or perirectal tissue
  - T4: tumour directly invades other organs or structures (direct invasion in T4 includes invasion of other segments of the colorectum by way of the serosa, e.g. invasion of the sigmoid colon by a carcinoma of the caecum) and/or perforation of the visceral peritoneum

Used with the permission of the American Joint Committee on Cancer (AJCC), Chicago, Illinois. The original source for this material is the AJCC Cancer Staging Manual, Seventh Edition (2010) published by Springer Science and Business Media LLC, www.springer.com.

- Regional lymph nodes:
  - N0: no positive nodes
  - N1: 1–3 positive nodes
  - N2: >4 positive nodes
- Distant metastases:
  - M0: no metastasis
  - M1: metastasis present

31. Answer: A

The anterior interosseous nerve ('volar interosseous' nerve) is a branch of the median nerve that supplies the deep muscles on the front of the forearm, except the ulnar half of the flexor digitorum profundus. It accompanies the anterior interosseous artery along the front of the interosseous membrane of the forearm, in the interval between the flexor pollicis longus and flexor digitorum profundus, supplying the whole of the former and the radial half of the latter, and ending below in the pronator quadratus and wrist joint. The anterior interosseous nerve is the most likely nerve in the upper limb to be damaged in supracondylar fractures of the humerus.

The functional status of the nerve may be tested by asking the patient to make an 'O' shape with their thumb and index finger. It is important to remember that displaced fractures of the supracondylar humerus can cause compromise to the vascular supply of the forearm by injuring the brachial artery.

32. Answer: B

Multiple endocrine neoplasia type 2 (MEN 2) is an autosomal dominant disorder caused by mutation in the *RET* proto-oncogene located on chromosome 10q11. MEN 2 can be subdivided into three distinct forms:

- MEN 2A (Sipple syndrome) is defined as medullary thyroid cancer (MTC) associated with phaeochromocytoma and primary hyperparathyroidism.
- MEN 2B is defined by phaeochromocytoma and MTC with Marfanoid habitus, mucosal neuromas and gastrointestinal ganglioneuromatosis.
- Familial MTC is the occurrence of MTC in 10 or more family members without the characteristic association of the MEN 2 syndrome.

MEN 1 is characterized by tumours of the parathyroid, pancreatic islets and anterior pituitary.

33. Answer: A

Humans typically have four parathyroid glands. The superior parathyroid glands are derived from the 4th pair of pharyngeal pouches and the inferior glands are derived from the 3rd pair, as is the thymus. As the embryo develops, the thymus separates from the inferior parathyroid glands and descends. This migration is extremely variable; the inferior glands are therefore more likely to be in an ectopic position. 15–20% of patients will have ectopic glands. Ectopic parathyroid glands are usually found in association with the thymus or embedded in the inferior aspect of the thyroid gland. If the glands are not found within the neck, the surgeon may have to explore the mediastinum (as guided by dyed or imaged localization) as they may be as low down as the aortopulmonary window, anterior mediastinum, posterior mediastinum, retro-oesophageal or prevertebral regions. However, even when the inferior parathyroid glands are ectopic, they tend to be bilaterally symmetrical making localization easier. This suggests that the 4th parathyroid gland of this patient is likely to be found within the neck, rather than in the mediastinum.

34. Answer: E

The tests performed in the scenario do not include serum amylase and so it will be difficult to confidently suggest pancreatitis; other possible diagnoses include perforated peptic ulcer and acute gastritis. The latter is a possibility but a decreased WCC would not regularly be expected. In the same way, insufficient information is available to diagnose septic shock or multiple organ dysfunction syndrome (MODS). It is, however, possible to make a diagnosis of systemic inflammatory response syndrome (SIRS), which is defined by the presence of two or more of the following:

- Temperature of more than 38°C or less than 36°C
- Heart rate of more than 90/min
- Respiratory rate of more than 20/min or $PaCO_2$ of less than 4.3 kPa
- WCC of over 12,000/mm^3, under 4000/mm^3, or over 10% immature (band) form

35. Answer: E

The popliteal fossa is a diamond-shaped region in the posterior aspect of the knee. It is bounded superomedially by semimembranosus and semitendinosus, superolaterally by biceps femoris, inferolaterally by the lateral head of gastrocnemius, and inferomedially by the medial head of gastrocnemius. The important contents of the popliteal fossa include the popliteal artery and vein, tibial nerve, common peroneal nerve, short saphenous vein, sural nerve, and the posterior femoral cutaneous nerve. The fossa is covered by the popliteal fascia, which is perforated by the short saphenous vein and the sural nerve. The sural nerve is the most superficial structure that is likely to be encountered when the popliteal fossa is explored during surgery. The sural nerve is formed by union of the medial sural cutaneous, and the peroneal anastomotic branch of the lateral sural cutaneous nerves. It then runs along the posterolateral aspect of the leg along with the short saphenous vein, lies lateral to the tendo calcaneus and lies in the area between the lateral malleolus and the calcaneus. It then runs forward below the lateral malleolus and continues as the lateral dorsal cutaneous nerve, along the lateral side of the foot and little toe, communicating on the dorsum of the foot with the intermediate dorsal cutaneous nerve, a branch of the superficial peroneal nerve. The sural nerve is the sensory nerve to the lateral aspect of the ankle, foot, and the lateral side of the 5th toe, so damage to the nerve may result in diminished sensation to these areas.

36. Answer: C

This patient is most likely to have intestinal tuberculosis. The classical features of intestinal tuberculosis include abdominal pain, nausea, weight loss, fever with night sweats, anaemia, and raised WCC and ESR. In addition, patients can also present with subacute intestinal obstruction secondary to small bowel adhesions. Although tuberculosis commonly affects the pulmonary system, it can affect a number of other systems in the body. Intestinal tuberculosis is common in tropical countries. Ileocaecal involvement is seen in 80–90% of patients with gastrointestinal tuberculosis. This is probably due to the abundance of lymphoid tissue (Peyer's patches) in the terminal ileum. The diagnosis of intestinal tuberculosis can be made from ultrasound examination or CT scanning, which may demonstrate mesenteric thickening, mesenteric lymph node enlargement, and, occasionally, ascites. The right apical fibrosis on this patient's chest radiograph suggests chronic (or reactivation of old) tuberculosis. South American blastomycosis is a systemic mycotic infection caused by the fungus *Paracoccidioides brasiliensis*. Yersiniosis is an infection caused by *Yersinia enterocolitica*.

37. Answer: B

The pericardium is a bilayered sac of connective tissue that invests the heart. The fibrous pericardium is a tough, non-distensible sac that encloses the heart and great vessels, fusing superiorly and blending into the central tendon of the diaphragm inferiorly. The serous pericardium, which consists of the visceral and parietal pericardium, reflects over the entire surface of the heart, forming a sac in which the heart can move as it beats. Where the serous pericardium invaginates between the left and right pulmonary veins and the inferior vena cava, it forms a blind ending sac called the oblique sinus. Similarly, it forms a transverse sinus when it drapes over the pulmonary trunk and the aorta on one side, and pulmonary veins and superior vena cava on the other. The surface markings of the right border of the fibrous pericardium run from the 3rd costal cartilage to the 6th costal cartilage on the right, behind the right lateral edge of the sternum. The inferior border extends from here to the left 5th intercostal space in the mid-axillary line (i.e. over the apex beat). The left border extends from the apex to the lower border of the 2nd left costal cartilage, 2 cm lateral to the left sternal edge.

The potential space between the two layers of parietal pericardium may fill with exudate, transudate, blood or metastases to result in a pericardial effusion. Cardiac tamponade is an emergency condition in which the effusion limits the contractile ability of the heart. If such patients in cardiogenic shock are left untreated, they will soon arrest (with a rhythm such as PEA—pulseless electrical activity) and die.

Pericardiocentesis can be performed as per Answer B, aiming the needle upwards and backwards towards the left shoulder tip, maintaining a negative pressure as it is advanced. This procedure should be performed with ECG monitoring, as a ventricular arrhythmia may indicate if the needle has been advanced too far.

38. Answer: C

Marjolin's ulcers are slow-growing, aggressive, well-differentiated squamous cell carcinomas that arise in previously traumatized, chronically inflamed or scarred skin. They usually occur in burns injuries, chronic wounds, chronic venous ulcers and as a result of osteomyelitis. The carcinoma spreads locally and is associated with a poor prognosis: 30–40% metastasize. Certain characteristics of Marjolin's ulcers include their slow growth (due to their relatively avascular nature); painlessness (due to the scars being devoid of nerve fibres); and without secondary deposits in regional lymph nodes (due to prior destruction of the underlying lymphatics). Despite the last point, lymphatic spread may still occur if the ulcer invades normal tissue surrounding the scar, as this would still have an uninterrupted lymphatic drainage.

39. Answer: A

The azygos vein is located on the right side of the body, it originates in the abdominal cavity and passes upwards through the diaphragm to drain into the superior vena cava at the level of T4/5. It drains the posterolateral thoracic and abdominal walls, parts of the right lung, mediastinum, and mid-oesophagus. The hemiazygos vein is located on the left side of the body. It ascends from the abdomen through the left crus of the diaphragm at T12 and crosses over to the right side to drain into the azygos vein at the level of T8/9. The hemiazygos vein drains the right posterior thorax, lumbar regions, lower oesophagus and parts of the mediastinum. The accessory hemiazygos vein is the venous confluence of right posterior 4–8th intercostal veins. It passes posterior to the oesophagus and thoracic duct to merge with the azygos vein at T8/9. It drains the right posterior thoracic cage and part of the left lung.

40. Answer: D

This patient is clearly ill and demonstrates Charcot's triad of ascending cholangitis (i.e. right upper quadrant pain, jaundice, and pyrexia with rigors). Although Charcot's triad occurs in less than a third of patients with ascending cholangitis (usually of bacterial aetiology), the majority of patients present with swinging fever and two-thirds are jaundiced at presentation. If Charcot's triad occurs together with hypotension and an altered mental status, the patient is said to demonstrate 'Reynolds' pentad'. Apart from urgent blood tests (e.g. FBC, U&Es, liver function tests (LFTs), group and save (G&S)), obtaining blood cultures and ultrasound evaluation of the biliary tree, are essential. These may then be followed by CT, ERCP (the definitive investigation in acute cholangitis to elucidate the cause and site of obstruction; it also functions therapeutically by allowing the removal of gallstones via sphincterotomy, or via stent insertion), or percutaneous transhepatic cholangiography (note that direct cholangiography is avoided due to the risk of worsening the ongoing sepsis). Antibiotic therapy is also imperative in infective cholangitis, and should be guided by microbial sensitivities. Note that in this question, the amylase level is not sufficiently high to attribute the clinical picture to pancreatitis over cholangitis.

41. Answer: D

The axilla is the space between the upper arm and the thoracic wall. Its anterior wall consists of pectoralis major, pectoralis minor, subclavius and clavipectoral fascia. It is bounded posteriorly by subscapularis, teres major and the tendon of latissimus dorsi. The medial wall is formed by the superior part of serratus anterior, and the lateral wall, by the medial border of the humerus.

The floor is formed by the axillary fascia running from the serratus anterior to the deep fascia of the humerus. Within the axilla lie several important structures that may be encountered during surgery. These include the axillary artery, axillary vein, cords of the brachial plexus, lymph nodes and fat.

Breast carcinoma spreads via lymphatics, and this lymphatic spread has been shown to be the single most important factor in the management of breast cancer. Several methods have been used to obtain information regarding the lymph node status, ranging from sentinel node biopsy, to sampling and axillary clearance. Anatomically, the nodes are said to be at one of three levels depending on their relationship to the pectoralis minor muscle:

- Level I: all nodes inferior to the inferolateral border of pectoralis minor. This usually comprises the lateral, anterior and posterior nodes. It is useful to note that the sentinel node (i.e. the first node to drain from that portion of the breast) is usually an anterior node.
- Level II: all nodes posterior to pectoralis minor. This includes the central nodes and some apical nodes.
- Level III: all nodes beyond the superior border of pectoralis minor. This includes the remaining apical nodes and infraclavicular nodes.

42. Answer: A

This patient's clinical presentation (i.e. acute onset, severe headache with nausea or vomiting) is typical of a subarachnoid haemorrhage. CT scanning of the head has a sensitivity of 90–95% in these instances and should be performed in all suspected patients. If CT is negative, lumbar puncture may be performed with specific identification of xanthochromia (i.e. at 12 hours post-onset). If xanthochromia is detected, a four-vessel cerebral angiogram should be performed urgently to identify active or potential bleeding sites and to plan subsequent intervention. In relation to this, magnetic resonance (MR) angiography is less sensitive and there are no advantages to performing an MR brain scan if the CT scan is negative. In addition, this patient demonstrates no overt evidence of infection and so antibiotics will not need to be commenced.

43. Answer: E

The carpel tunnel is an osteofascial compartment formed by the concavity of the carpel bones and the flexor retinaculum. The flexor retinaculum attaches to the scaphoid and trapezium on the radial side, and the hamate and pisiform on the ulnar side. The contents of the carpel tunnel include options A–D and the tendon of the flexor carpi radialis.

The palmar cutaneous branch arises from the median nerve at a point proximal to the flexor retinaculum, and supplies sensation to the thenar eminence. As it passes outside the tunnel, it is not compressed under the flexor retinaculum, thereby preserving the sensation to the thenar eminence, if the median nerve lesion is truly within the carpel tunnel and not located more proximally.

44. Answer: C

Similar to the patient in this scenario, central cord syndrome traditionally occurs to those with pre-existing cervical canal stenosis. It is characterized by a greater loss of power in the upper (rather than the lower) limbs, with varying degrees of sensory loss. In contrast, anterior cord syndrome, which is usually the result of interruption of the unpaired anterior spinal artery, is characterized by the loss of motor function below the level of injury, loss of pain and temperature sensation, and preservation of fine touch and proprioception. Posterior cord syndrome is caused by interruption of the posterior spinal arteries and is much rarer; it results in loss of fine touch and proprioception, with sparing of temperature and pain sensation. Brown–Sequard syndrome is caused by hemisection of the cord, resulting in ipsilateral loss of motor function, vibration and proprioception; with contralateral loss of pain and temperature sensation.

45. Answer: E

The adrenal cortex comprises endocrine cells that produce glucocorticoids (from the zona fasciculata), mineralocorticoids (from the zona glomerulosa), and androgens (from the zona reticularis). Adrenocortical adenomas are well-encapsulated, benign tumours measuring up to 2 cm in diameter. They present in up to 10% of the population, and approximately 15% of such tumours are functional. Due to the oversecretion of specific hormones, they may cause Cushing's syndrome, Conn's syndrome, and feminization in males or virilization in females. In contrast, adrenocortical carcinomas are aggressive tumours that can extend into local vasculature or spread via lymphatic and haematogenous routes. These may also cause endocrine dysfunction via the oversecretion of hormones.

In contrast to this, catecholamines (e.g. noradrenaline, adrenaline, and dopamine) are produced by neuroendocrine cells of the adrenal medulla. Phaeochromocytomas arise from this region; note the '10% rule' of this tumour: 10% are extra-adrenal, 10% are multiple, 10% are familial, and 10% are metastatic. The tumour itself may present in all ages of any race but its peak incidence is in the third/fourth decades of life, with equal incidences between the genders. As in this case, hypertension (either sustained or paroxysmal) is the usual presenting feature. The catecholamine excess may present acutely as a hypertensive crisis, with features such as headache, palpitations, tachycardia, sweating, anxiety, panic attacks, tremor, nausea and vomiting, and fever. They may be diagnosed by measuring urinary free catecholamines, and treated with antiadrenergic drugs prior to surgical resection.

In contrast, neuroblastomas are paediatric tumours that tend to be aggressive and lead to elevated levels of catecholamine precursors (e.g. vanillylmandelic acid, homovanillic acid, vasoactive intestinal peptide).

46. Answer: A

Breast cysts are one of the most frequent reasons for referral to the breast clinic. They are considered to be an aberration of normal development and involution (ANDI) with a prevalence of about 7%. Breast cysts are classically seen in perimenopausal women, although they may be seen in younger women, or older women on hormone replacement therapy. Fibroadenomas are benign tumours (and hence not associated with lymphatic spread) originating from the breast lobule and show proliferation of both epithelium and connective tissue—another form of ANDI. They are considered to be an aberration of lobular development. Some of the recognized risk factors for the development of a breast cancer include nulliparity or first pregnancy after the age of 30 years, late menopause, early menarche, a past history breast cancer, the presence of a first-degree relative with breast cancer, and prolonged exposure to 'unopposed' oestrogen (e.g. oral contraceptive pills and hormone replacement therapy). Invasive ductal carcinoma accounts for about 80% of all breast cancers. In simple mastectomy, both the breast tissue and nipple–areolar complex are excised.

47. Answer: A

The history, signs and symptoms of this patient are suggestive of acute cholecystitis. Acute cholecystitis is more common in females over the age of 40 and those with a high BMI. Gallstones are the commonest cause for acute cholecystitis. Obstruction of the common bile duct due to stones leads to the stasis and subsequent infection of bile, resulting in an acutely inflamed gallbladder. Other risk factors for acute cholecystitis include alcohol abuse and tumours of the gallbladder (which may mechanically obstruct biliary outflow). The signs and symptoms of acute cholecystitis include constant right hypochondrial pain exacerbated by inspiration, nausea and vomiting, and pyrexia. The rise in temperature is frequently mild to moderate; a very high temperature with or without chills and rigors may suggest the more serious diagnosis of acute cholangitis. A tender, inflamed gallbladder may be palpable in some patients. Likewise, jaundice may or may not be present. The differential diagnoses for acute cholecystitis include acute pancreatitis, peptic ulcer disease or perforated peptic ulcer, appendicitis, acute infective hepatitis and pleurisy.

Note that unlike for biliary colic (in which the pain waxes and wanes), the pain of acute cholecystitis is typically constant. Both conditions are complications of gallstones, which may be classified as follows:

- Complication of gallstones within the gallbladder:
  - Biliary colic
  - Acute/chronic cholecystitis
  - Mucocoele
  - Empyema
  - Carcinoma of the gallbladder
- Complication of gallstones within the biliary tree:
  - Acute pancreatitis
  - Ascending cholangitis
  - Obstructive jaundice
- Complication of gallstones outside the biliary system:
  - Gallstone ileus

48. Answer: B

Ulcerative colitis is an idiopathic, acute-on-chronic inflammatory bowel disease involving the mucosa and superficial submucosa of the colorectum (and occasionally, the terminal ileum— 'backwash ileitis'). Although it can affect any age group, it is most commonly seen in younger patients aged between 20–40 years. Patients may have a familial tendency towards the disease, and an association with human leucocyte antigen (HLA) B27. Macroscopically, ulceration of the mucosa (and superficial submucosa) occurs and almost invariably involves the rectum, extending proximally in a symmetrical, circumferential, and uninterrupted pattern. This may affect only parts of the colon, or its entire mucosal surface. It is known that 50% of patients with the disease have total colonic involvement. Microscopically, mucosa-centric disease is observed (i.e. compared to Crohn's disease, in which transmural inflammation of the bowel wall is observed), with pathological hallmarks such as goblet cell depletion, inflammatory cell infiltrate, crypt abscesses, and mucosal ulcers. The redundant mucosa between ulcers forms pseudopolyps, and the mucosa is friable and tends to bleed easily on contact (e.g. during colonoscopy). This is in contrast with Crohn's disease, where skip lesions and granulomas can be observed. In ulcerative colitis, the chronic disease process eventually causes shortening and thickening of the bowel wall, with associated haustral loss. The natural progression of the disease typically involves relapses and remissions.

49. Answer: A

The annual incidence of symptom recurrence in patients treated for thyrotoxicosis is easily calculated and one should not be distracted by the recurrence rate provided for the untreated population. In the group treated with carbimazole, there were 490 recurrences (i.e. 7% of 7000).

In the group receiving propylthiouracil, there were 990 recurrences (11% of 9000). Thus, there were 1480 recurrences amongst the treated population (n=16000) over a 5-year time period. The annual incidence of recurrence in the treated population is therefore derived by the total proportion of recurrences in this cohort over the 5-year period (i.e. 1480/16000) divided by 5 (years), to give an annual incidence rate of 1.85%.

50. Answer: C

Primary hyperaldosteronism is the excessive secretion of aldosterone independent of the renin–angiotensin system. Unilateral adrenocortical adenomas secreting aldosterone account for over 50% of cases (Conn's syndrome). Idiopathic bilateral hyperplasia accounts for 30% of cases. Hypertension is usually asymptomatic. Symptoms of hypokalaemia are rare but patients may experience muscle weakness, cramping, intermittent paralysis, headaches, polydipsia, polyuria and nocturia. Blood tests may reveal a hypernatraemic, hypokalaemic alkalosis. Calculating the ratio of serum aldosterone to renin is the screening test of choice (i.e. aldosterone is elevated and plasma renin is suppressed.) CT or MRI may be used for tumour localization. Sampling of aldosterone and cortisol concentrations from the adrenal vein may be used to demonstrate unilateral hypersecretion of aldosterone, if this is suspected. If the cause of Conn's syndrome is found to be an adenoma, surgery is usually attempted after 4–6 weeks of spironolactone therapy (e.g. 300 mg/day). If adrenal hyperplasia is found to be the cause, spironolactone or amiloride are generally adequate to control symptoms.

INDEX

Key: ▦ denotes question, ▨ denotes answer

abdominal anatomy 163
abdominal aortic aneurysm repair 2, 5, 18
abdominal compartment syndrome 14
abdominal pain 2, 5, 9, 62, 69, 73, 75, 101, 102, 105
    child 15
    diagnosis 208
    elderly 11
    hypercalcaemia 160
    intussusception 57
    pneumatobilia 171
    pregnancy 15
abdominal ultrasound, target sign 105
abdominal wall, congenital defects 68, 84–5
abscess 185
    breast 176
    ischiorectal 216
    retropharyngeal space 154
    subphrenic 24
ACE inhibitors 155
achalasia of cardia 80
Achilles tendon reflex 131, 148
acid reflux 70
action potential, non-nodal cardiac cells 130
activated partial thromboplastin time (APTT) 5
acute ischaemic event 181
acute (adult) respiratory distress syndrome 106, 122
Addisonian crisis 52
adhesive capsulitis (frozen shoulder) 18
adrenocortical adenoma 224
alcohol abuse 10, 75, 135, 202
    alcohol intake 39
alcoholic liver cirrhosis 39, 129
alcoholism 2, 131
aldosterone 226
    Conn's syndrome 60
ampulla of Vater 57
Amyand's hernia 121–2
anaemia 69, 86
anal canal 19, 83–4, 127
anatomical snuffbox 191, 210
aneurysm, abdominal aortic, repair 2, 5, 18
aneurysmal expansion, Laplace's law 21
angiogenesis, neovascularization 78
anion gap, metabolic acidosis 101

ankle reflex 12
anorectal continence 143
anorexia nervosa, nutritional management 131
anterior cord syndrome 223
antibiotics, dog bite 109, 124
anticoagulants 58
antidiuretic hormone 36, 52, 63
antiplatelet agents 52
antireflux surgery 97, 114
antithrombin III 181
aortic dissection 58, 68
    classification 85
aortic regurgitation 198, 217
aorto-enteric fistula 89
appendicitis 26–7
    pregnancy 15, 29
ARDS 106, 122
arteriovenous difference 210
artery, identification 61, 101, 102
artery of Adamkiewicz 21
ascending cholangitis, Charcot's triad 222
atelectasis, basal 9
atherosclerotic plaque 142
atlanto-axial fracture-dislocation 142
atrial fibrillation 38, 162
atrial septal defect, left-to-right shunt 123
atropine 41
    sinoatrial node 56
auriculotemporal nerve 53
autonomic nervous system 66, 129
axilla 222
    anatomy 65, 149
axillary artery 78, 82
axillary nerve 114, 187
azygos vein 222

back pain 14
bacterial peritonitis 29
bariatric surgery 192, 212
Barrett's oesophagus 157, 175
Barton's fracture 213
basal cell carcinoma 36
Battle's sign 54, 176
benign prostatic hyperplasia (BPH) 36, 52

bile salts 58
bile secretion 9, 24
2,3-bisphosphoglycerate (2,3-BPG) 210
bladder cancer, smoking 144
bladder malignancy 35, 144
  haematuria 13
blastomycosis 221
bleeding
  circumcision 5
  nasal septum 101
  nostril and ear 39
  oesophageal varices 39, 145
  prophylaxis prior to surgery 98
  tympanic membrane 158
bleeding risk, warfarin 53
bleeding tendency, assessment 130
bleeding time, haemostasis 81
blood, carbon dioxide 219
blood pressure, critical care 49
blood sample, analysis problems 16
body mass index (BMI) 97
Boerhaave's syndrome 58, 149, 152
Bohr effect 184
bone, metastasis 49
bone cysts 49
bone mineralization 218
bowel disorder 99, 101
bowel function 46
bowel perforation 47
bowel protusion 128
bowel resection 162
bowel tumour, prognosis 171
brachial artery 181
  injury 144
brachial plexus 43, 57, 175, 185
  injury 119
breast abscess 176
breast cancer 154, 170, 224
  management 193, 205
  risk factors 137
breast cysts 224
breast disease 104, 207
breast lumps 72, 132, 196
breast surgery, haematoma formation 212
breast swelling 159
breast trauma 215
breastfeeding 176
Breslow's thickness 152
bromocriptine 186
bronchial diameter, adrenaline and 146
Brown–Sequard syndrome 224
bupivacaine 87
  with adrenaline 71

calcitonin 218
calcium homeostasis 159, 177, 199
callous formation, pressure areas 124
Calot's triangle 8, 23, 171

carbon dioxide 219
  transport in blood 200
cardiac action potential, non-nodal cells 147
cardiac cycle 39, 54
cardiac tamponade 221
cardiorespiratory dysfunction 23
carotid endarterectomy 52, 93, 110
carotid sheath 11
carotid stenosis 37
carpal tunnel 223
  decompression 183
  nerve injury 164
  structures 206
  syndrome 185
case–control study 60
catabolic adrenergic–corticoid phase 49
catecholamines 224
cavernous sinus 185
cell cycle 10, 25
central cord syndrome 223
cerebral aneurysm 23
cerebral ischaemia 155
cerebral perfusion 67
cerebrospinal fluid 6, 21
  drainage 5
cervical nodes 151
cervical spine, fractures 126, 142
Charcot's triad, ascending cholangitis 222
cheek injury 138
cheek swelling, lymph node tumour cells 134
chemoreceptors 55
chest drain 41
  safe triangle 55
chest infections, ventilation 163
chest pain 68
  polymyalgia rheumatica 44
chest trauma, tension pneumothorax 204
chest wall bruising 100
choking 57
cholangitis 188, 222
  Charcot's triad 222
cholecystectomy 9
  elective 3
cholecystitis 224
cholecystokinin 149
chondrosarcomas 49
ciliary muscles 146
circumcision, bleeding 5
cirrhosis 39, 56
coagulation factors 178
coagulopathy 38
Colles' fracture 58, 213
colloids 215
colon, lymph nodes 31
colon cancer 48
  Dukes' staging 187, 199, 218
  TNM staging 200, 219
colorectal adenomatous polyps 188

compartment syndrome 176, 211, 214
congenital malformations 144
Conn's syndrome 224
    aldosterone 60, 226
consent 30, 35
continence 143
convulsions 69
coronary blood supply 130, 147
Corrigan's sign 217
corticosteroids, sepsis 181
cranial nerves 185
cricoarytenoid muscles 143
Crohn's disease 75, 77
    fistulation 44
crush injury 14, 175
Cushing's syndrome 224
cyanosis, causes of 108
cystic fibrosis, meconium ileus 59, 150

De Musset's sign 217
dead space 175
deep vein thrombosis 68
    transoesophageal echocardiography (TOE) 19
dental pain, infection 137
dental treatment 16
Dercum's disease (adiposis dolorosa) 81
desmopressin 115
diabetes insipidus 216
diabetes mellitus
    day surgery 21–2
    type I 7, 37
    type II 6
diabetic foot 109
diaphragm 195
    motor innervation 214
    raised hemidiaphragm 100
    rupture 117
diarrhoea
    child 15
    enteral feeding 128, 145
1,25-dihydrocholecalciferol 218
diplopia 186
dislocations 111
    hip 143
    Monteggia fracture-dislocation 80–1
diverticular disease 86
dog bite, antibiotics 109, 124
dopamine agonist therapy 186
Down's syndrome, duodenal atresia 145
drivers, consent 30
Dukes' staging, see colon cancer
dumping syndrome 176, 182
duodenal atresia 145
duodenal ulcer 9
duodenum
    CT scan 166
    key structures 56, 184
    mass 11

Duroziez's sign 217
dysphagia 63
    oesophageal cancer 156

ear, bleeding 39, 158
elbow swelling, nerve injury 168
electrolytes, 24-hour requirements 142
emesis, emetic centre 55
enteral feeding, diarrhoea 128, 145
epididymitis 55
epigastric pain 131
    elderly 32
    heavy drinking 202
epiphysis fractures 45
    Salter–Harris classification 59
epiploic foramen 56
episiotomy 86
    mediolateral 70
erythropoietin 210
Ewing's sarcoma 49
exomphalos 144
expiratory reserve volume 175
extensor retinaculum 10
extracellular compartment 19, 214
extraocular muscles 1, 17
eye muscles 186

facial mass 76
facial nerve anatomy 180
facial nerve injury, parotid surgery 53, 179, 185
facial nerve symptoms 161
familial adentomatous polyposis (FAP) 172, 188
fat malabsorption 51
fat-soluble vitamins 51
femoral artery 193
    palpation 212
femoral canal anatomy 165
femoral epiphysis, osteonecrosis 50
femoral neck, fractures 4, 9
femoral nerve anatomy 26
femoral sheath 183
femur
    deformity, blood loss 164
    fractures 45
fertility, restoration 168
foetal haemoglobin 115
foetus, red blood cells 98
fever 9
    joint pains and night sweats 16
fibroadenoma 88, 224
fibroepithelial tumour 72
fine needle aspiration 6, 10
finger drop 50
finger extension, motor function 33
fistula 66, 74
    fistula-in-ano 50
    Goodsall's rule 50
fluid, 24-hour requirements 142

fluid replacement, in children 117
fluid therapy, postoperative period 48
fluids
    distribution 195
    maintenance 126
FNA biopsy 22
FNAC 147
foam cells 125, 141
follicular carcinoma 96, 113
foramen of Winslow 56
foreign body, choking 57
Fournier's gangrene 153
fractures
    bone fragments 95
    cervical spine 126, 142
    compartment syndrome 113
    femoral neck 4, 9, 20
    femur 45
    Gustilo-Anderson classification 107, 123
    hip, elderly 4
    humerus 104, 128, 144, 201
    left tibia 96
    mid humeral and nerve damage 104
    pelvis 5
    pin placement 3
    ribs 100
    Salter–Harris classification 45, 59, 94, 95
    skull 54, 176, 197
    Smith's 194, 213
    tibia 3, 32, 192, 195, 196
    tibial plafond/pilon 19
    ulna 64
    wrist 45
    zygomatic 155
Frey's syndrome 37, 53, 191, 210
functional residual capacity 175
furuncle 185
    sensory loss and headache 167

gallstones 25, 38, 54, 154, 188
    Mirizzi syndrome 150
gastrectomy 182
    complications 164
gastric acid secretion 70, 86, 133
gastric cancer, metastatic 203
gastric secretion 149, 150
gastrin 149
gastrinomas 162, 181, 189
gastro-oesophageal reflux 97
gastrointestinal disease 101, 108, 132, 136, 172, 203, 205, 208
gastroschisis 145
genital pain 136
glioblastoma multiforme 20
glossopharyngeal nerve 177
glucagon 50
glucocorticoids, proteolytic state 49
Goodsall's rule, fistula 50
graft loss 60

Graves' disease 216
growth hormone-producing tumours 185
gunshot injury 12
gustatory sweating 210
Gustilo-Anderson classification, fractures 107, 123
gut hormones 132
gynaecomastia 170, 186

haematemesis 38, 96, 129
haematoma
    extradural 4
    periorbital 39
haematuria 144
    bladder cancer 13
haemorrhage risk, warfarin 53
haemorrhagic proctitis 57
haemorrhagic shock 182
haemorrhoids 4
haemostatic activity 65
Haldane effect 184
Hartmann's solution 142
head injury 4
head and neck lymphatic drainage 151
headache 8, 138
    sensory loss 167
hemiazygos vein 222
hernia 106, 107
    repair 6
hip
    fractures 4
    traumatic dislocation 143
hip dislocation 126
hip pain, child 34
hip replacement
    nerve supply 63
    revision 10
hip surgery 25
    approaches 80
Hirschsprung's disease 145, 173
HLA antigen 77, 92, 156
Horner's syndrome 34, 50
human leukocyte antigen (HLA) 77, 92, 156
humerus, fractures 104, 128, 144, 201
Hunter and Hess scale, pathology grade 107
hydrocephalus 155
hydronephrosis 53, 161, 179
    bilateral 161
hyperacute rejection 124
hyperaldosteronism 46, 60, 226
    primary 209
hypercalcaemia 59, 161, 177, 178, 211
    abdominal pain 160
    causes of 160
    hyperparathyroidism 134
hypercapnoea 182
hyperchloraemic acidosis 216
hypercholesterolaemia 37
hyperkalaemia 178

hyperparathyroidism 45, 59, 161, 177, 178, 211
   hypercalcaemia 134
   parathyroidectomy 135
   tertiary 184
hypertension 7, 37
hypokalaemia 216
hypomagnesaemia 180
hyponatraemia 9, 24
hypothalamus, ADH secretion 52
hypovolaemic shock 5, 217
   classification 198
hypoxic pulmonary vasoconstriction 182

iliac fossa pain 12, 26–7, 70
iliohypogastric nerve 118
immobilization 178
   physiological changes 160
infection, dental pain 137
infective endocarditis 30
inferior mesenteric vein 54
inferior vena cava 73, 88
inflammatory bowel disease 225
information, patient's rights 51
informed consent 35
inguinal canal, spermatic cord 154
inguinal hernia 7, 122
   triangle of Hesselbach 23
inguinal lymph nodes 55
   drainage 40
inguinoscrotal hernia 213
inspiration/expiration 22
insulin 33, 50
interosseous membranes 28
interosseous nerve 219
intersphincteric fistula 83
intervertebral disc 14, 28
intestinal tuberculosis 221
intra-abdominal pressure 28
intracellular compartment 19, 214
intrinsic factor-dependent receptors 58
intussusception 57, 121
iron deficiency anaemia 210
ischaemic heart disease 66, 69, 83
ischioanal fossa 197, 216

jaundice 150, 154
   obstructive 11, 150
Jefferson fracture 142
jejunal biopsies 65, 82
jejunum, structure 99, 116
joint capsule exposure 10
joint pains 16

keloid scar 27–8, 106
   treatment 13
knee, popliteal fossa 151
knee joint 62
knee reflex 12

lactate dehydrogenase, non-Hodgkin's lymphoma 156
large bowel, obstruction 116
laryngeal muscles 143
laryngeal nerve 176
   choking 57
laryngopharynx, injury 43
Law of Laplace 6
Le Fort classification, maxillofacial trauma 55
leg pain 158
leg swelling 14
leg ulcer, unresolved burn 204
Legg–Calvé–Perthes disease 50
limb penetrating injuries 33
limping child 34, 50
Little's area 117
   nasal septum 101
Littre's hernia 121
liver disease, alcoholism 129
liver function tests 42
liver surgery 42
loin pain 38
lower motor neuron lesions 180
lower urinary tract symptoms (LUTS) 52
Ludwig's angina 154
lung cancer, smoking 34
lung volumes 157
lymph nodes
   axilla 222
   colon 31
   excision 149
   inguinal 55
   metastasis of colon cancer 48
   neck, classification 115
   primary site 13
lymphatic drainage, thyroid gland 135

McBurney's point 12
Mackler triad 152
macrocytic anaemia 58
magnesium 180
   homeostasis 161
maintenance fluid regimen 100, 126
malabsorption syndrome 51, 65
malignancy
   histological changes 48
   necrosis 4
   non-histological features 31
   rectal 7
malignant melanoma, ultraviolet light 146, 152
Mallory–Weiss tear 113
Marfan's syndrome 61, 78–9
Marjolin's ulcers 222
mastoid process 39
maxillofacial trauma, Le Fort classification 55
Maydl's hernia 121–2
meconium ileus 59, 133, 150
median nerve 185
medications, stopping 52

medullary artery of Adamkiewicz 150
medullary respiratory centre 112
melaena 11, 38
   warfarin 53
meningeal artery 29
meningitis 8
mesenteric infarction 26
mesenteric ischaemia 79, 88
metabolic acidosis 117–18
   high anion gap 101
metabolic alkalosis 216
metacarpophalangeal (MCP) joints 178
metaplasia 1, 17–18, 175
metastasis
   bone 49
   gastric cancer 203
   lymph nodes 48
micturition reflex 146
middle cranial fossa 121
Mirizzi syndrome 150
mitral area, pansystolic murmur 16
Monteggia fracture-dislocation 80–1
motor function, limited finger extension 33
mouth ulcers 12
multiple endocrine neoplasia type 2 (MEN 2) 183, 220, 212
multiple organ dysfunction syndrome 185
Munro-Kelly doctrine 84
muscle necrosis 176, 211
myocardial infarction 58
myofibroblasts 93, 110

nasal septum, bleeding 101
nausea, chronic 40
neck dissection 98
neck lump 6, 69, 96, 102, 201
neck pain, and arm weakness 100
necrotizing enterocolitis 46
   neonates 59
necrotizing fasciitis 153, 211
needle types 74, 89
neonates
   abdominal wall defects 68, 84–5
   necrotizing enterocolitis 59
neovascularization 78
nerve identification 102, 157
   after injury 105
nerve injury 33, 132, 136
   paralysis of upper limb 103
   popliteal artery surgery 202
   tumour operation 125
neuralgic amyotrophy 116–17
neuroblastomas 224
neurology and neurosurgery 206
nipple discharge 120
nitric oxide (NO) action 37
nitric oxide synthetase (NOS) 53
non-Hodgkin's lymphoma 156
non-nodal cells, cardiac action potential 147

non-steroidal anti-inflammatory drugs (NSAIDs) 49
nostril and ear, bleeding 39
null hypothesis 189
numbness, leg 12

obstructive jaundice 11, 150
ocular muscles 170
oculomotor nerve 146
oesophageal adenocarcinoma 140, 156
oesophageal atresia, tracheo-oesophageal fistula 80
oesophageal varices 39
   bleeding 39, 145
oesophagus, perforation 148
oliguria, postoperative period 48
omental foramen 56
omphalocoele 144
opioid agonists 92
osmolality, serum 3, 19
osmotic pressure 19
osteomyelitis 174, 189
osteonecrosis, femoral epiphysis 50
osteopenia 151
osteosarcoma 49
otorrhoea 54, 176
oxygen delivery 67, 191
oxygen–haemoglobin dissociation curve 163, 182, 210
   right shift 166

pain, rating scale tests 173
paired t-test 189
palliative care 77
Pancoast syndrome 104, 120
Pancoast tumour 50
pancreas
   arterial supply 67, 84
   endocrine secretions 50
pancreatectomy, physiological effects 35
pancreatic polypeptide 50
pancreatic tumours 181
pancreatitis 10, 18, 90
   Glasgow-Imrie scoring 188
pansystolic murmur, mitral area 16
Pantaloon hernia 121–2
papillary thyroid carcinoma 119, 216
paraesthesia, upper limb 162
parathyroid adenoma 135
parathyroid gland 167, 201, 220
   hyperparathyroidism 45, 59
   renal colic 192
parathyroid hormone (PTH) 217
parathyroidectomy, hyperparathyroidism 135
parenteral nutrition 62
parotid gland 7, 22
   tumours 91, 151
parotid surgery, facial nerve injury 53, 185
parotidectomy 37
partial thromboplastin time (APTT) 147
pathology grade, Hunter and Hess scale 107

patient's right to information 51
pelvis, fractures 5
peptic ulcers 32, 49, 74, 89, 113, 165, 172, 183, 189, 220, 225
perianal abscess 34
perianal pain 66
periorbital haematomas 39, 54, 176
peripheral vascular disease 37
peritoneal carcinomatosis, malignant ascites 123–4
peritoneal cavity infection 86
Perthe's disease 34
phaeochromocytoma 103, 119, 220
phyllodes tumour 87
Pierre Robin syndrome 126, 142
piriform fossa 177
    nerve supply 159
pleural effusion 9
pneumatobilia, abdominal pain 171
pneumococcal vaccine, splenectomy 196
pneumothorax 41
polydipsia, polyuria 166
polymyalgia rheumatica, chest pain 44
popliteal artery aneurysm 95
popliteal artery surgery 202
popliteal fossa 87–8, 112, 133, 151, 220
portal hypertension 39
portal vein 54
portal venous system 39
porto-systemic anastomoses 54
posterior cord syndrome 223
posterior interosseous neuropathy 50
postoperative pain, rating scale tests 173
postoperative period, oliguria 48
postural changes 179
pregnancy
    abdominal pain 15
    appendicitis 15, 29
Prehn's manoeuvre 40, 55
pressure areas, callous formation 124
primary biliary cirrhosis (PBC) 56
proctitis 57
projectile vomiting 197
prolapsed intervertebral disc 14, 28
prostate, high riding 5
prostatic hyperplasia (BPH) 52
protein C 49, 111, 178, 181
    deficiency 94
protein S 178
    activation 111
proteolysis, catabolic adrenergic–corticoid phase 49
prothrombin complex concentrate (PCC) 53
prothrombin time 147
pseudocyst of pancreas 24–5
pterion region bruising 15
pudendal nerve 129, 146
pupil dilation 15
pyelonephritis 91
pyloric stenosis 16, 29–30, 216

pylorus of stomach 181
    absence 182
pyuria, sterile 75, 90

quadriceps tear 79
Quincke's sign 217

radial artery 218
radial nerve 50, 120
radiation proctitis 57
radioulnar joint 64
Raynaud's disease 83
rebound effect 184
rectal bleeding 70
rectal examination 42
recurrent laryngeal nerve 153
red blood cells 98
    foetal 98
refeeding syndrome 113–14, 148
rejection, post-transplantation 60
renal artery stenosis 155
renal colic 192
renal dysfunction, postoperative period 48
renal function 31, 80
renal transplantation 94, 140, 201
renal trauma 90
renin 118–19
renin–angiotensin–aldosterone system (RAAS) 102, 139, 155
respiration control 95
respiratory acidosis 216
respiratory alkalosis 178
respiratory frequency 146
retroperitoneal fibrosis 179
retropharyngeal abscess 154
rhinorrhoea 54, 176
ribs, fractures 100
Richter's hernia 122
rotator cuff 87
Royal Marsden classification, testicular cancer 13, 27

safe triangle, chest drain 55
safety precautions, surgical practice 44, 58
Salter–Harris classification, fractures 45, 59, 94, 95
saphenous nerve 90
scapula, winging 187
scars
    hypertrophic 106
    wound healing 122
scrotal bruising 5
scrotal lump 194
scrotal oedema 55
secretin 149
self-harm 200, 218–19
sensory loss, shoulder 100
sepsis
    corticosteroids 181
    steroids 181

systemic inflammatory response syndrome (SIRS) 125, 141, 167, 184, 220
septic shock 33
serum osmolality 3
sharps injury 58
short saphenous vein 199, 217
shoulder
   abduction, and elbow extension 100
   adhesive capsulitis 18
   pain 2, 9, 94, 97
   sensory loss 100
sickle cell disease 189
sinoatrial node 147
   atropine and 56
Sipple syndrome 220
Sister Mary Joseph nodule 186
skin lumps 64
skull, fractures 54, 176, 197
small bowel
   anatomy 116
   obstruction 118
Smith's fracture 194, 213
smoking 95
   bladder cancer 144
smooth muscle relaxation, nitric oxide synthase (NOS) 53
sodium overload 142
somatostatin 50
spermatic cord 138
   inguinal canal 154
spinal accessory nerve 153
spinal cord
   arteries 150
   blood supply 5
spirometry 175
splenectomy 139
   pneumococcal vaccine 196
   time of vaccination 194, 213, 215
squamous cell carcinoma 67, 222
squamous metaplasia 175
starch-iodine test 211
sterile pyuria 75, 90
steroids, sepsis 181
stomach, secretion 70, 86, 133, 149, 150
stretch receptors 55
study methodology, case–control study 60
subarachnoid haemorrhage 8, 122–3, 155, 223
submandibular gland 87, 141
submandibular space, infection 154
subphrenic abscess 24
Sudeck's atrophy 58
sural nerve 217, 221
surgical practice, safety precautions 44, 58
'Surviving Sepsis' guidelines 49
sweating 16
   auriculotemporal nerve 53, 210
sympathetic trunk 25–6
systemic inflammatory response syndrome (SIRS) 125, 141, 167, 184, 220

t-test 189
temporal lobe lesion, with necrosis 4
tendon reflex 131, 148
tendons 10
   anatomical snuff box 191
tension pneumothorax, chest trauma 204
terminal ileum, bile salts 58
testes, undescended 156, 213
testicular appendage 119
testicular cancer 55
   Royal Marsden staging 13, 27
testicular descent 193
testicular mass 13
testicular pain 40, 55
testis, undescended 139
thoracic diaphragm 195
thoracodorsal nerve 187
thrombolytic drugs 58
thrombus formation 159, 177
thyroarytenoid muscle 143
thyroid gland 85, 89
   anatomy 73
   bleeding 73
   lymphatic drainage 135
   lymphatic vessels 152
thyroid medullary carcinoma 165
thyroid papillary carcinoma 119, 216
thyrotoxicosis 209, 225
tibia
   fracture nailing 195
   fractures 3, 32, 192, 195, 196
tidal volume 175
TNM staging, colon cancer 200, 219
TPN, metabolic complications 79
tracheo-oesophageal fistula, type 64
tracheostomy 186
   bilateral vocal cord paralysis 169
transient ischaemic attack 37, 53
transitional cell carcinoma, bladder cancer 27
transplant, see renal transplantation
transplant immunology 109
transplant nephrectomy 94
transplantation, types of rejection 47, 60
transpyloric plane 181
trauma
   classification 76
   major, multiple organs 33
   psychological effects 32
traumatic dislocation, hip 143
tuberculosis 221
tumour markers 93, 110–11
tympanic membrane, bleeding 158

ulcerative colitis 77, 91, 225
ulcers, peptic, see peptic ulcers
ulna, fractures 64
ulnar canal 183
ulnar claw 178

ulnar nerve 121
ulnar paradox 178
ultrasound scan 38
ultraviolet light
    exposure risk 129
    malignant melanoma 147
umbilical discoloration 2
umbilical nodule 169
undescended testes 156
ureteric patency 179
ureteric stones, impaction 38
urethral injury 20–1
urinary bladder
    anatomy 35
    children 51
urinary tract stones 53
urinary tract symptoms 36

vaccination
    splenectomy 213, 215
    time of 194
vagotomy 183
    physiological effects 165
varicose veins 217
vascular occlusion 181
ventilation, chest infections 163
viral gastroenteritis 100
Virchow's triad 178

vitamin B deficiency 148
vitamin B12 deficiency 58, 183
vitamin D 177
vitamin K 53
vocal cord abduction 127
vocal cord paralysis, tracheostomy 169
voice hoarseness 135
vomiting 2, 10, 11
    child 15
von Willebrand's disease 20, 98, 130

warfarin 68, 85
    haemorrhage risk 53
    melaena 53
    stopping 52, 53
Wharton's duct 71
Wolffian duct remnant 103
wound healing 1, 8, 17, 61
    phases 24
wrist, fractures 45
wrist anatomy 25
wrist deviation 50
wrist injury, self-harm 200, 218–19

xanthochromia 223

Zollinger–Ellison syndrome 189
zygomatic fractures 155

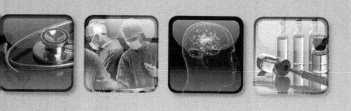
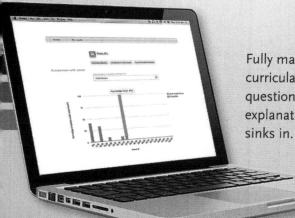

Printed and bound by CPI Group (UK) Ltd, Croydon, CR0 4YY